Say Little, Do Much

Studies in Health, Illness, and Caregiving

Joan E. Lynaugh, Series Editor

A complete list of books in the series
is available from the publisher.

Say Little, Do Much

Nurses, Nuns, and Hospitals
in the Nineteenth Century

SIOBAN NELSON

PENN

UNIVERSITY OF PENNSYLVANIA PRESS

Philadelphia

10 9 8 7 6 5 4 3 2 1

Published by
University of Pennsylvania Press
Philadelphia, Pennsylvania 19104-4011

Library of Congress Cataloging-in-Publication Data

Nelson, Sioban
  Say little, do much : nuns, nurses, and hospitals in the nineteenth century /
Sioban Nelson
    p.   cm. — (Studies in health, illness, and caregiving)
    ISBN 0-8122-3614-9 (cloth : alk. paper) — ISBN 0-8122-1783-7 (pbk. : alk. paper)
    Includes bibliographical references and index.
    1. Nursing — Religious aspects — Christianity. 2. Monastic and religious life of women.
3. Hospitals. 4. Sisterhoods. 5. Caring — Religious aspects — Christianity. I. Title. II. Series.
RT85.2.N455   2001
610.73′09 — dc21   2001033028

Contents

Chapter 1

"Say Little, Do Much"

Veils of Invisibility — Nursing Nuns

Some years ago at a North American nursing conference I delivered a paper on religious nurses and their impact on the nursing profession and the health care system. When I had finished, a woman stood to make a statement. She told the conference that she was of Boston Irish Catholic stock. She had worked as both a bedside nurse and a senior administrator at a number of Catholic hospitals owned and managed by sisters. Yet when she undertook her MBA and focused her major paper on women in senior health care management, she had found none. The literature told her there were none; she analyzed this deficiency from a feminist perspective and duly received a high grade. After hearing my paper she realized her error — the women were there, she'd even been working for them at the time. Yet, somehow, she had not been able to see them.

In what follows I focus on this blind spot. I look closely at religious nurses, their work, and its impact, aiming to integrate the history of religious and secular nurses into the story of the emergence of professional nursing. The intention is neither critical nor celebratory. The fact that religious nursing is argued to have been formative of professional nursing in profound and far-reaching ways is not intended to provide a rationale for the "return" to a religious or spiritual basis for nursing practice. It is historical observation. Nor are the religious nurses, with their powerful vocational imperatives, blamed for subsequent dilemmas in the professionalization of nursing — for its poor pay, its lowly professional status, its gendered character. Again, the vocational origin of respectable nursing is historical observation — it cannot be escaped.

Neither are nineteenth-century religious nurses argued to be feminist in any way — latent, nascent, or crypto. Religious life was not about individuals but about communities of women. These women did not care for franchise or working conditions. They were on God's mission, and their spiritual training enabled them to turn hardship and adversity into spiritual exercises in obedience and humility. Necessity made them mothers of invention. Moreover, in the United States a good proportion of these women were European. The battles and preoccupations of their Protestant sisters were a world away from their daily lives as immigrant nuns.

But despite the eradication of self through total obedience striven for by religious women, despite their spiritual practices performed to achieve Christian perfection through this erasure, and finally, despite their obedience to clergy and the narrow confines of religious life, these women constituted a powerful social movement. They were singleminded missionaries whose faith in God's will and belief in the miraculous enabled them to achieve far more than any group of individual women could ever have accomplished. They were the means to the creation of a Catholic world in the New World, and the foundations they laid for the work of all women in the pastoral domain has never been subject to the scholarly scrutiny it deserves.

I approach this subject matter as a nursing historian of Irish Catholic background, a background that I believe equipped me to recognize traces of Catholic culture, even when removed from its doctrinal context. As a student nurse (armed with a history degree) in a public secular hospital, I was often struck by the religiosity of nursing training. The weighty moral framework and conventual model of practice under which so many programs operated were, in my view, unpleasant reminders of my convent schooling. But I was even more struck by a general lack of recognition of this legacy, even as we registered nurses in Australia in the 1980s were still called "sister" and in some hospitals expected to wear veils.

Furthermore, my Irish sensibilities were offended by the ostensible Englishness of nursing history. How did the story of modern nursing and hospital reform become an English one? In Australia the old nursing schools all proudly laid claim to their Nightingale heritage, and the Imperial flag-waving that once upon a time accompanied this allegiance included the exclusion of Irish Catholic girls. Catholic girls had their own hospitals — St. Vincent's or Mater Misericordia — hospitals seldom mentioned in the nursing histories. But it seemed to me that at least in these hospitals the title "sister" and the veils made sense — their heritage openly acknowledged, not bizarrely rescripted as an English secular invention.

Unlike the triumphant Nightingale nurses whose story obscures them, religious nurses, Catholic nuns, Anglican sisters, and deaconesses are difficult to see and discuss — particularly in a collective sense. To overcome some of the difficulties entailed in crossing the confessional boundaries (the divisions between Christian religious sects or groups that define them as Roman Catholic, Methodist, Lutheran, and so forth) that still dictate our understanding of these women, I adopted the generic term "vowed women." This notion allows us to speak collectively about those women who separated themselves from the rest of the world to live in a community according to a set of religious precepts. Technically the deaconesses did not take vows — though they were consecrated and "set apart." Anglican sisterhoods were not supposed to take vows, but they did. Catholic women were all vowed. The "active" communities, however, whose work took them beyond the convent walls, took what was termed "simple" vows; lifelong solemn vows belonged only to women bound to the cloister and "dead" to the world.[1]

The term vowed women emphasizes the fact that these were simply women who took a voluntary vow. Second, vowed women produced vowed labor. It was the vowed labor of these women that built so much of the health care system that we take for granted today. Their labor was a phenomenal resource for Christian churches, most notably the Roman Catholic Church — it created Catholic institutions and shaped Catholic life in the New World.

The story of nursing addressed in this book concentrates on the English-speaking world of North America, Britain, and Australia. This awkward categorization represents the best educated and best paid nurses in the world today. These were all ostensibly Protestant countries which, until the Catholic diaspora of the nineteenth century, were dominated by Protestant values and anti-Catholic sentiment. They thus provided a consistent and particular milieu for the work of the Catholic sisterhoods. It was a milieu that expressed strong reservations over the entry of Protestant women into the world and into professional life. It was a world that was fraught with anxiety over the rising profile of Catholicism and the large numbers of immigrant Catholics. It was a world where social reform movements occupied the intellectual energies of many. And finally it was a world that held romantic notions of Sisters of Charity and Gothic fantasies about Rome, convents, and nuns.

For its part the Catholic Church had to build its institutions and minister to its immigrant millions in an English-speaking world — an alien world for the church when only a tiny proportion of its nineteenth-century followers even spoke English. The nursing nuns who built a Catholic empire in the English-speaking world were largely immigrant women. They were part of a vocational wave of European women who were building institutions and creating services for the poor. They were doing all this long before the emergence of the modern hospital and scientific medicine. But when these trends did appear the sisters were already old hands at a new game.

Care of the sick as a serious and skilled activity is argued to have emerged in seventeenth-century France with Vincent de Paul's Daughters of Charity. The opening up of the pastoral domain as the site of expertise and government has been well examined by scholars in the fields of poor law, psychiatry, and prison reform.[2] However, the role of pious women in this government of the poor has received little attention. The achievements of these women in France were of direct relevance to the subsequent development of nursing in the English-speaking world. In particular, the connection between these French events and the Irish Catholic Church is argued to be of major significance. The Irish diaspora brought a flood of women to the New World as novices and nuns, and also produced the first and second generation of convent entrants. This is a complex story involving Catholic emancipation in Britain and Ireland; the resurgence of the Irish Church; the Irish diaspora and mass migrations of German, Italian, and Polish Catholic communities to the previously Protestant strongholds of North America, Australia, and mainland Britain (the United Kingdom minus Ireland); and political turmoil, such as the Nativist movement in the United States. The care of the sick occurred in the context of these religious and social conflicts, and the work of the nursing nuns was part of, and significant to, the broader goals of the Catholic apostolic mission.

Of course the first women to be nursing and building hospitals in the New World were the women of New France—Jeanne Mance and Marguerite D'Youville, founders of the Hôtel de Ville in Montreal and the Grey Nuns respectively. The contribution of these Canadian religious nurses to the development of the nursing sisterhoods in Canada and the United States is immense. But the story in Canada is truly distinctive when it comes to the notion of the English-speaking Protestant world— because Canada was two countries, one Catholic and one Protestant. The tensions and dynamism that characterized the work of Catholic women in the Protestant English-speaking worlds of Australia and the United States were very different from the tensions between Catholic French Canadians and English-speaking Canadians—tensions much complicated by issues of sovereignty and national identity. For this reason the Canadian situation warrants special investigation and has not been covered in the current research. I do, however, deal in depth with one group of French Canadian women, the Daughters of Providence, missionaries in the Northwest of the United States.

In the nineteenth-century social landscape of Australia and North America, Ireland, and Britain, Catholic nuns were everywhere—abroad in the world like no other women. They ran corporations, dealt with national governments, journeyed on fact-finding missions—crossing the country, indeed the world, in search of recruits, funds, and ideas. They dealt with banks and businessmen with a lawyer's mind, mastered the tendering process for private and state contracts with a mixture of faith and business acumen, dealt with boards of notaries and hostile bishops as a matter of course. These women did not speak from platforms at temperance meetings, they did not write memoirs, they did not express a political or sexual critique of contemporary society. Importantly, neither did these women seek the path of individual progress and personal development, but embraced anonymity. They mobilized the ancient techniques of the cloister to "eradicate" self and become the mere expression of their holy rule. They were institution builders, workers for the poor and for their church. As St. Vincent de Paul had admonished them, they said little and did much.[3] They were, as we will see, "Marthas" — hardworking, resourceful, and indefatigable.

The aim of this work is not to claim territory for religious women but to eradicate the divide that separates these women from their non-vowed sisters, and to resituate the emergence of modern nursing within the religious and pastoral domains of nineteenth-century society. In reality, the nineteenth-century nursing innovators were all religious women. The very notion of "secular" meant something quite different in the nineteenth-century context.[4] It meant "nonsectarian" — not formally affiliated with a religious sect, not "without religion." The distance between Catholic, Protestant, and secular women was writ large in the nineteenth century. This religious and social distance discursively situated secular nurses as the "new wave" of nursing reformers — a positioning that was of major importance in the Nightingale story. At the same time as the work of the vowed nurses was ignored or trivialized, always depicted as a preparatory stage to real nursing, the religious and vocational ethos of the Protestant reformers was erroneously endowed with a purely secular basis.

However, the historiographical problem confronting the study of religious nurses has been not just with the issue of religion, but with the usual focus on secularization (as the starting point of nursing). I would argue that this focus on secularization has obscured the mechanisms activated by nineteenth-century women to colonize new territory — territory that was to become gendered professional territory. Also obscured is the relationship between vocational ethos and the emergence of a role for women as part of a professional work force. One of the barriers to making visible and rethinking the nursing nuns has been the idea that these women were "pre-professional." Professions cannot include vowed women — the nuns are not independent, they are obedient and follow whatever path is decreed for them by their superiors. Doctors and lawyers are professional. Nursing may or may not be a profession, depending on the definition used. However, a religious woman — even if she runs the largest public institution in a city of five million, holds higher degrees, and plays a leading role in professional associations — is never professional. The barrier in essence is the tacitly accepted view that there is a division between the world of religion and the world of work. Almost by definition, then, secularization becomes the only means to professionalization. By contrast, what is proposed here is that nursing emerged as a hybrid religious and professional practice. Its continuing ambiguous and ambivalent fit with models of professions is a legacy of those origins.

Finally, it needs to be made clear that, while this particular story of nursing has European origins, it took on a distinctive gloss in the New World. For the Catholic sisterhoods, Protestant hostility and the impoverished state of the Catholic Church, combined with the wider community's desperate need for the skills and expertise of the sisters, worked to produce a new variation of the nursing religious sister. This was not the Catholic nursing sister of Europe — the sister-nurse of the New World was a new creature. To live by her wits in the New World she had to be professional and accountable; she had to be innovative and entrepreneurial; finally, she had to understand the politics and economics of her domain to be self-funding. She, in turn, had a major impact on the way nursing in North America and Australia came to achieve a high level of professionalism in the twentieth century. O'Connell points out that at the time of the Second Vatican Council (1962), the American church had 950 hospitals with 156,000 beds and admitted 16,000,000 patients per year.[5] This was the result of the efforts of these nineteenth-century women.

The series of five case studies presented here does not constitute the basis for a comparative analysis of religious nursing over the course of a century, in three continents and from four confessions (Roman Catholic, Anglican, Lutheran, and Methodist). Rather, this collection of essays is designed to convey the sense that nursing and hospital foundation was part of a gendered international movement — a movement that to a great extent was neither English nor Protestant.

Chapter 2 examines the way nursing history, the history of women, and nineteenth-century religious history have dealt with the religious communities of women. It argues that these women have fallen through the gaps in contemporary scholarship. Religious women are dealt with seriously only by "insider" histories. They have not received serious consideration in the histories of women and philanthropy, they are seldom included in professional nursing histories, and their "professional" contribution to English-speaking nineteenth-century society is generally of only tangential interest to historians of religion. Concepts such as the women's sphere and secularization are revisited to explore what is argued to be a set of discursive evolutionary assumptions that set the basis and the limits of nursing history. The Vincent de Paul Daughters of Charity are discussed, and their impact on the subsequent rise of the nineteenth-century religious nursing — Catholic and Protestant — examined.

In Chapter 3 the American "take" on this Vincentien Daughter of Charity is explored. Of importance to this discussion were the extremes of response the nursing nuns were capable of evoking. As one of the most visible symbols of Catholicism and foreign power (Rome), the "un-American" identity of the nuns caused them a great deal of difficulty. However, episodes such as the cholera epidemics, when they volunteered to nurse the sick, and later their heroism during the Civil War made them complex and unstable figures in the American psyche — vilified and romanticized. But despite the social and political difficulties faced by the communities of nursing women in the United States, Catholic vowed women managed to found an extraordinary number of hospitals right across the country. The work of Mother Seton of course features here. Her Sisters of Charity were founded in 1809, the earliest non-French version of the Vincentien vision.

The Old World of London and the New World of the northeast American cities were not such different universes by the end of the nineteenth century as they had been when the century began. Over the course of the century rural America had been filled with cities, choked with industry, and swamped by immigrants. The Catholic Church, filled with immigrant congregations, took enthusiastically to its role of unsettling Protestant certainties. In New York, Toronto, and London the defenders of the Reformation found themselves in a pluralistic world of Catholics, Jews, and liberals. In England, the passage of the Catholic Emancipation Act in 1829 signaled the beginning of decades of debate, riot, and confusion over the role of the established church (Anglicanism), the rise of secularism, and the colonial designs of the Catholic Church for the souls of England.

Chapter 4 takes up this story through the Sisters of Mercy at Bermondsey in the East End of London. This community played a significant role in nineteenth-century nursing history, providing a team of nurses to accompany Florence Nightingale to the Crimea. Mother Mary Clare Moore, the mother superior of the Bermondsey convent, went on to become a confidante of Nightingale. But it is the period prior to the Crimean events that is the focus of the chapter. Founded in 1838, this convent was the first to be established in England since the Reformation. The work of the sisters involved home visitation and epidemic nursing. It was not until after the Crimean War that their public standing was so boosted that they were able to open a hospital — the first Catholic hospital in England since the Reformation. So this community of women were very much in the front line of the reestablishment of Catholicism in a very hostile Britain. They were also well established in Britain prior to the great famines in Ireland and served the burgeoning and increasingly desperate Irish poor. By the second half of the nineteenth century the Catholic nursing orders began to share the stage with communities of Protestant women, some vowed, others not, who too had answered a call from God to nurse the sick poor. This chapter looks at the commonalities between religious nurses — their vocational imperative, their strong commitment to an "active" life, and their powerful sense of the need that they were meeting. It argues the importance of the religious sisterhoods in establishing the groundwork to the Nightingale reforms.

The complexity of work, gender, and religion as it was played out in Victorian England permeated to the boundaries of the empire. In Chapter 5 I turn to the story of professional nursing in colonial New South Wales. In 1868 a team of Nightingale-trained nurses arrived in the colony. But long before the Nightingale sisters disembarked at Sydney Cove, a group of French-trained Irish Sisters of Charity had been nursing the sick in their homes, and in 1857 they established a widely supported hospital, St. Vincent's. This juxtaposition, in a small remote colony, of English Nightingales and Irish nursing nuns in the city's only two hospitals continues the story of Catholic Emancipation, Irish politics, Anglican tensions, and women's work. The Sisters of Charity and the Nightingale nurses were both victims of sectarian bigotry as each "community" of women overstepped the bounds of female authority while struggling to establish an independent domain — a hospital run by women. This chapter, then, provides a case study of issues of competence, professionalism, religion, sectarianism, and colonial politics.

That strange bedfellows are born of the exigencies of frontier life is nowhere better illustrated than in the complex arrangements of Irish, French, and Québecois women that are featured in Chapter 6. To some extent the story of the frontier sisterhood is the story of all the sisterhoods writ large. The poverty, the oppression, and the inventiveness that characterize successful communities of religious women, particularly nursing communities, are in evidence whether one looks in New York City or Dawson City. That said, there was something distinctive about this experienced group of women with a firm identity and confidence in their rule and life, taking on the enormous challenge of working, not among communities of immigrant poor, but in the male world of mining towns, logging camps, railroad camps, forts, and mission settlements. It was a world impenetrable to ladies without protection of veil and vow.

Commercialism and business acumen were the skills developed by the successful sisterhoods in the sink or swim world of the North American west. The northwest and the southwest provide counterpoints for our examination of the phenomenon of vowed women in the wilds. Quite different women, very different religious communities, and different social and political contexts reveal remarkable consistencies in mode of adaptation and successful establishment.

Between the wilds of the west and the factories of the east lies the midwest. This episode of American settlement is distinctive. It does not have clear parallels with settler societies in Australia or with industrial Europe. It is an American story of cultural pluralism, ethnicity, and settlement. For despite the great dominance of Irish in the American Catholic Church, they were only the first wave, the English-speaking wave, and the group well practiced in tribal politics. The next largest group of Catholic immigrants to the United States in the nineteenth century was German. It was a German community in exile from persecution. Its goal was continuity of community and tradition, continuity of liturgy and prayer, and continuity of language. These imperatives were in stark contrast to those of the Irish Church which had been in expansionist mode throughout the century. The German-American story of nursing sisterhoods is also distinctive in that it introduced to North America a successful Protestant sisterhood of nurses—the deaconesses. Chapter 7 sets out to examine these women, connected by culture and language rather than religion, and explores their impact on the American health care system.

The final chapter brings together the collection of essays to explore the emergence of a "professional vocation" through the work of the nineteenth-century religious nurses in Britain, North America, and Australia. The work of women within these predominantly Protestant countries was affected by social trends such as the secularization of nursing and teaching, the growth of a female workforce, and the development of military nursing. Thus, just as the religious nurses pioneered this professional space, secular women began to join them in their work, and the religious women, too, had to adapt and respond to a changing professional climate. It is this interplay between the religious and the secular world that is explored in the final chapter.

The pioneering of new worlds of energy and competence for women through piety and community was a nineteenth-century phenomenon. Through the tumult of diaspora and the rapid establishment of institutions for the provision of care to immigrant poor and new settlers, Catholic vowed women, alone on the stage, stepped out to make their mark. Others soon followed. By the late nineteenth century this hybrid field of gendered pastoral work had become crowded with Protestant vowed women and secular reformers. The twentieth century heralded a hardening of the Catholic Church's attitudes toward communities of women. Through progressive decrees, culminating in the promulgation of canon law in 1917, the sisters were placed under direct clerical supervision, increasingly bound to their convents, and denied the possibility of independent action. At the same time as the Vatican was closing in, the worldly professions in which sisters were engaged were demanding higher levels of training and professional development—placing the women in an untenable position. In the twentieth century the Anglican sisterhoods too, after decades of relative freedom within the church were gradually brought under the administrative control of the bishops. For its part, the deaconess movement, which began as a nursing movement, steadily increased its pastoral role within the various Protestant confessions, eventually forsaking nursing work for other forms of ministry.

The nineteenth-century rise of nursing by religious women was therefore the product of a specific and time-limited set of contingencies— religious, cultural, and political. These contingencies generated a remarkable field of possibility for communities of vowed women — one they did not pass by.

Chapter 2

Martha's Turn
Vowed Women and Virtuous Work

> *Jesus came to a village where a woman named Martha made him welcome in her home. She had a sister, Mary, who seated herself at the Lord's feet and stayed there listening to his words. Now Martha was distracted by her many tasks, so she came to him and said, "Lord, do you not care that my sister has left me to get on with the work by myself? Tell her to come and lend a hand."* *But the Lord answered, "Martha, Martha, you are fretting and fussing about so many things; but one thing is necessary. The part Mary has chosen is best; and it shall not be taken from her."*
>
> *— Luke 10: 38–42, New English Bible*

> *In Martha we see the active earnest, practical life which is wanted in this working for God; and a readiness to do and toil for others; an eagerness and fervor of spirit which carries one out of oneself; a restlessness to be up and doing, which the need without and the love within unite to claim.*
>
> *— S. B. Mansell, 1863[1]*

The spiritual paths open to women over the centuries of Christian practice were shaped by the popular New Testament story of the sisters Martha and Mary. Mary sat at the feet of Jesus and washed his feet in expensive oils. Martha fussed, providing food for the apostles and followers, and criticized Mary's selfishness. She spoke out irritably to Jesus, asking for Mary's help. But Jesus praised Mary's singular, unworldly devotion, and criticized Martha's mundane and temporal preoccupations. From this story two paths for women were delineated. Mary's path was the prestigious path of prayer and withdrawal from the world and its concerns — blessed by Jesus himself. Martha's path was that of the lowly housewife or the drudge, unable to separate herself from worldly matters. But after centuries of the cloister and devotion to Mary's path to perfection through prayer, finally it was Martha's turn. In the nineteenth century pious women on both sides of the confessional divide followed the inspiration of the Daughters of Charity to attend to their spiritual perfection through work in the world. The nineteenth century, with its social dislocation, poverty, immigration, and epidemics, welcomed them. It was a time for deeds — for Martha's work, not Mary's prayers.

In this chapter we examine this nineteenth-century opening out of opportunities for pious women and the manner in which they moved their work into the public domain. We also look closely at the invisibility of these women, both in the nineteenth-century context and to contemporary historians of women, particularly nursing historians. Vowed women, it will be argued, have failed to generate intellectual interest because their conservatism, the submission of individuality inherent in vowed religious life, and their embrace of gender constraints combine to constitute a life antithetical to contemporary values. Paradoxically, however, it is this very triumvirate of attributes — conservatism, submission, and asexuality — that empowered these women to be pioneers and innovators. The origins, background, organization, and training of the sisterhoods warrant discussion here, as, despite the specificity of each community, there are general elements to the life and training of nineteenth-century vowed women. The chapter ends with the place of these women in the story of nursing and the challenge they present to the Nightingale version of nursing history.

The Power of Religious Identity

Religious identity allowed women to present and assert themselves in private and public ways. It enabled them to rely on an authority *beyond the world of men* and provided crucial support for those who stepped beyond accepted bounds.[2]

When Nancy Cott made this observation in 1977 in *The Bonds of Womanhood,* she was referring to New England Protestant women and to the enabling dynamic that grew between religious fervor and the extension of feminine responsibility from the home to the charitable and, finally, humanitarian domain of public philanthropy and social action. Cott argued that through submission to religious ideals these women practiced a radical form of self-assertion. This self-assertion empowered women to challenge gender constraints, to "define self and find community."[3]

Cott's work on Protestant New England forms part of an extensive corpus of scholarly writings on the Protestant women whose efforts, in the first part of the nineteenth century, intimately intersected with the subsequent rise of political and social movements in which women, for the first time, played a major part.[4] From the abolitionists to the Christian Women's Temperance Society, women claimed the high moral ground by virtue of their sex, found the voice to comment on the ills of society and to lobby politically for social change.[5] The female suffrage movement was

built on the political consciousness that followed for a good many campaigners, and represented the culmination of nearly a century of political training and organizational experience for women. Not surprisingly,
the links between these nineteenth-century women's activities and the
political and social history of twentieth-century women make the earlier
world of female political and social action of great interest to contemporary women historians.[6]

However, Cott's comments are equally true for the other, less overtly
political side of the confessional divide. Catholic women, too, relied
on an authority beyond the world of men to find self and community.
Through piety, philanthropy, and a commitment to the social apostolate,
thousands of nineteenth-century Catholic women in the Old and New
Worlds mobilized to form religious communities of vowed women.[7] In
these communities women worked. They spent their lives establishing
the social institutions that were to become critical to nineteenth- and
twentieth-century society. In so doing, they pioneered the professional
paths that eventually opened to all women.[8] They were women who,
to paraphrase Cott again, "practiced a radical form of self-assertion"
through submission to religion.

It is surprising, then, to find relatively little scholarly interest in the enormous work of the Catholic sisterhoods. Maria Luddy's study of women and
philanthropy in nineteenth-century Ireland is typically dismissive:

While Protestant and Quaker women developed an independent and secular tradition of philanthropic involvement which removed itself, within the first three
decades of the century, from clerical influence, Catholic women did not do so. In
societies organized by Catholics the clergy exerted a powerful control over the
direction taken by women philanthropists, seen particularly in the formation of
female religious congregations, and the impact of such influence shaped the
conservative nature of Catholic social action among lay and religious.[9]

Perhaps one problem for contemporary scholars is that Catholic
women engaged in public social action collectively — obscuring their individual social identities behind habit and veil. More than this, the religious way of life pursued by Catholic women actively eradicated individuality.[10] In its ideal form, membership in a community involved the
surrender of individual will, loss of birth name and identity, and indifference to place and one's work in life.[11] Vowed women espoused submission of individuality, unlike the working class labor activists or the activist
middle and upper class women so beloved by historians. Activist women
reflect historians' own values of individuality and self-actualization without gender constraints. Vowed women embraced gender constraints and
turned them to their advantage.

A further problem with Catholic vowed women and their place in history is that it has been difficult to see them simply as women. It seems that there were (and are?) three categories of human beings: men, women, and nuns. This sleight of hand recategorized pious women who undertook voluntary vows, wore distinctive clothes, and lived apart from society — a recategorization that served important functions. The original purpose of this assertive asexuality had been to protect women from male interference.[12] In the nineteenth century, when women set apart as "brides of Christ" left the confinement of the cloister for the first time to work in the world, they brought the separation of the cloister with them. Cloaked in its mystique, and rendered invisible by their political conservatism, their obedience to authority, and their submergence of individuality, the sisters managed to create a place for themselves in but not of the world. The legacy of this categorization is the continued elimination of sisterhoods from consideration when thinking about women and work, women and the professions, and women and skill. Nowhere is this erasure more evident than in the case of nursing.

Of all the female professionals, the nurse alone can claim a precise precursor in the nursing nun. Indeed, in the two pivotal events for nineteenth-century nursing, the Crimean War and the American Civil War, nuns not only nursed alongside other women, but provided the inspiration for many other women to come and do likewise. They were also competent and experienced. In the Crimea, Florence Nightingale's right hand were the Sisters of Mercy from Bermondsey, London, while over 600 nuns nursed on both sides in the American conflict.[13] Nursing, too, unlike teaching and social work, remains to this day a sharply gendered practice, with few men choosing it as a career.[14] The contribution of nursing nuns to the overall professional development of nursing is evident in the training schools they conducted, in their involvement in professional associations, and in their participation in the development of the discipline in the university sector.[15] But even more impressive than their intellectual or ethical impact on the nursing profession has been their impact on the health care system as a whole. In the area of service delivery, Catholic women stand apart. In the United States, Canada, and Australia these women have been both major health care providers and working nurses since the early nineteenth century.

The intention here is not to laud the sisters and their contribution to nursing and the health care system, but rather to question the analysis that sets the limits of history in a way that renders these women invisible and colors the past (and therefore the present) in a particular way. Why is there a blind spot in relation to religious women — even in nursing, where the results of the sisters' efforts sit, clear as beacons, in major inner city real estate portfolios in almost every major town and city in the United States, Canada, Australia, and New Zealand? The "Church" did not buy these properties and build these major hospitals — small communities of hardworking women did. These women were often immigrant, often Irish. They neither sought attention nor received it. They did not care for suffrage or politics. They did not perceive their "work" in secular terms. Thus the nursing sisterhoods have been of little interest to scholars from women's history and nursing alike.

Invisibility

Margaret Susan Thompson agrees that Catholic women have fallen through the gaps in historical scholarship. She charges that, by neglecting the contribution of these women, scholars "help perpetuate incomplete and highly inaccurate perceptions of religion's practice and significance."[16] Until recently, religious women have been dealt with seriously only by "insider" histories.[17] But religious histories, even ones sympathetic to the sisters, commonly reinforce this invisibility. For instance Marvin O'Connell describes the Sisters of St. Francis's association with the Mayos in Rochester, Minnesota (of Mayo Clinic fame) in terms that remove the sisters' agency and initiative. He describes the hospital as opening "under the supervision of Mayo," even though the sisters raised all the capital, and owned the hospital, and Mayo had to be entreated to support them.[18] Even George C. Stewart, Jr.'s *Marvels of Charity*, while it lauds the nuns and their contribution to American society, at times still reinforces the passivity of the sisters and the guiding hand of their male confessors (pastors and priests).[19]

The situation is improving. Jo Ann McNamara's *Sisters in Arms* gave women's religious life in the Catholic Church its own history and its own mark.[20] Recent texts such as Mary Peckham Magray's *The Transforming Power of the Nuns* closely examined the impact of the Irish sisterhoods, and reconceptualized Ireland's famous "devotional revolution" of the second half of the nineteenth century as the sisters' achievement, not their genesis.[21] Susan O'Brien's detailed work on the impact of French sisters in Victorian England also emphasized the importance of the sisters' introduction of their highly refined "female decorative arts" into the stark Puritan aesthetic of England.[22] In American history a cadre of women historians have tapped the rich archival sources to write the stories of Catholic women pioneers. For instance, Carol Coburn and Martha Smith have written of the Sisters of St. Joseph of Carondelet and brought to the field a thorough account of the challenges the sisters faced and their contribution to the Catholic community.[23] Suellen Hoy's work charts the major contribution of Irish women to religious life in North America.[24] Canadian scholar Elizabeth Smyth has examined the marginal position of Catholic sisterhoods, particularly with respect to their work in the field of education, and highlights the existence of a professional identity among religious women.[25]

This growing corpus of scholarly work has been concerned with the scope and impact of the sisterhoods. For instance, Coburn and Smith cover the range of apostolic work, with some emphasis on education.[26] Smyth's work on the influence of the sisterhoods, too, focuses on education.[27] Joan Lynaugh, Jean Richardson, and Bernadette MacCauley have provided analyses of nursing by sisters in Kansas City, Buffalo, and New York City respectively.[28] And Kathleen Joyce's research synthesized these local studies into the historical background to her largely twentieth-century review of religious hospitals in the United States. Barbra Mann Wall moved this project further by undertaking a comparative analysis of two communities, the Sisters of the Incarnate Word and the Sisters of the Holy Name in the west and midwest.[29]

To be sure, Catholic women were not the only nineteenth-century religious women to formalize community and to live apart yet in the world. Scholars of Victorian England such as Martha Vicinus, Susan Casteras, and more recently Susan Mumm have provided details of the intricacies and diversity of religious community among Anglican women.[30] While there is some discussion of the nursing work to which several of these communities were devoted, with the exception of Judith Moore's work these references remain tangential to the central focus of these scholars on the women's community life.[31] The deaconesses, particularly the German and American deaconess movements, have yet to receive such detailed exposition.[32] This omission is quite startling, given the primary significance attached to Kaiserswerth, Germany in the early development of Protestant nursing communities, and its influence on Florence Nightingale's vocation to nurse.

Women and "Good Works"

But who were these vowed women and how were they formed? In the Catholic Church, technically speaking, religious women who nursed were not "nuns" but sisters in a community of religious women. The term nun is an ancient one and implies solemn vows. Traditionally, solemn vows were lifelong, and vowed women were bound to remain enclosed in their convent. They could not engage in apostolic work — nursing, orphanage work, or teaching. The legal status of the many nineteenth-century sisterhoods was as confused as the terminology. In the nineteenth century the Catholic Church did not formally recognize the non-enclosed sisterhoods, and up to 1900 each application for papal approval was dealt with on a case-by-case basis. This led to quite a degree of variation from one community to the next. Communities of women could be contemplative, which meant withdrawn from the world and devoted to prayer — such as the Carmelites. Others were restricted in what was permitted; for instance, sisters might be allowed to teach, but the girls needed to enter the convent grounds as the women were not allowed to leave, as was the case with the Ursulines. Other communities were quite unrestricted in their pastoral activities and engaged in any kind of work (prison visiting, asylum work, rescue of women) such as the Irish Sisters of Charity, the Sisters of Mercy, and the original Daughters of Charity of St. Vincent de Paul. Each community, then and now, is defined by its rule — a guide to the sister's identity as a member of this community, and the charism (the special works such as nursing or care of the elderly) that the holy foundress had established the community to pursue. Not all sisterhoods engaged in nursing, much less founded hospitals, but for some this work was central to their charism.

A final point. Catholic communities of women in the nineteenth century were part of an international and an internationalizing church. Catholic women were caught up in the great diaspora that led to the establishment of the Catholic Church in the English-speaking world — in Britain as well as in the settler societies of North America and Australia. German, Italian, and Polish Catholics also emigrated in great numbers. In the nineteenth century 91 of the 119 communities established in the United States were "European or Canadian in origin."[33] But the communities established on local soil or imported from Europe were not static in this changing world. Irish communities assumed Australian or American identities, German communities became American. But most commonly American and French communities were filled with Irish and German women — especially Irish women.[34] It all depended on immigration and recruitment patterns. This nineteenth-century flood of active women followed a path pioneered in seventeenth-century France by the Daughters of Charity. Given that so many nursing communities were formally, or in spirit, linked to this French vision of a nursing sister, it is worth examining what was so radical and innovative about the Daughters of Charity of St. Vincent de Paul.

Counter-Reformation Piety

In seventeenth-century France, the laity (or ordinary believers) established nationwide secular societies to spread the missionary zeal of the Counter-Reformation — the radical movement that was the Catholic Church's response to the challenge of Protestantism.[35] Vincent de Paul (1576–1660) was able to harness this zealous piety of the well-born into formal charitable foundations and open a huge reservoir of feminine energy and talent.[36] Vincent de Paul's achievement was remarkable in that he succeeded where so many others had failed: he was able to institute and formalize an active (uncloistered) form of religious life for women. In 1617, in collaboration with Louise de Marillac, he founded a national lay society: the Ladies of Charity (Dames de la Charité). The Ladies of Charity proved successful in the provinces visiting the poor and working among the sick. However, in the cities, the enormous popularity of the movement among the aristocracy proved problematic. In ancien régime France, the social distance between the poor and the ladies of the court, of whom the Paris confraternities of the Ladies of Charity were comprised, was so great that Louise de Marillac organized humbler women to perform the tasks of care of the sick or poor on behalf of the devout ladies of her society. In 1630 she began taking countrywomen into her home and hiring them out as nurses to the Ladies of Charity. The Daughters of Charity (Filles de la Charité) emerged as a solution to the problems of class and piety when, in 1633, Louise de Marillac received Vincent de Paul's permission to offer these humble women spiritual as well as practical instruction in the work of the Charités.[37]

The Daughters of Charity represented a new form of religious life. Extending the tradition of tertiaries, the unvowed category of religious affiliate that emerged in the twelfth century and most notably produced groups of women such as the Beguines, the Daughters were not a religious order in the strict sense of the term.[38] The religious state was precisely defined in the seventeenth century as the avoval of *perpetual* poverty, obedience, and chastity. What is more, the medieval law of *clausura* (cloister) for women religious had been reaffirmed at the Council of Trent, and the Counter-Reformation church would tolerate no exceptions. Pious women had a single vocational path — withdrawal to the cloister. As a result of these constraints, the Daughters of Charity were *soeurs* not *religieuses*, they took only private annual vows, and their rule was not written until the society was well established.[39]

Ever conscious of their precarious position, Vincent de Paul instructed the Daughters of Charity on what to say if questioned by a bishop:

If he asks you who you are, and if you are religious, tell him no, by the grace of God; that it is not that you do not have high esteem for religious, but if you were like them you would have to be enclosed, and that as a result you would have to say good-bye to the service of the poor. Tell him that you are poor Daughters of Charity, and that you are given to God for the service of the poor, and that you are free to retire or to be sent away.[40]

The second distinction between the Daughters of Charity and traditional religious was that the Daughters were overwhelmingly of humble origins. As many as 80 percent of the early recruits were illiterate.[41] Thus the dowry requirement for convent entrance and the traditional literate religious life of liturgical devotion and prayer would simply have been beyond them. As a consequence of their modest background, the spiritual life of the Daughters of Charity was developed and nourished by other, less traditional means. The selection process for Daughters of Charity was rigorous. The disposition of the recruits was scrutinized and they were only accepted into the order to become one of "Christ's militia" if they were strong of body and mind, above reproach in moral/sexual deportment, and able to work. In return, the order provided for its members in equally pragmatic terms. It offered the successful recruit "a steady wage, free accommodation, clothing, security, a modicum of comfort in illness and old age, a decent burial, and also the sense of social promotion that membership of such an esteemed community entailed."[42] This "esteem and social promotion" should not be underestimated as an important attraction, along with the economic security that went with membership. According to demographic data used by Jones, approximately 7 percent of women in seventeenth-century France were unmarried.[43] The prospect of a secure existence for women without financial independence was slight. As Daughters of Charity these women were free from those material concerns. But of course the Daughters of Charity were more than just workers: they were a religious phenomenon. The Daughters represented a powerful combination of asceticism and pious service for common women. Throughout the seventeenth and eighteenth centuries the phenomenon of these pious women workers continued to grow. Communities of women were inspired by the Daughters of Charity, and the social apostolate for women that this form of religious life provided began to be noticed in Protestant countries.

The anticlerical French Revolution put an end to the monumental growth of these communities, and while some went to the guillotine, the redesignated "citizen nurses" generally continued their work, honoring their contracts with municipal authorities and leaving martyrdom to the highborn Carmelites.[44] Under Napoleon the nursing sisterhoods, alone of the Catholic religious communities, were fully and immediately restored, successfully resisting the Emperor's urge to unify all communities into a single national nursing body.[45]

Nineteenth-Century Catholic Revival

The anticlericalism expressed during the Revolution continued to be a feature of nineteenth-century political life. From the 1848 revolutions throughout Europe to the Paris Commune in 1871, Garibaldi's Risorgimento in Italy, Bismarck's Kulturkampf in Germany, and the Third Republic of France, Catholicism was viewed as the enemy of nationalism, liberalism, and socialism. Despite, or perhaps because of, its embattled state, in France female piety surged to an extraordinary level of intensity. Hundreds of thousands of women (compared to a few thousand men) heard God's call and rushed to join religious communities.[46] In 1878 there were 135,000 religieuses in France, seven for every thousand French women.[47] The Irish church, too, a close companion of the French church, was about to begin the greatest comeback in Christian history — going from almost nonexistent at the turn of the century (due to the efforts of the British to suppress the Catholic Church under the Penal Codes) to the jewel in the crown of the Catholic Church's English-speaking empire by 1900.[48]

Women played no minor part in this Irish Catholic rebirth; between 1841 and 1901 the number of Irish nuns increased eightfold while the Irish population halved.[49] This figure does not include the export of nuns to the rest of the United Kingdom and the New World. For not only did the Irish church provide enormous numbers of priests for missionary posts throughout the world but, as Suellen Hoy has pointed out, Ireland provided a hothouse for English-speaking female religious recruits. These recruits were obtained both through direct measures (recruitment drives) and through the establishment of novitiates for overseas missions, training schools for bright girls without dowry prospects, and sodalities — parish societies. For instance, St. Brigid's Missionary School in Kilkenny (1884–1958) trained over 1,900 young women for convents, primarily in Australia, New Zealand, and the United States.[50] By mid-century Germany was also undergoing a Catholic revival, with communities of religious women providing the impetus and energy behind the rebuilding and reassertion of a German Catholic identity.[51] Cut short by Bismarck, this work yielded fruit for the New World as millions of Germans abandoned Europe and headed abroad.

Becoming a Nun

I have a particular reason for wishing to be under St. Vincent. I have an obligation to him.
—*Florence Nightingale, 1852*[52]

In the nineteenth century as today, there was no single training that all Catholic sisters underwent. There were and are, however, important traditions — a repertoire of possibilities — that the foundresses drew upon to create a particular community of women religious. The principal traditions for nursing communities were the Rule of St. Vincent de Paul,

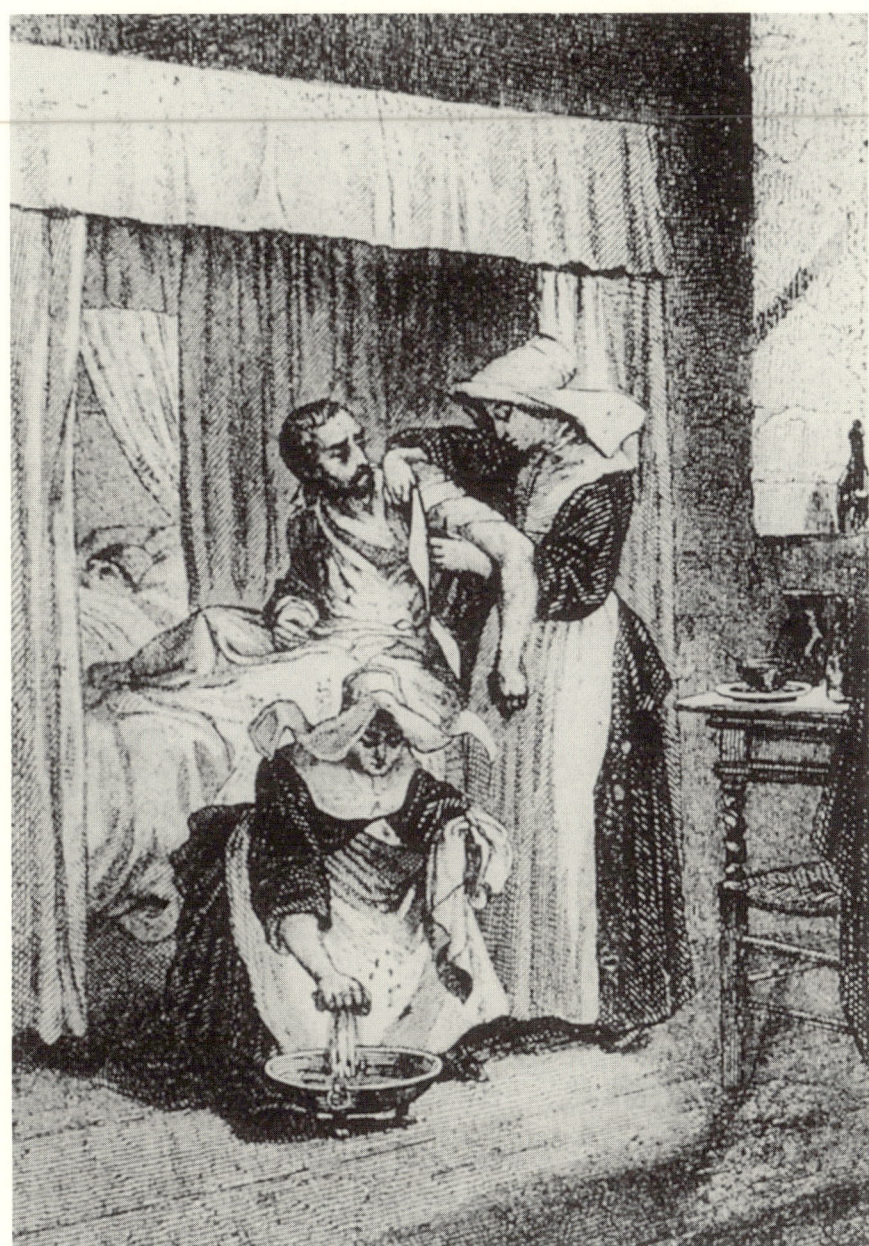

Figure 1. *Sisters of Charity*. Wood carving, Casimir Tollet, from *Les Edifices hospitaliers*, 1892. Two nuns wash and bandage a man in a French hospital ward, possibly a military hospital. Courtesy of National Library of Medicine, Bethesda, Maryland.

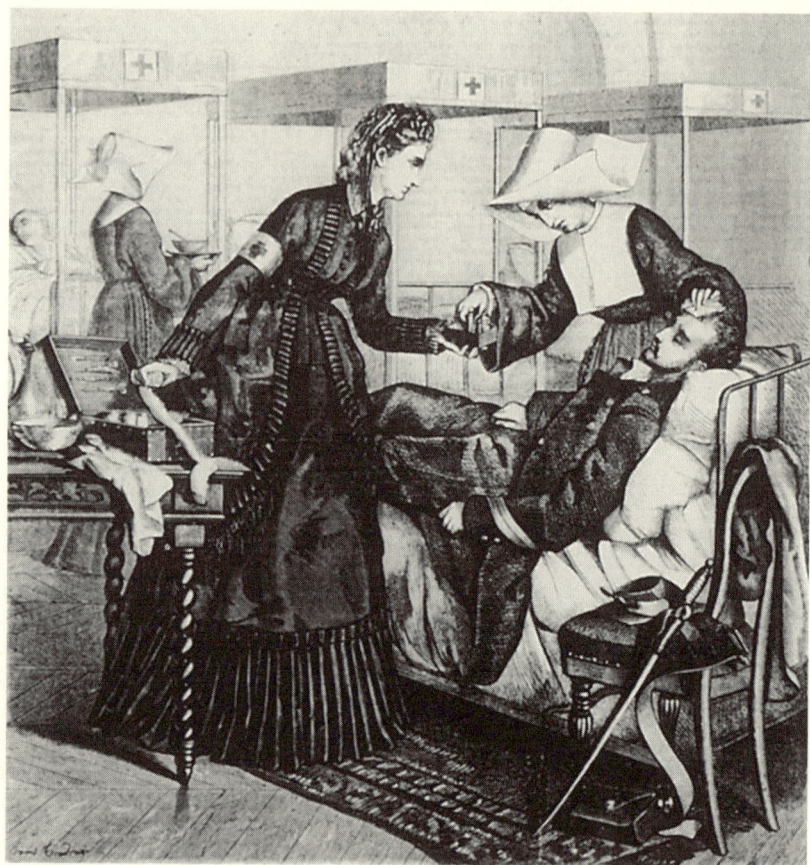

Figure 2. *L'Ambulance*. Anais Coudour, France, 1870. Interior of a Red Cross hospital ward during the siege of Paris. wounded soldier being helped by a nursing nun and a Red Cross nurse. Courtesy of National Library of Medicine, Bethesda, Maryland.

the Rule of St. Augustine (this hospital code dates back to the Crusades and the hospitalers), and the Rule of St. Francis. The Vincentian model was the most influential on nineteenth-century nursing communities of Catholic and Protestant women. This rule was developed in seventeenth-century France. With it a new mode of religious life for women emerged where for the first time the active apostolate (or good works) was the core of their spiritual life.[53] What Vincent de Paul and Louise de Marillac created with the original Daughters of Charity was a rule for women where "work" was central.[54] Work dominated over prayer, over daily offices. These women's very religious life was defined by a pragmatic attention to the needs of those around them, as distinct from an ascetic spiritual life of prayer. The impact of this initiative is hard to overstate. It provided the model for countless Catholic communities and the ubiquitous St. Vincent Hospital; influenced Lutheran Theodur Fliedner in Kaiserswerth, founder of the deaconesses movement; moved Quaker Elizabeth Fry, prison reformer and founder of the group of Protestant women who called themselves the Sisters of Mercy; and inspired all the Anglican sisterhoods and, of course, Florence Nightingale.

To join a religious community in the nineteenth century a woman commonly needed a dowry. Although humble communities such as the French Daughters of Charity did not have a dowry requirement, in the first half of the nineteenth century in Ireland, when elite women dominated the convent movement, the minimum sum was £500–600. By the second half of the century it had dropped to £200–300.[55] Lay sisters, who formed a servant class in convents, did not require a dowry. However, the Catholic diaspora radically altered the opportunities available to women without dowries. To attract women on "missions," that is foundations in non-Catholic countries such as Australia and North America, the dowry requirement was commonly waived. In the United States, too, the distinction between lay sisters and choir sisters came to be considered undemocratic and was abandoned by communities.[56]

The religious training of women in the nineteenth century is difficult to investigate or compare. The rule of each community, the designated prayers and suggested readings, novitiate training, retreats, and special devotions, all depended on a constellation of factors — such as the inclination of and influences on the foundress. An important influence was the foundress's confessor. Here the man's own religious training was highly significant. If he were a Vincentian (a member of the male order of priests established by Vincent de Paul), then this influence was likely to be pronounced. If he were a Jesuit, then the spiritual exercises of Ignatius Loyola would be important. The foundress of a community also relied on her own strong spiritual call — what God was demanding of her. Her rule was developed in collaboration with sympathetic clergy, who would assist its smooth passage through the Vatican. For instance, the rule of the Irish Sisters of Charity had a strong Jesuit influence. Mary Aikenhead had been unable to undergo her novitiate training in France (due to war) and had gone to York in England instead. The Bar Convent at York was the Institute of the Blessed Virgin, founded by Mary Ward, the so-called female Jesuit. Later, the rule of the Irish Sisters of Charity was formulated with the assistance of a Jesuit priest.[57] A similarly complex story could be told of every community, as each rule has its history and its own set of religious traditions that it calls upon to shape the women who enter the community.

The training of novices was (and is) the responsibility of the novice mistress. The novice mistress was the most significant person in the community after the mother superior. She was commonly in that role for many years, and could be responsible for an entire generation of novices. The novice mistress assisted novices to achieve spiritual perfection through attendance to the rule and the study of the life of the holy foundress. Novices worked on spiritual exercises recommended by the foundress, and in obedience to the novice mistress and the mother superior. Common texts for study in the nineteenth century were the *Imitatio Christi* and the Life of St. Teresa of Avila.[58] Vincent de Paul provided explicit guidelines for nursing sisters in his "Conferences," lessons he held in a workshop format.[59] These classes were faithfully recorded by Louise de Marillac and subsequently published and translated. The Conferences were widely used by nursing communities.[60]

In addition to the novice mistress, the confessor for the community played an important role in the religious life of the sisters and might or might not be involved directly in the formation of novices. As their confessor he was responsible for providing spiritual guidance to sisters (during confession), for conducting religious services for them, and often for holding retreats for them. Retreats were a time when each member of the community examined herself, her work, and her obedience to God, and then reaffirmed her vows. The question of confessor was often a vexed one. Sisters went to great lengths to have control over the selection of their confessor, one who fitted in with their tradition and offered them spiritual guidance sympathetic to their rule.[61] As archbishop of Dublin, Paul Cullen drily remarked about the sisters: "Although after their fashion they will do nothing but as they will be told, still, they know how to manage so as to be told what they wish."[62]

Just as there was and is great variance in religious rule, there was also a variety of organizational models of religious life. In the nineteenth century, religious communities of women not subject to the cloister rule were a new phenomenon outside France and New France. Rome did not proclaim any general rule or guidelines for these new communities, and each carved its own path in adaptation to local needs, while at the same time praying for formal recognition from Rome, termed Papal approbation.[63] The Vincentian mode of organization revolved around the motherhouse.[64] All recruits were trained centrally in the Paris head office or motherhouse. This practice ensured that every Daughter of Charity received identical training, was shaped under the experienced eye of the novice mistress for the entire community, and was sent into the field from Paris to a region away from her home. In this way recruits were transformed from simple provincial women into Daughters of Charity. This centralized organization also made the Daughters relatively independent of church politics and the machinations of bishops. In financial terms it meant that they could allocate their resources centrally and strategically, as opposed to being swept up in each bishop's plan for charitable works in his diocese.

It also meant that the community had to have organized structures to reinforce the links between the sisters, who worked in pairs in regions far from their homes and far from Paris. The Daughters of Charity established elaborate communication networks, written reports of conferences with Vincent de Paul, newsletters, retreats, and annual visits to maintain their spiritual life in such difficult isolation. For instance, when one member died her fellow sisters would participate in a collective obituary process. All the glory and individual credit denied in life was granted in death and used as a means to strengthen the Daughters' collective bonds and to reinforce the heroic nature of their calling. In the nineteenth-century New World, these mechanisms kept alive strong links between women isolated by many thousands of miles. They provided sisters with guidance in their pioneering endeavors and nourished new foundations with recruits trained at the motherhouse in Cologne, or Emmitsburg (Maryland), or Cork, or Montreal.

Instead of following the motherhouse model, some communities constituted each house separately. In this case legal jurisdiction for the community came not from a central body but from the diocese where the community resided. The Sisters of Mercy were (and are) one such group. As an international community they maintained strong links within their organization, but remained fully under the jurisdiction of their local bishop. However, whether communities of women are motherhouse or diocesan in organization, conflicts with men dominate nearly all their stories. Whether the problem was the theft of the sisters' money by priests or bishops, or punishments such as the denial of sacraments and interference with their rule, the women frequently struggled against heavy odds to keep their work going and their communities intact. Communities with a motherhouse structure remained free to quit a diocese where a bishop or one of his clerics made their lives a misery;[65] diocesan communities did not have this option. Yet, despite the plentiful tales of oppression, as Thompson points out, "nuns were in a seller's market."[66] When every bishop needed the energy and skill of the sisters to help develop his diocese, it made sense to woo rather than bully. Moreover, as the sisters became more experienced in both their work and their organization, they knew how to manage situations that their predecessors did not.[67]

The nineteenth-century Catholic Church was distinguished by the variety of form and structure of religious life. There were large communities with many convents or houses all ruled by their motherhouse, there were large communities with each house a separate entity operating within its diocese; there were also communities that started off one way and split, changed, and merged over time. For instance, when Mother Seton founded the American Sisters of Charity in 1807, these women operated under a motherhouse structure. Mid-century the New York Sisters of Charity and the Sisters of Charity of Cincinnati split to become diocesan communities. The American Sisters of Charity then merged with the French community, becoming a branch of the Daughters of Charity of St. Vincent de Paul. Thereafter the Sisters of Charity of Cincinnati formed other foundations well beyond the diocese of Cincinnati.[68]

The communities of sisters that were highly successful as nurses tended to be of the motherhouse structure, though not exclusively so. The large communities of Daughters of Charity, Sisters of Charity, Sisters of St. Joseph, and Sisters of Providence all became major health care providers. The motherhouse structure fostered skill development, and the Catholic Church understood and valued both training and experience. The spiritual training of the sisters equipped them to lead, to establish new communities, and to recruit and train new members. It was what separated the sisters from the rather motley group of enthusiastic amateur secular nurses that began to appear following the Crimean War and the Civil War.

Protestant Apostolic Call

For a Protestant woman the situation was very different. For her, God's call was to the place into which she had been placed by God — the family home as a daughter, a wife, a mother. Good deeds reflected God's blessings and redemption was a matter of acceptance of God's will. In a radical shift in perspective, virtuous Protestant women in the nineteenth century extended the bounds of the domestic sphere to encompass the social needs of those around them. This reframing of the female realm of influence gave permission for women to re-site their energies beyond their own four walls.

As the nineteenth century wore on, possibilities for Protestant women slowly emerged. The first such possibility came out of Germany's Catholic Rhineland. This region had been absorbed into Protestant Prussia with the Congress of Vienna in 1815. The work of the Daughters of Charity from the newly established motherhouse in Strasbourg began to be noticed, and among Lutherans too there arose a movement for a social apostolate.[69] For Lutheran women the most significant event was the revival of the female diaconate by Pastor Theodur Fliedner at the small Rhineland town of Kaiserswerth in 1838.[70]

Fliedner was both driven by the vocational call to be of service to the poor and needy and stirred by the success of the Daughters of Charity in evangelizing among the poor. His work marked a radical break for Lutheran women that moved them into the public sphere. Such was the success of the deaconesses that within a few decades they transformed the social institutions of Lutherans in northern Europe. Deaconesses from Switzerland to Norway took over the management of hospitals, nursed, and worked among the needy.

In Britain, too, women were called to serve God through work with His needy. But again it was not clear how this could be achieved. Debates in and outside of the pulpit raged on the vexed question of a "Protestant Sister of Charity."[71] Consensus was never to be reached on the subject, but the full gamut of options found expression in Victorian England, ranging from the deaconesses and bible missioners to female religious communities scandalizing Protestantism with vows and habits.[72]

Rewriting Nursing History

Institutional reform in Britain and institutional foundation in the New World were situated within a broad program of social reform. Education, sanitation, housing, the ordering of public space, epidemic control, and prison, asylum, and workhouse reform were all part of the sweep of activities pursued in the nineteenth century by good citizens and the state alike. The overpopulated cities and vast numbers of immigrants from Ireland and the Continent, coupled with the enormous prosperity of industrial Britain and Northeast America, established the imperatives of social reform. It is here that the modern professional nurse appeared.

Professional nursing in its modern form emerged in tandem with major transformations in the management of the health of populations, in the delivery of health care, and, indeed, in the care itself. The history of professional nursing is a story of these nineteenth-century scientific and moral imperatives. Under their impact, by the early twentieth century, unified training and registration procedures were in place in Britain, the United States, Canada, Ireland, New Zealand, and Australia.

The traditional view of these developments is an evolutionary one. Broadly speaking, the trajectory for the emergence of professional nursing goes as follows: The predecessors of the modern nurse were the well meaning but untrained Catholic nursing nuns. In post-Reformation Europe nursing had fallen into ignoble hands — servants and fellow patients. The reformist nurses, personified in the figure of Florence Nightingale, established trained secular nursing as a career for respectable women. Ostensibly, Nightingale's involvement in hospital reform began with the establishment of the Nightingale Fund.

According to legend, Nightingale deployed these funds to establish a model training school of nursing at St. Thomas's Hospital in London. St. Thomas's personified what became known as the Nightingale system:

all-powerful matron, elite corps of students, training undertaken by ward sisters, nurses resident in nursing home. St. Thomas's graduates, so the tale tells, passed out into elite positions as matrons of key hospitals in Britain and throughout the world. Through her tireless correspondence, Nightingale continued to be intimately involved in their achievements. Moreover, in addition to her work at St. Thomas's, where she was directly involved with the nurses, Nightingale was a key adviser on all matters concerning hospitals in Britain till the end of the nineteenth century.

The impact of the Nightingale legend is as important as the true story. The legend makes Nightingale the inventor of the trained, elite nurse and the modern safe hospital. But the Nightingale Fund's reputation depended as much on what it was perceived to have achieved as what it actually did.[73] The authoritative biography of Nightingale by Thomas Cook was published in 1913, a mere three years after her death. The sources were provided to Cook by Sir Henry Bonham Carter, literary executor, lifelong friend, relative and adviser of Nightingale, and secretary of the Nightingale Fund from 1861 to 1914. Many of the figures discussed by Cook were still alive, and the glories of Nightingale's achievements were charted in high relief. Monica Baly found that all the subsequent works on Nightingale had used Cook as a primary source and barely reexamined the original documents.[74] This explains the remarkable consistency of the Nightingale legend. Of course it was very important for Nightingale's reforms to have credibility. As Baly puts it, "Although the concept of nurse training had been accepted, it was still necessary to hammer home the message."[75] Henry Bonham Carter had a vested interest in the "steady progress toward the light" theory of history.

Contrary to the official view, Baly reveals that not many of Nightingale's graduates went on to reform the British hospital system, though a few certainly did.[76] Nor was her model training school the actual application of a Nightingale vision; rather, Nightingale lost many a battle for control of the school, and the hospital, the training program, and the nurses it produced seldom pleased her. But perhaps the actual story is less the point than the emblematic significance that Nightingale came to assume for nursing.

Early historians of Nightingale, and of the development of the profession, to a great extent looked uncritically at the Nightingale legend, sharing the reformist agenda. It was expedient to portray nursing as a unified, educated profession evolving from religious ignorance to sophisticated expertise. These hagiographies shaped modern nursing's sense of itself. Their discourse overshadowed earlier developments in nineteenth-century nursing, overstated the iniquities of the past, and overlooked the work of other reformers. More recently, however, Nightingale's views on women, class, medical authority, and nursing education disappointed a generation of revisionist historians who blamed the elitist and feminized nineteenth-century reworking of the nurse for many of the contemporary trials of the nursing profession.[77]

But history always tells us about the present, about what we choose to study and care to reveal about our collective past. The study of nursing nuns has offered nothing to the professional project that until quite recently so expended nursing's historical energies. For other historians the picture again lacks nuns. They are, after all, hard to see through the wall of forthright women with opinions on issues that still matter to us — such as politics and feminism. English historian Anne Summers has been a lone voice since the 1980s, exploding the notion of secularization and professionalization. Her work emphasizes the role of philanthropy, religion, and class in the gentrification of nursing.[78] Her research on the Protestant nurses reveals the important groundwork performed by religious nurses in England in raising clinical and professional expectations of nurses in the lead-in to the Nightingale story.[79]

For nursing hagiography in nineteenth-century Protestant England to set out to create nursing anew, with scant reference to the Catholic Church, is of course perfectly understandable. In that sectarian context, secular nurses were women who were not members of religious communities — but they were not without religion. F. B. Smith attributes Nightingale's success in the Crimea partly to the fact that Nightingale negotiated this particular minefield so well. "Miss Nightingale had the advantage in the government's view by being safely Protestant but otherwise religiously neutral."[80] Summers agrees. She argues that so-called secular nursing was more often than not Protestant nursing.[81] In fact, the emergence of the image of nursing as secular provided the means through which Protestant women were able to commit themselves to a recognizably Catholic form of life and avoid the sectarian repercussions. But to depict the nineteenth-century reformers as nonreligious is to misunderstand the religiosity of the civic reform movement.

Religious Women as Nurses

Even if the importance of the Catholic and Protestant nursing sisterhoods in the emergence of nursing as a respectable path for women is granted, it still does not answer the question whether the nuns were competent nurses. The verdict on the nursing competence of the St. John's House Sisterhood in London by Summers, Moore, and Helmstadter is certainly positive.[82] For the Catholic sisterhoods, the story is varied and complex. Nightingale at times thought they were good nurses, while at other times she thought not. Her report on Italian nursing nuns was highly critical; however, she had a great deal of time for the "dear Daughters of Charity" she found in Turkey.[83] She was dismissive of her enemies — the Irish contingent of Sisters of Mercy in the Crimea, but lauded her allies — the (also Irish) Sisters of Mercy from Bermondsey.[84]

The nursing sisterhoods all engaged in home nursing — this is often overshadowed by hospital nursing. The clinical and social impact of this work by sisterhoods is difficult to determine. Nonetheless, Magray's examination of Irish records reveals a remarkable level of coverage by nursing nuns. She estimates that in 1850 seven Dublin convents visited ten thousand patients. By extending this figure to include household members the figure she estimates is 78,000 people came into direct contact with a nursing nun.[85] Even if a more modest estimate of the range of influence of the sisters is made, as a group of women working with the sick poor, their corporate knowledge of the conditions of the poor and the medical and apothecary needs of the sick must have been considerable.

Paradoxically, nursing nuns were criticized by Dorothy Dix and her nurses for kowtowing to medicine,[86] whereas they were opposed in France for refusing to recognize medical authority as supreme.[87] A common criticism arises out of restrictions imposed by their religious rule on the care of men, the care of pregnant women, and treatment of venereal disease. Again there was a wide range both in rule and in its application. After all, army nursing involved the exclusive care of men, and epidemic nursing was not possible without attending to the cleanliness of patients — cholera nursing scarcely seems suitable for the modest. In fact, men always represented the majority of nineteenth-century hospital patients. Sisters at the frontier certainly delivered babies, although nineteenth-century women in childbirth would not expect to be admitted to hospitals, other than specific "lying-in" institutions.[88] Catriona Clear in her landmark work on Irish nuns maintains that they were not full nurses. She asserts this position even though she cites evidence from a medical officer that the sisters did perform all the nursing at the hospital — except for the care of men with venereal disease.[89] Clear see.ms unaware that no respectable nurse would have performed such care, nor would she have been expected to. Secular nurses well into the twentieth century received assistance in the intimate care of men through male nurses, orderlies, and dressers.[90] The final familiar criticism raised by Clear is that the "daily timetable of spiritual examination" interfered with the sisters' ability to be effective nurses. Again, there was a wide range of community expectations of their sisters, expectations that have changed over time. Daughters of Charity, for instance, have never had in place religious duties that take them away from the bedside. In general, though, as we will see, the twentieth century brought pressure from Rome on religious women to devote themselves to a fuller daily prayer regimen.

In the nineteenth century, long before diplomas or training registers, these religious women nursed. They tended the sick, cared for the dying, assisted at surgery, and ran apothecaries. They knew the sick and the poor of their cities and towns. They took over during epidemics, and set up well organized hospitals — sites of philanthropy and medical practice. In this way, the vocational wave of energized pious women translated itself into a new form — the religious nurse. The Marthas of the nineteenth century kept quiet but they did not keep still. Beneath the attention of men of power, unnoticed or dismissed by women with voice and ideas, driven by vocational ideals that obeyed God's call, they went to work.

Chapter 3

Free Enterprise and Resourcefulness

An American Success Story —

The Daughters of Charity in the Northeast

> *The Sisters of Charity will have the free and undisturbed management of the internal economy of the institution. The Sister-Servant is authorised to name Physicians, to hire servants and dismiss them; to admit patients & discharge them; to procure necessary provisions and make ordinary expenditures for the establishment; and to receive money coming from pay-patients, donations or otherwise. . . . Building or considerable repair must be sanctioned by the Board.*
>
> *— 1857 By-Laws for the regulations of the Trustees of the Rochester St. Mary's Hospital of the Sisters of Charity.[1]*

In the second half of the nineteenth century Catholic hospitals, owned and conducted by communities of vowed Catholic women, were playing a major role in hospital foundation in the United States. In fact, Catholic sisters founded a total of 299 hospitals between 1829 and 1900.[2] The Protestant pride and rampant anti-Catholicism of the period could lead one to assume that the United States was the country least likely to support the work of Catholic women through taxes levied on the hardworking Protestant majority. One would be wrong. In fact, unlike Britain, where Protestant dominance was never breached by a Catholic hospital system, or Australia, where the large Catholic community produced a network of fine public hospitals owned and conducted by communities of women religious with virtually no government aid in the nineteenth century, in the United States the spirit of free enterprise paradoxically functioned to support the sisters' efforts. Throughout the country the sisters were able to provide the best value for money in the care of the indigent sick, to compete for public tenders to secure these monies, to gain contracts with insurers, railroad and mining companies, federal government, and army. They attracted excellent doctors, collaborated with medical schools, and ran teaching facilities. Importantly, in return for their private patients, they opened up hospital practice to private medical practitioners excluded by the medical boards of competing hospitals. They thereby established private hospital care as the province not of the rich but of the modest. By the end of the century patient fees were what supported Catholic hospitals. They created the prototype for the modern twentieth-century hospital and laid the foundation for the twentieth-century dominance of private institutional and medical care in the U.S. health care system. The success of the sisters' nursing work, far more than their work with schools or orphanages, is the story of the sisters coming to understand the particularities of the American political and economic climate to run the best businesses in the market. America respected that.

An Active Path for American Women

Finding their place in the United States was a challenge for the Catholic sisterhoods. As one of the most visible symbols of Catholicism and foreign power (Rome), the "un-American" identity of the nuns caused them a great deal of difficulty. However, the cholera epidemics of the first half of the nineteenth century, when they volunteered to nurse the sick, and later their heroism during the Civil War, made the nun a complex and unstable figure in the American psyche — vilified and romanticized. In this chapter I examine the impact of Catholic women on the health and welfare of nineteenth-century Americans, and their role in shaping the American health care system. I look closely at the Daughters of Charity of St. Vincent de Paul, the largest single community of Catholic nursing women, as major health care providers for both the nineteenth and the twentieth centuries. The importance of the Daughters' epidemic nursing, their role in the care of immigrant communities, their work during the Civil War, and, finally, their relationship with medical men, are all important elements of their story — and of the story of American nursing. The Catholic nursing sisters, most particularly the Charities, developed a successful model of hospital service provision for the American public. These women created the health services (to use a modern term), building their major institutions through a combination of simple faith and sophisticated skill. It is the interplay of these attributes, faith and skill, that needs to be understood if we are to appreciate how the sisters, as modest vowed women, achieved so very much.

The Daughters of Charity are important for another reason. They represent the first Anglophone adaptation of the model for an "active" religious life for women developed by Vincent de Paul and Louise de Marillac.[3] We examine how this distinctive path for women, which emerged during the Counter-Reformation in seventeenth-century France in response to massive social dislocation and widespread poverty, found such easy application among pious nineteenth-century American women, desperate to make a difference to the suffering that surrounded them.

Catholicism in the United States

Around the world the Catholic Church was on the rise in the nineteenth century. And its progress was remarkable. In 1820 no Catholic could hold public office in Britain, the Church had only a tiny presence in the United States, Australia, and Canada, and its missionary activities in the East and Africa were only beginning. By the end of the century, it had survived trials of fire to achieve such a position of defensive certainty that papal infallibility had been proclaimed; the Catholic position in Britain was vastly expanded, with prominent British converts leading the English church; in the United States the church was filled with immigrants to become the country's largest congregation; and the Irish church was the star in the English-speaking church's crown, providing thousands upon thousands of priests, nuns, and brothers for the newly established English-speaking Catholic world.[4]

But it was not only Catholicism that adopted a tone of strident and overbearing confidence in the nineteenth century. In the United States the First and Second Great Awakenings stirred religious passions of an evangelical kind.[5] Many hundreds of thousands of souls were "saved" at revival meetings that swept the country. Meanwhile, the rising numbers of immigrants, industrialization, and the rapid rate of social change in the cities unsettled American confidence in the nation's capacity to assimilate all the newcomers and still retain its traditions. In the centers that received the million Irish paupers who fled the famine after 1845, such as Boston, New York, and Philadelphia, the social dislocation caused by the tide of such poor, desperate, and ignorant peasantry flooding into the city slums led to a major backlash. In the decade before the Civil War, nativist sentiment and the political movement known as the "Know-Nothings" set out to counter "foreign" influences. Anti-immigrant feelings frequently spilled over into violence. Anti-Catholic riots took place across the country; the worst unrest was in Philadelphia in 1844, where churches and houses were burned and fifteen people killed. In Louisville in 1855 twenty were killed and hundreds injured in Know-Nothing riots.[6]

The fears produced by Protestant renewal and the flood of pauper Catholic immigrants were further inflamed by the extraordinarily popular salacious tales of escaped nuns. The traveling road show of "escaped nun" Maria Monk (with baby), whose "awful disclosures" of her convent life were such a bestseller, provided a type of Puritan pornography that revealed nuns as sex slaves for priests, with abortion and infanticide as common practices, and with unwilling girls made captive in an international white slave trade.[7] It was good business for speaking-tour promoters and booksellers, and it spawned an entire genre of "discovered documents" such as plans of secret passages between convents and monasteries, secret diaries, confessional documents, and testimonials of "escaped" nuns and "reformed" priests.[8]

The main target of such hostility and fevered imagination was the convent nun — the sister away from the world and enclosed by high walls behind which unspeakable acts were thought to be commonly perpetrated. The active working sister, whose daily tasks brought her into contact with the poor and infirm, whose hospital provided care for all, was conspicuously absent from these accounts. However, with passions running high, the distinction between active sisters and enclosed orders was certainly not clear to an angry mob, and the convent and the habited woman became the direct target of arson and intimidation. Even convents filled with schoolchildren or orphans were on occasion surrounded and threatened. The Ursuline convent burned to the ground in 1834 in Charlestown, Massachusetts was the home of sisters and schoolchildren.[9]

Given the climate of hysteria, it must have been unsettling for the pious American woman to feel called by God to dedicate her life to work with His needy. For her, as with her English counterpart, this call was a recognizably Catholic one. Protestants were convinced that the Catholic Church preyed on the impressionable minds of wealthy women. They suspected machinations by the nuns who conducted schools for wealthy American girls. Worse still were priests (perhaps the dreaded Jesuits), who were believed to charm and lure women to "surrender" to Catholicism.[10] The image of seduction is important, for it offered the central motif of many Protestant anxieties around Catholicism and around the relationship between the priest/confessor and the young woman/nun.[11]

More reasoned fears were expressed by Catharine Beecher. In her American Women's Education Association 1856 annual report, she warned that the best and the brightest of Protestant women might be driven to convert to Catholicism "for the power it gives them to throw their energies into a sphere of definite utility under the control of high religious responsibility."[12]

Elizabeth Seton and the Daughters of Charity

The story of Elizabeth Seton is one such conversion story. Elizabeth Ann Seton, first American-born saint and founder of the Sisters of Charity in 1807 (later called Daughters of Charity), began a movement of women, the American Charities as they were known, who established an extensive network of fine hospitals throughout the country. Elizabeth Seton's path to Catholicism, her rejection by family and society, and the difficulties she and her children suffered have been well recorded. What is of interest here is that her call to Catholicism and her call to serve the poor were synonymous. This Vincentian impulse had no Protestant parallel in the first decade of the nineteenth century, and it demanded of Elizabeth that she carve the way for American women. The Napoleonic wars made the affiliation of the American Charities with the French Daughters impossible, so the path was created as an American one, led by an American-born former Protestant.

The American Sisters of Charity began nursing in the first American medical teaching hospital when they took over nursing at the Baltimore Infirmary in 1823. The opportunity to work at the Baltimore Infirmary, which was affiliated with the University of Maryland, was the best clinical introduction to modern medicine and hospital management available at the time, and was to serve the sisters in good stead for further hospital work.

The rule of the Daughters of Charity, formulated by Vincent de Paul and Louise de Marillac, provides guidelines for the sisters in the "exposed" area of hospital work. Their training focuses on the dual material and spiritual benefits their nursing work brings to the sick poor and gives them clear guidance on ways to maintain their "interiority" away from the protection of the convent walls and grille.[13]

The success of the sisters at hospital management and nursing built more success. They were experienced nurses in established hospitals right at the beginning of the wave of hospital foundation that accompanied urbanization and industrialization. The Sisters of Charity, therefore, were perfectly placed to become experts in the field. Their competence and energy made them much in demand. However, as their energies produced great assets for the needy church, their independence became increasingly irksome to many bishops. This tension came to a head for the American Charities in New York in 1846.

Motherhouse Versus Diocese

> *We were like anxious spectators, standing on the shore, watching a shipwreck, hoping and fearing, wondering which of the strugglers would be saved, which would not,*
>
> — *Sister of Charity, Troy Hospital, 1891*[14]

In 1845 Bishop John Hughes of New York declared that he felt the Sisters of Charity required some "modification to their system." The specific difficulty that infuriated Hughes was the care of boys. The care of boys over the age of seven was proscribed by the rule of the American Sisters of Charity (in conformity with the original French community rule).

Hughes needed sisters to care for boys and girls in the rapidly expanding parochial school system. He wanted fifty-two sisters, a sixth of the national congregation, to belong to his diocese alone.[15] The response of the Sulpician priest superior of the Sisters of Charity at their motherhouse in Emmitsburg, Maryland[16] was that "we consider this step of yours as calculated to inflict a deep and dangerous wound on the community, and if the example be imitated, and every bishop in the Union had the same right, I would consider it mortal."[17]

In 1846 the individual Sisters of Charity in New York City were forced to make a choice — stay in New York in a breakaway community within the diocese, or leave New York and remain part of the original community under the Emmitsburg motherhouse. Thirty-three of sixty-two women chose to remain in New York at the institutions they had worked so hard to establish. They became the Sisters of Charity of St. Vincent de Paul, of New York.[18] This community established St. Vincent's Hospital in 1849 and went on to be led by Bishop Hughes's sister, Mother Angela Hughes.

The division of the community and the risk of further splintering as other bishops made claims on the sisters to become purely diocesan workers, led the community to strengthen its independence by seeking unification with the community in France. In 1858 the American Sisters of Charity became part of the French order, the Daughters of Charity of St. Vincent de Paul, as the American province of this international community of women. This un-American move was unacceptable to some Sisters of Charity, and in the end five independent communities formed.[19]

This time of turbulence was a decisive event in the history of religious women in the United States. The increasingly powerful bishops, as both community and political leaders, were unsympathetic to religious workers, male or female, who were not under their complete jurisdiction.[20] The Daughters of Charity were a very important community of women, with extensive resources and more than 300 members prior to the 1846 split. The bishops wanted their energy and resourcefulness, but wanted it as their own, a tool for their ministry, not in a collaborative and negotiated relationship. One element of the problem was that the bishops were particularly irritated by the fact that sisterhoods with a motherhouse system, such as the Daughters, were guided by priests not subject to episcopal authority.[21] Moreover, it is scarcely surprising that the patriarchal bishops were inclined to interpret independent behavior by the sisters as evidence of male influence. They appeared to be threatened by the perceived male usurpation of their diocesan authority.[22]

Clergy were consistently blind to the independent authority women exercised within their own organizational structure. This blindness has been shared by historians who rely on the correspondence between men on sisterhoods' business, interpreting the formal silence of the women as literal silence, rather than understanding the protocols involved in ecclesiastical correspondence — which is hierarchical and legalistic.[23] It is no surprise that a bishop would write to the male superior (priest) of the Daughters. This does not, however, imply that the mother superior had no views or influence on the matter. Moreover, the issue of misogyny among the clergy, though undeniable, should not be overstated. The Christian Brothers, as a nondiocesan male lay community (non-priests) were also in constant conflict with priests and bishops.[24] In fact, Jesuits, with their politics and their independence, were probably more detested by diocesan clergy than by Protestants! The issue here is about power. The bishop was a prince of the church in his realm. Those who lay beyond his influence and control were a constant thorn in his side.

The American Context

Despite the split of 1846, the Daughters of Charity continued to build and manage hospitals throughout the country, establishing forty-four hospitals between 1823 and 1898. (See Table 1 for a list of hospitals established or managed by this community in the nineteenth century.) According to Sister Armiger, whose 1947 thesis examined the nursing work of the Daughters of Charity in the Eastern Province, "the purposes for which these hospitals were founded can be reduced to three in order of frequency: 1) pestilence; 2) lack of hospitals in various localities; 3) the requirements of medical education."[25] In what follows I examine the development of hospitals by the Daughters of Charity of St. Vincent de Paul according to Armiger's precepts plus an additional one — the Civil War.

We look specifically at five hospitals conducted by the Daughters of Charity: the Buffalo Hospital of the Sisters of Charity, Buffalo, New York, founded in 1848; St. Mary's Hospital, Troy, New York, founded in 1850; St. Mary's Hospital, Rochester, New York, founded in 1857; Providence Hospital, Washington, D.C., founded in 1861; and St. Joseph's Hospital, Philadelphia, managed by the Daughters of Charity in 1859–1947. These hospitals are a sample of those conducted by this small group of women, in what became the Northeast Province of the Daughters of Charity, over the twenty-year period 1848–68. The discussion focuses on the development of expertise and personnel among the Daughters and their growing corporate experience as they responded to the diverse needs and challenges of conducting hospitals.

Pestilence

It has been well noted that it was epidemic nursing that first brought the nursing work of the sisters into prominence. It must have seemed to the

TABLE 1. HOSPITALS ESTABLISHED OR MANAGED BY THE DAUGHTERS OF CHARITY, 1823–1900

1823	Baltimore Infirmary
1827	~~Baltimore Marine Hospital~~
1828	St. Louis Mullanphy Hospital, now De Paul
1833	Maryland Hospital, Baltimore
1834	Charity Hospital, New Orleans
1838	Richmond Medical College Infirmary
1840	St. Vincent's, Mount Hope
1844	St. Vincent's, Donaldsonville, Louisiana
1845	St. Vincent's and St. Mary's, Detroit
1846	Washington Infirmary, Washington, D.C.
1848	Sisters Hospital, Buffalo, New York
1848	St. John's Infirmary and St. Mary's, Milwaukee, Wisconsin
1850	St. Mary's Hospital, Troy, New York
1852	Hôtel Dieu, New Orleans
1852	City Hospital, Mobile, Alabama
1855	Providence Hospital, Mobile, Alabama
1856	Charitable Institution and St. Vincent's Hospital, Los Angeles
1856	St. Vincent's de Paul, Norfolk, Virginia
1857	St. Mary's, Rochester, New York
1858	St. Vincent's Institution, St. Louis
1859	St. Joseph's, Philadelphia
1860	St. Francis de Sales Infirmary, Richmond, Virginia
1861	Providence Hospital, Washington, D.C.
1861	Providence Retreat, Buffalo, N.Y.
1862	St. Agnes, Baltimore
1863	Carney, Boston
1864	St. Joseph's, Alton, Illinois
1865	Louisiana Retreat, De Paul Sanitarium, New Orleans
1866	St. John's Hospital, Lowell, Massachusetts
1869	Providence, St. Joseph's, Chicago
1869	Providence Hospital, Detroit
1870	Michigan State Retreat, Detroit
1870	St. Joseph's Retreat, Dearborn, Michigan
1871	St. Mary's, Evansville, Indiana
1874	St. Mary's, Saginaw, Michigan
1875	St. Vincent's, Baltimore, Maryland
1876	St. Marie Louise's, Virginia City, Nevada
1881	St. Vincent's Infirmary, Indianapolis, Indiana
1885	St. Vincent's Hospital Women and Children's, Philadelphia
1892	St. Mary's, Hôtel Dieu, El Paso, Texas
1895	St. Paul's Sanitarium, Dallas, Texas
1896	Leper Home, Iberville, Louisiana
1898	St. Thomas's Sanitarium, Nashville, Tennessee
1898	St. Vincent's, Birmingham, Alabama

sisters that God sent such a pestilence to open the heart of the world to His true church, and the sisters were front line soldiers in this fight with the devil and the world. As Charles Rosenberg makes clear, sensible nurses abandoned their posts when the epidemics struck.[26] There is no doubt that the sisters received the invitation to epidemic nursing with both great fervor and great trepidation.[27] Nonetheless, they not only held firm but took up the challenge. Some were fearless. Many of course were terrified and prayed to God for courage.[28] In the confusion and desperation that struck the cities in the midst of an epidemic, there was something extraordinary in the heroism and calm with which the sisters volunteered to nurse in the cholera, smallpox, yellow fever, typhoid, and diphtheria hospitals. It was the most visible and corporeal of actions. Their distinctive dress, their calm demeanor, their pious acceptance were all ancient and powerful Christian motifs that stood now in stark contrast to the panic, desertion, and plundering of a city in the grip of an epidemic. It was the type of behavior that had astounded the Romans during the plagues of the third century, and its impact was no less powerful during the nineteenth-century waves of cholera.[29] And in the Unites States, too, where many people still interpreted epidemics as divine retribution, the actions of the sisters, the power of their faith, and their heroism touched many.[30]

The epidemic nursing of the sisters also provided the city authorities with something of a fait accompli. What could they do with those hospitals once the epidemic had subsided? The epidemic could return at any time; there were still no nurses to speak of; the sisters had earned the respect and trust of all and were well entrenched in the hospital. To throw them out would be at the very least ungrateful and graceless. It was a hand played well by the sisters in Ireland and in the United States. By these means — through initiative and then by default — they acquired the management of a great many public institutions, from the Charity Hospital in New Orleans to St. Vincent's Hospital in Norfolk, Virginia.[31]

The Church's position in these cities and towns laid waste by epidemics was critical. So many of the dead and dying were the Church's own. It was the poorest who suffered the most, and the poor were the immigrant Irish in the slums of the industrial north.[32] So not only were the sisters serving the poor and dying, they were making sure that Catholic souls were restored to God. For a nineteenth-century pauper, to find oneself a cholera victim in the care of a nun, perhaps from one's own homeland, must surely have been a powerful incentive to return to the faith of one's birth. As the Annals record, many a prodigal soul affirmed the evangelical mission of the sisters in those circumstances.

In Buffalo the cholera epidemic of 1849 was the first big test of the

Daughters and their hospital, and they managed to bring about a great success. The sisters rose to the occasion to demonstrate such heroism, devotion, and care that praise poured in from all quarters.[33] Bishop Timon of Buffalo expressed in his correspondence the belief that "the service of the sisters during the cholera epidemic earned them respect and acceptance among Protestant community elites."[34] The sisters were also praised by the *Buffalo Medical Journal* for their "astonishing" dedication.[35] But it was more than dedication that made them a success. Their outcomes were excellent. The survival rates for their cholera patients were dramatically better than those of the temporary municipal pest house — a mortality rate of only 39 percent, compared to 53 percent for the county hospital.[36]

The yellow fever in Virginia, in the summer of 1855, provided another heroic stage for the Daughters of Charity. As soon as the epidemic took hold, the sisters volunteered and sent three women from Emmitsburg to Portsmouth, where they took over the naval hospital. Later another group came from Baltimore to nurse at Norfolk. In addition to the eulogies that filled the press on the devotion and heroism of the sisters, the yellow fever epidemic delivered the Church two rewards. First, a Know-Nothing Senator, Robert M. T. Hunter, publicly retracted his previously stated position on Catholics. Hunter is quoted in the *Washington Sentinel* as saying:

But fellow citizens, I went a little too far, when I said it was proposed to proscribe Catholics from all offices in this country. There are some offices, which sons and daughters of the church are still considered competent to discharge, I mean the offices of Christian charity, of ministration of the sick. The Sisters of Charity may enter yonder pest-house, from whose dread portals the bravest and strongest man quails and shrinks; she may breathe there the breath of pestilence which walks abroad, in that mansion of misery, in order to minister to disease where it is most loathsome, and to relieve suffering where it is most helpless.[37]

Second, one philanthropic victim of the epidemic willed her mansion to the sisters for a hospital. Ann Plume Behan had contracted yellow fever nursing her slaves.[38] Her beneficence allowed the sisters to open the Hospital of St. Vincent de Paul, Norfolk in 1856.[39]

It was the sisters who excelled at inspiring such sentiments, and the Church was eager to exploit the opportunities they brought for rapprochement with state authorities, even the chance of some state funds in return for the sisters' efforts. The dearth of suitable women in the community at large to manage and staff a hospital was the key. The nursing work of the sisters constituted a trump card in the Church's hand. It provided a crucial mechanism by which the church negotiated itself from the margins to the center of social and political influence in a city.[40]

Lack of Hospitals

In upstate New York, the cities of Buffalo, Rochester, Troy, and Albany, swamped with immigrant poor and fearful of epidemics, were the pioneering towns for the sisters and their nursing services.[41] The frontier town of Buffalo burgeoned through the 1840s and 1850s to become America's largest inland port. Westward expansion and the Erie Canal made Buffalo the key intersection between northeast and northwest—between New York City and Chicago. It attracted workers and immigrants as they traveled west; it also found itself the terminus for many tired and sick immigrants who could go no further. Thus industrialization, expansion, and immigration brought both wealth and poverty to Buffalo. The newcomers during the middle decades of the nineteenth century were Irish and German—a great many of them Catholic. The poor and indigent were largely Irish Catholic.

According to Buffalo historian David Gerber, the good citizens of Buffalo were disinclined to philanthropy—particularly philanthropy toward Irish Catholics. The only two institutions in the city in 1840 were the orphanage and the poorhouse. Neither of these institutions permitted priests to visit—their secularism barely disguised anti-Catholicism.[42] These conditions were similar to those in New York City and in the other towns of the industrial northeast. However, Buffalo was a new city—not a Philadelphia or a Boston with a powerful old ascendancy to contend with. Important, too, was the fact that its first bishop was John Timon, no Irish firebrand such as New York's John Hughes, but an American-born Vincentian. Timon had no desire to antagonize American sensibilities against the Church; as a Vincentian missionary he had worked in Protestant and frontier communities. At the same time he was the son of Irish immigrants, aware of the culture and background of the poorest of his diocese, and his Vincentian training made him more a European Catholic than men such as Hughes.

Gerber shows how the Catholic Church was able to dominate local charities largely by default because the prejudices of Buffalo Protestants against Catholics "stemmed public and private efforts to care for the needy."[43] Jean Richardson further argues that the sisters stepped into the breach provided by a disorganized medical profession.[44] The sisters promptly availed themselves of state and county funds for capital expenditure and ongoing patient care to found a 100-bed hospital in 1848. Private patients supplemented this funding. Within the year a severe cholera epidemic had commenced and the sisters offered their hospital to the city.

The hospital at Buffalo was atypical of hospitals established by Catholic women at this time. First, it began as a large-scale civic institution (100 beds). Second, it was publicly funded. In addition to the maintenance money for the care of the indigent, there was money for county patients, money for the care of sick almshouse inmates and immigrants from the State Commission of Emigration, and private patient funds.[45] Capital costs were supported by fund raising and substantial state endowments. In 1848–51 the state accounted for 41 percent of the sisters' income.[46] It is something of a surprise that, in the home of Know-Nothing-nominated President Millard Fillmore, the 1851 application for $14,000 in state appropriation should go unchallenged.[47] But political pragmatism meant the accommodation of the immigrant vote. Richardson argues that "in addition to funding an inexpensive means to provide for the poor, the growing importance of Catholic votes prompted state politicians' generosity toward Catholic charitable institutions."[48] Moreover, Timon was extremely careful to stay clear of provoking anti-Catholic sentiment. In his diocese the sisters were expressly forbidden to proselytize and ordered to "refrain from speaking of religion to Protestants inside and outside the hospital, unless Protestants broached the subject themselves."[49]

The Daughters of Charity continued to found hospitals in the Northeast, following the new settlements. St. Mary's Hospital in Troy, New York was established in 1850 precisely because of the problem with starving Irish immigrants sick with "ship fever" (typhus).[50] The Rev. Peter Havermans worked among the temporary shelters the city had set up for the immigrants and requested sisters from Emmitsburg to run a hospital.[51] In Rochester Sister Hieronymo O'Brien, veteran of the 1855 yellow fever epidemic in Norfolk, Virginia and one of the original Buffalo hospital sisters, accepted the invitation to open a hospital, another St. Mary's, in 1857.[52]

In 1859 Sister Ursula Mattingly, founding sister servant of the Sisters Hospital, Buffalo and former sister servant of St. Mary's, Troy, took charge of St. Joseph's Hospital, Philadelphia. St. Joseph's had also been set up in response to the needs of Irish immigrants. Unlike Troy, Philadelphia was not without hospitals, but the successful members of the Irish community considered it important to have a third hospital to provide for their own. Ten years later, the Daughters of Charity took over the hospital from the Sisters of St. Joseph. The hospital then changed from a debt-ridden troubled institution to a standard Daughters hospital that ran without interference and made money. Gail Casterline may have missed the critical point in the handover of St. Joseph's to the Daughters. She states:

In August 1859 the board voted to divest itself of the internal management of the hospital by leasing it to the Sisters of Charity. The abrupt dismissal of the Sisters of St. Joseph is puzzling, but apparently their replacements had closer ties to the hierarchy and [Rev.] Wood referred to the new superior, Sister Ursula Mattingly, as an "old acquaintance."[53]

What Casterline fails to appreciate here is that, despite "old acquaintances," in bringing Sister Ursula Mattingly to the helm of a hospital in trouble, the board was calling in one of the most successful and experienced hospital nurses in the country. The key issue for St. Joseph's was the terms of the Daughters of Charity contract. They would not enter into an arrangement with the hospital under the terms with which the Sisters of St. Joseph had been forced to work — a high level of medical and board member interference. The Charities' contract stipulated full independent management of the institution. In this way costs dropped, care improved, and the diocese's problems with the hospital were solved. The management of the Daughters of Charity was also considered something of a "selling point" of the hospital. Note the advertisement of late 1859:

St. Joseph's Hospital — I would call the attention of all whom it may concern to the advertisement of St. Joseph's Hospital in another column. This hospital has recently been leased to the Sisters of Charity, under whose sole management it now is. Strangers visiting this city who may be taken ill, and all other persons needing kind care and tender nursing of a home, as well as the most skillful medical attendance the city affords, will find them all in this admirable institution. Sister M Ursula Mattingly is the Mother Superior of the house. Several important changes have occurred in consequence of the lease referred to above. The Medical Faculty of the Hospital, formerly elected by the Board of Corporators are now appointed by the Sisters of Charity. This necessity required an entire new organisation of the Medical Faculty, which received its appointment on Tuesday Sept 13th, and is now constituted as follows.[54]

In another city full of poor Irish, Boston, the case of Carney Hospital (founded in 1863) shows the difficulties that existed for the sisters without any state or major philanthropic support in the service of the desperate poor. Wealthy Irishman Andrew Carney unfortunately died before his will was finalized, and the hospital was denied its bequest.[55] Without a major benefactor, and in anti-Catholic New England, the hospital's claims for state support were rejected. Moreover, in 1848 the patients were destitute: "Not a single person now receiving care and support is able to pay one cent. The only way I have of keeping our doors open to the poor is by sending our sisters out every day to solicit aid."[56]

In 1892, when the hospital was nearly crippled by its debt, the legislature declared that no money would be given to institutions not wholly under state control. The disappointment brought testimonials of the importance of the Carney from such disinterested parties as the Hebrew Benevolent Society.[57] So infuriated was the *Boston Post* that it established a subscription to make up the $10,000 — a quarter of the amount was raised in a week.[58]

As the sisters established and conducted hospitals throughout the Northeast they encountered a variety of contexts — from well-funded Buffalo to desperate Carney in Boston. The sisters learned to avoid inflaming Protestant anxieties and to build friendships in the broad community. They also learned to make their hospitals vital to local medical interests.

Requirements of Medical Education

It was not only the epidemics that opened the door of public institutions to the sisterhoods. Their reputation brought important friends. The nursing nuns in the early to mid-nineteenth century were often, by experience or reputation, able to develop good working relationships with doctors. These relationships fostered the idea that collaborate ventures could be established to improve the care of the poor. In this manner hospitals were founded by the sisters in succession across the northeast.

The original hospital contract that began the Daughters in their nursing work is an historic one — with the first teaching hospital in the United States. In 1823 the Sisters of Charity agreed to work in the Baltimore Infirmary with a group of doctors from the Medical Faculty at the University of Maryland. It was an acute institution with three physicians and four surgeons and a special ward for eye diseases, plus one ward for sailors.[59] The contract for the sisters' service was carefully negotiated to allow them appropriate privacy and living conditions.[60]

The role of insurance levies in funding hospital foundation is evident even in this early example. The financing of the contract for the sisters was made possible in part by the 1798 federal law that taxed every merchant seaman twenty cents per month to underwrite the care of sick and disabled seamen. The Baltimore Infirmary housed one of many marine wards, funded by this tax, that sprang up around the country and eventually led to the construction of federal hospitals at major ports.[61]

The promotion of private medical practice, and its increasingly significant role in the United States health care system, is also part of the success of the sisters. The sisters were critical to the development of medicine, particularly in Buffalo, where the sisters provided clinical facilities for two fledgling medical colleges. In Buffalo the sisters established close links with the Niagara University Medical School, providing the school with its clinical facility, and in 1849 admitted medical interns — the first Daughter of Charity hospital to do so.[62] However, the issue of medical residents remained problematic for the sisters, who terminated and restored the resident program on several occasions throughout 1849–56. The sisters terminated their relationship with the Buffalo

Medical College in 1883, becoming the teaching hospital for the Niagara Medical School until 1898.[63] At that time the aging sister servant, Sister Florence O'Hara, completely reorganized medical departments within the hospital in order to accommodate new specialties and opened those positions to physicians not affiliated with Niagara University Medical School. When the entire faculty of the university resigned in protest, she accepted their resignations. The university lost its teaching facility and was subsequently forced to close down.

The sister servants who succeeded Sister Florence continued the work of reorganizing medical services within the hospital and the hospital's relationship to medicine in Buffalo. In 1899 Sister Blanche Hooper reviewed the performance of doctors in the light of the number of private patients they were bringing to the hospital. Those doctors who failed to bring private patients were sacked.[64] Finally, at the end of 1899, Sister Felicita McNulty abolished the medical board and renegotiated all contracts for the year 1900. She brought matters under control through mandated monthly staff meetings, at the first of which she appointed the chairman of the committee (no elections!) to create bylaws, a constitution, and a procedure for selection of medical appointments.[65] Importantly, she renegotiated the terms under which doctors could charge their private patients, making it more profitable for private medical practice.[66] Private patients continued to provide the most stable and profitable income sources for the sisters. By 1903 private patients accounted for over three times more revenue than county and city patients.[67]

Even at St. Joseph's, Philadelphia, which began as a philanthropic response to the suffering first wave of Irish famine victims, patient fees were essential for the hospital. Despite the predominance of Irish-born patients (83 percent of the 1850 admissions were born in Ireland and the figure remained high for the next five decades), throughout the nineteenth century St. Joseph's relied on patients who could pay their way. "As early as 1850, 78 percent of St. Joseph's inpatients paid board fees, and the ratio of pay-to-charity cases continued to be one of the highest of any hospital in the city, averaging anywhere from 50 to 80 percent paying patients through 1900."[68] Thus it was not the destitute victims of the Irish famine that supported St. Joseph's through these years; in fact, poor Irish still filled the beds in the city's other hospitals throughout this period — representing 48 percent of patients at the Quaker Pennsylvania Hospital.

Prominent Philadelphia doctors played a significant role in the establishment of St. Joseph's. Gail Casterline argues that disaffection with the restricted opportunities for medical practice in Philadelphia's existing hospitals may have been a factor. Dr. William E. Horner and a Dr. Keating had been part of a controversial mass resignation from the Blockley Almshouse when medical teaching was discontinued on the wards.[69] As a progressive collaboration between medicine and philanthropic Irish citizens, St. Joseph's began its operation with medical school affiliation and resident medical officers. However, when the Daughters of Charity assumed control of St. Joseph's in 1859, this arrangement ceased, as the sisters felt it incompatible with their rule to share the hospital with undisciplined medical students at night. In 1880 the sisters allowed the reintroduction of medical students to the hospital — but under their own terms.[70] That good behavior was a requirement of the arrangement is hinted in the Annual Report of 1897 where the sisters comment: "It is a pleasing duty to record the gentlemanly deportment and self-sacrificing labors of the resident doctors. The best wishes and kindliest feelings of the Sisters and all connected with the Hospital follow them in their future labors."[71]

This opportune association between private medicine and the success of hospitals by the end of the nineteenth century can even be seen in the way St. Joseph's promoted its school of nursing. One of its attractions was argued to be the hospital's "open" policy for private patients. This meant that nurses had the opportunity to build good relations with a large number of private practitioners, relationships that would assist them in establishing a thriving private practice when they completed their hospital training:

The advantages of the school to its pupils are those afforded by its work of charity in the wards, as also in the experience gained in the care of private patients in the many rooms devoted to their use. Many of these patients still remain under the care of their home physicians, thus assuring for the nurses a professional acquaintance outside the hospital staff, who do not forget the skillful, conscientious nurses when the same nurses enter their independent profession outside the hospital.[72]

Medical training, and the open policy of accommodating private medicine, brought funds to the hospital and supported nurses. These medical associations also made the institution financially viable and clinically important to the development of both the medical profession and private nursing in Philadelphia.

The Civil War

In the history of both nursing and of the Catholic sisterhoods, the American Civil War is commonly cast as the defining event, the rupture between the old and the new.[73] For the sisterhoods this is true in a literal rather than a figurative sense. For during the Civil War many Catholic women volunteered to work in the hospitals and cared for the wounded on both sides. The Daughters of Charity nursed in twenty-five different areas during the war; they served in military hospitals and prisons, in tents and improvised hospitals, and turned their existing hospitals over to the care of soldiers.[74]

Keen to seize the opportunity, the clergy volunteered the services of nuns from all rules and communities from all over the United States. Altogether some 600 women from twenty-one communities (or roughly 20 percent of nurses overall) nursed soldiers on both sides.[75] For some orders this was a logical extension of their religious life and their vow to serve God's poor and sick. These women turned their experience and skill to the job at hand and arrived as ready-made experienced nurses and hospital mangers. For other sisters it was a radical departure and one toward which they may have been reluctant.[76]

Despite the charges of proselytism made against a number of sisterhoods, the war increased the standing of both the sisters and the church to a remarkable extent.[77] The horror and hostility with which sisters had previously been met by non-Catholics was lessened and, more important, their utility in the acute hospital setting was confirmed in the minds of government, doctors, and the military. Nursing skill was one important element of this success. However, of great importance, too, was the discipline and reliability the sisters offered, not as a group of enthusiastic amateurs, but as a disciplined corps — something the army related to and admired.

Although it is a commonplace that the sisters were the unsung heros of the war (after all, their memorial at Washington was not built until the twentieth century), there was, in fact, a great deal of direct appreciation and recognition of their contribution to the nation. The annals of each community record the laurels received by their war nurses. Lincoln, Grant, and Jefferson Davis all sang the praises of the nursing nuns.[78] In fact, in 1874 President Ulysses S. Grant requested that a Dominican nursing sister, Mother Josephine, a veteran of the Battle of Perryville, Kentucky, unveil the Lincoln Monument at Springfield, Illinois.[79] The war also meant that many thousands of men were grateful for the efforts of the sisters, less suspicious of their habits and veils, and well aware that the skillful attendance of an intelligent nurse made all the difference between life and death.[80]

In the decades following the Civil War, the number of communities involved in hospital foundation continued to climb, until it peaked in the 1890s at fifty-nine communities that established eighty-nine new hospitals between 1890 and 1900.[81] The Civil War also provided the sisters with tangible opportunities to establish new institutions and consolidate existing ones. For instance, in Washington, D.C. in 1861 the Daughters of Charity volunteered to serve the wounded soldiers wherever the government required them. At the same time the Washington Infirmary was

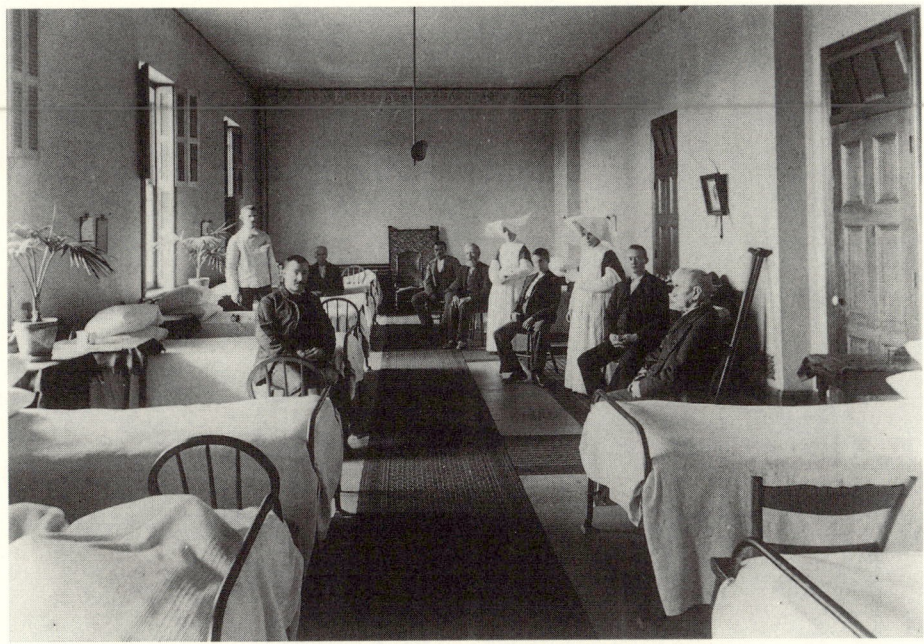

Figure 3. St. Joseph's Hospital, Philadelphia. Male surgical wards, 1880s. Reprinted with permission of the Daughters of Charity Archives, Albany, New York.

redesignated as a military hospital and closed to the public. The Daughters of Charity were then approached by a group of Washington physicians to establish a civilian hospital.[82] The rate for ward patients was $4.00 per week, private rooms available at extra cost, and "All members of the medical profession of the District (had) an equality of privilege."[83] Immediately following the war the hospital continued to enjoy federal and public support and was granted a congressional appropriation of $30,000 for a new building, and annual funds for the care of the indigent in the District of Columbia.[84]

St. Mary's Hospital, Rochester, New York, was another hospital whose fate was caught up with the Civil War. This institution was established in 1857 by Sister Hieronymo O'Brien, one of the sisters who began the sisters' Buffalo hospital. In contrast to the relative prosperity of the Buffalo foundation and the Providence Hospital in Washington, in Rochester the sisters slept on pallets of straw through their first winter with little more than their habits for covers.[85] County funding for poor patients was hard to come by in Rochester, and Sister Hieronymo fought a running battle with the Board of Supervisors of County Welfare.[86] In 1859 friends

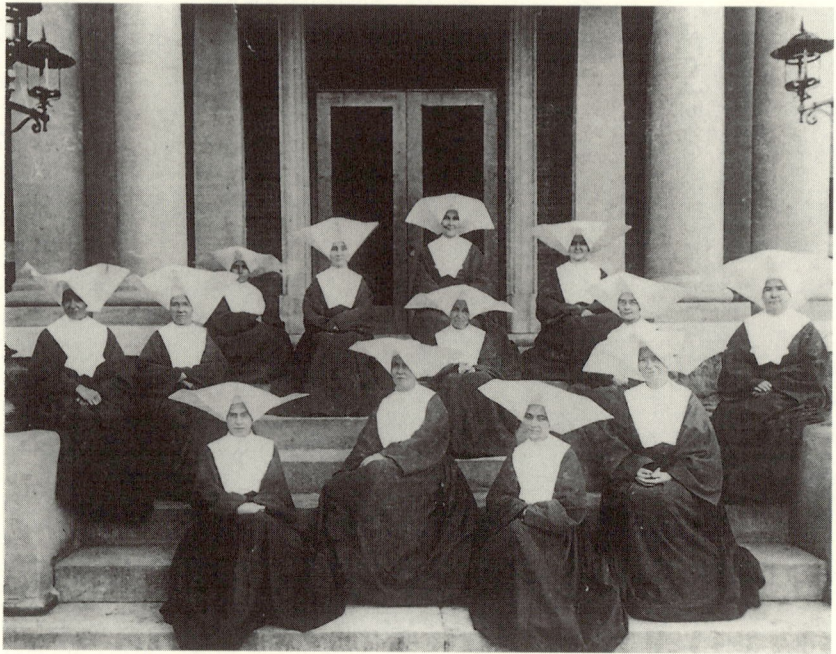

Figure 4. Daughters of Charity of St. Vincent de Paul, St. Vincent de Paul Hospital, Birmingham, Alabama, about 1906. Courtesy of the Center for the Study of Nursing History, University of Pennsylvania.

of the hospital petitioned Washington to authorize a department at St. Mary's for the care of sick seamen and bargemen on the Erie Canal. The hospital ward was formally named "Marine Department of the Hospital of the City of Rochester."[87] In 1861 Sister Hieronymo was denied aid from the state legislature and her county payments were refused by the Board of Supervisors.[88]

As the only hospitals in western New York, Sisters Hospital in Buffalo held the federal navy contract and St. Mary's, Rochester, with much relief, secured the army contract. (As legend has it, however, Sister Hieronymo had to go to Washington in person in 1864 to force the federal government to pay her their debt of $30,000.[89]) Estimates vary, but between three and five thousand soldiers were treated at St. Mary's over the course of the war at the rate of $5.50 per week.[90] Following the war, in an effort to maintain demand, Sister Hieronymo advertised the hospital (briefly) as an "Invalid Retreat." She promoted the hospital as providing farm fresh food, fresh milk, baths, and the "best medical team in western New York." The nurses were described as possessing "skill and fidelity"; the choice of doctors was one that "patients can make . . . to suit themselves."[91]

The American context, then, provided the Daughters of Charity with a "market" for their skills. The place of the Daughters of Charity in the forefront of nineteenth-century American nurses was created by the waves of epidemics and the nursing skills the sisters developed in the care of infectious patients; by the lack of hospitals throughout the country during this antebellum period; by urbanization, industrialization, and immigration — which led to an overwhelming demand for nurses and hospitals in both new settlements and older cities; by the steady improvement in medical knowledge and the need for medical training and facilities for private medical practice, and the subsequent need for better educated and disciplined nurses; and finally, by the Civil War, which produced many friends for the sisters and created funding opportunities for their hospitals. The Daughters of Charity did not create these conditions, but neither they did miss the opportunities these events afforded them to consolidate their position in American society, and to realize their vocation to serve the sick and the poor.

The sisters' ability to respond so positively to the social and political challenges of nineteenth-century America depended on their organizational structure and training. A combination of their motherhouse structure, their organization and training, and their distinctive sense of apostolate made them hospital builders par excellence.

Organization and Training

Elizabeth and Emily Blackwell, the first female medical graduates and practitioners in the United States, grasped the true secret of the Daughters of Charity. Commenting on their experience of the French Daughters of Charity they declared:

Anyone who has seen much of these sisters in actual work, . . . will soon perceive that the practical success of these orders does not depend upon religious enthusiasm, but upon an excellent business organization. Religious feeling there is among them, and it is an important aid in filling their ranks and keeping up their interests; but the real secret of their success is the excellent opening afforded by them for all classes of women to a useful and respected social life.[92]

Despite the Blackwells' sanguine views as to the value of religious fervor, their observation that the sisters excelled in "business organization" is well made. What they may not have understood, as secular outsiders, was that the sisters' acumen was not a simple byproduct of religious fervor or the outpouring of previously frustrated female talents, but the result of training. Not every community was successful at hospital work, whereas others were famous for it. What was it about the Daughters of Charity?

After 1858, communities of Daughters of Charity in the United States were managed in conformity with the conventions set down by France. The relationship between dioceses and the motherhouse became increasingly formalized, and the motherhouse took the lead in ensuring that the communities were clear about their properties, their institutions, and their relationship to the diocese. All property deeds were held by the motherhouse at Emmitsburg (safe from domineering bishops!), and all hospital boards were taken over from local diocese and community members and transferred in toto to the sisters. Moreover, the sisters also began to express reluctance to become involved with any foundation they did not own and independently administer, preferring to avoid difficulties and maintain their independence.

Emmitsburg began to offer clear guidelines for the sisters as corporate citizens, providing "Forms of Meetings," so that "the sisters may more easily see how meetings should be conducted."[93] A letter from the Director at Emmitsburg to the community at Troy in 1875 clearly shows the strong role that the motherhouse took in rationalizing processes for the sisters.

I have been thinking seriously for some time, what method to adopt to prevent any irregularity in holding meetings of the various Corporations. . . . Irregularities in recording minutes of meetings, or omission of the same, when required by law, might render the Corporation illegal; and in case of a lawsuit, the property held by such Corporations might be lost to the Community. That such irregularities occur I have evident proof, having found the minutes of meetings not signed by the proper Officer [Sister] or rather not signed at all, rendering such meeting perfectly illegal; and, in some instances, the annual meeting — *always necessary* — omitted. Other irregularities may render the meetings illegal and destroy the legal existence of the Body Corporate.[94]

The letter goes on to provide the sisters with a step-by-step guide to corporate process, ending with the postscript:

Having received the minutes of meetings from some but not in proper shape, observe to the letter the following: Write minutes neatly on single leaf of foolscap paper, enclose it into a large envelop, by itself, and address it to Mother Euphemia.

Not all the sisters' foundations were remiss in this way. At St. Mary's Hospital, Rochester, directors' meetings were carefully minuted from 1857 to1949. Incorporation took place in 1857 and the detailed minutes reveal the financial workings of a major corporation. The meetings of the

President (sister servant), treasurer, and secretary (two other sisters), discuss matters such as the purchase of gas stock or the decision to pay off the floating debt.[95] The sisters as individuals were all named on the mortgage documents, boards of trustees elections, deeds of incorporation, architect contracts, and so forth.[96]

The "excellent business organization" noted by the Blackwells was underpinned by rigorous religious training. This training shaped the women in their relation to work, to each other, and to God. It provided them with the faith that, as instruments of God, great things would be achieved by the lowly to His glory. It also provided them with a network of what would today be called "mentors," to assist the individual woman to develop skills for God's purposes and to maintain her religiosity.

The organization of the Daughters of Charity is centered around the motherhouse. All new members of the community complete their training at that motherhouse. For the American Daughters of Charity this meant that every single nineteenth-century sister was trained at Emmitsburg, Maryland. The sisters' spiritual "formation," as it is called, was therefore consistent and the result of tried precepts. Women who did not demonstrate the correct personal and spiritual attributes would be evident to the novice mistress and be brought to the attention of the superioress of the community and the confessor. These individuals were highly experienced in training women and allocating them their duties within the organization, aware of their strengths, weaknesses, and potential.

But what of the "interiority" of the nursing nun? What was it that her spiritual formation strove to create? It may be difficult for the secular mind to accept, but the level-headed and pragmatic qualities of health care provider and skilled nurse coexisted, in the nineteenth-century vowed woman, with a miraculous view of human existence that guided her work and decision-making. The Catholic nun was never alone; in addition to her religious community, her life was enriched and empowered by the community of saints and an unwavering certainty that God would work through her to achieve His goals. In this frame of mind she buried holy medals on land the sisters coveted for hospital extensions,[97] she wrote angry letters to St. Joseph when debts mounted, she bargained with the Blessed Virgin, offering statues and chapels to repay her efforts on their behalf.[98] It was a resourceful and positive interiority that equipped the nineteenth-century nun to keep going, to build on successes, and to learn from errors.

The skills of new recruits, once training was completed, were honed by strategic placements. The motherhouse structure meant that a community was organized like an army or a corporation. It was a highly centralized structure, independent of the bishop or the diocese. This structure allowed for centralized strategic decision-making. Did they think they should build another hospital in this or that state? Should they decline this invitation because the bishop was hard to work with? Who would be a good person to send on this difficult assignment? Who needed more guidance and would benefit from working with a more experienced individual?

Submission and obedience, two essential attributes instilled during spiritual formation, made the sisters completely acquiescent to the directives of their superiors. This enabled the motherhouse to apply the human resources of the community expeditiously, according to their centrally determined need. In this way, experience was consolidated. For instance, Sister Ursula Mattingly was sent from Buffalo (1848–55), to Troy (1855–59), to St. Joseph's, Philadelphia (1859).[99] Sister Rosaline Brown, one of the Buffalo pioneers, established St. Mary's Infant Asylum and Maternity Hospital in 1854, then in 1860 founded Providence Retreat (for the mentally ill) at Buffalo.[100] Sister Hieronymo O'Brien, a veteran of the yellow fever epidemics, helped found the hospital in Buffalo (1848–57) and was "Chief of Staff Sister Nurses" there.[101] She went on to establish St. Mary's, Rochester in 1857. Sister Mary de Sales Taylor is another example of a woman with an impressive curriculum vitae. In 1852 she became superior at St. Mary's Hospital, Detroit. Under her leadership the sisters nursed 359 cholera victims during the 1854 epidemic. She established a mental asylum, and in 1869 she opened Providence Hospital, Detroit, for mothers and babies. She is eulogized in the annals for "an ability to plan and execute . . . united to a shrewdness that mastered every detail of complex business affairs. In business she had the inflexible methods of a businessman."[102]

In addition to obedience, the sisters' training also equipped them to lead, to establish new communities, and to recruit and train new members. Nightingale's much quoted "For what training is there to compare with that of a Catholic nun?" was precisely about this point.[103] The Catholic Church understood and valued both training and experience. Some of these women established three or four hospitals from nothing. They knew how to raise loans from individuals — many of their mortgages were from "friends."[104] They understood the way government worked and what funds were available from the county or state. They established good relations with the medical profession and were the beneficiaries of nursing contracts through private corporations. Basically, they knew how to do business, how to raise money and build support, how to deal with clergy and the medical profession. They did this their entire working lives, without the distraction of family cares, and with utter commitment and professionalism, training a new generation of sisters in their wake.

Conclusion: An American Success Story

Thus, through religious training, centralized administration, and skill building, the sisters were remarkably well suited to take on the complex task of hospital foundation and nursing. Not only did these women show what could be done, what diligent and disciplined women had to offer the community in the field of health care, but hospital foundation work provided a platform from which the Church could increase Catholic stocks in the broader community. The hybridity of their role as service providers, government fund holders, key connection points between the church and the state made them perhaps the most visible members of the Catholic Church to the non-Catholic community.

The impact of Catholic women on the health and welfare of nineteenth-century Americans was extraordinary. The sisters worked at the "coal-faces" of epidemics, battlefields, and immigrant slums. But what is most astonishing is that the sisters transformed these desperate responses to overwhelming social need into opportunities for the development of health care services to the American public. With political knowhow, and in partnership with private medicine, they turned their efforts into self-sustaining, even profitable enterprises. All the while they walked a careful path of obedience and independence on the bishop's soil.

Chapter 4

Behind Enemy Lines
Religious Nursing in England — Conflicts and Solutions

Like their sisters in Ireland, France, Germany, and the United States, pious nineteenth-century English women felt the call to serve God through work with His needy. The most famous nurse of all time, Miss Florence Nightingale, was one such woman. Nightingale's call to serve God occurred in 1837, when she was just seventeen.[1] The extraordinary impact of Florence Nightingale on the development of nursing training during the second half of the nineteenth century has effectively over-shadowed earlier events.[2] To understand how nursing in England became synonymous with Nightingale's own project and how it eclipsed all other narratives in the history of nursing, it is necessary to examine the conditions underlying the professionalization of the care of the sick. These conditions, it will be argued, are less the product of medical and scientific arrangements of the period than the result of a vocational wave of godly women. It is this vocational wave, its impact on nursing, and the problems it caused for Protestant England that are the subject of this chapter.

According to Catholic legend, the first nursing mission in England and Scotland was begun by the Irish Sisters of Mercy in 1838 at their Bermondsey convent in the East End of London.[3] Catholic Emancipation in 1829 was the critical event that stimulated not only the foundation of the first convent in England since the Reformation, but the foundation of the Irish Sisters of Mercy in 1831.[4] I begin with a discussion of the position of Catholics in Britain, the impact of Catholic Emancipation on the Church in Ireland and England, and the political implications of a re-vitalized Catholic Church with both English and Irish elements. We move then to examine the Bermondsey story, what it tells us about tensions between Irish and English Catholic notions about the place of work in the spiritual life of women. The chapter then turns to a distinctively English solution to the problem of Protestant women called to serve God through an active life. The importance of formal nursing in the many Protestant sisterhoods that emerged in nineteenth-century England will be examined. Finally, the limitations of both the Catholic and Protestant nursing communities will be addressed, and the astonishingly successful Nightingale solution to these problems discussed.

In 1829 the final Catholic Emancipation Bill reversed a policy that had barred English Catholics from public life, from a military career, and from attending university.[5] In Ireland the Penal Code was even more severe, affecting inheritance and civil rights.[6] But despite such severity Catholicism had been eradicated in neither England nor Ireland. The history of Catholicism in each country in Britain is quite distinct, and here we can only allude to the dominant issues. In England the Catholic Church existed in rural pockets, protected by powerful recusant aristocratic families. Within the estates of these families masses were held in private chapels. It was not a public religion. The church had no formal hierarchy—no bishops or parishes. It retained a pre-industrial flavor of aristocratic devotion, strong European links through visiting clergy, and a largely rural sense of social obligation.[7]

With Catholic Emancipation in Britain—that is, the relaxation of prohibitions against Catholic religious practice and against Catholics entering public life—came a Protestant panic that three hundred years of English Reformation would be swept away in a Catholic assault. The furor that raged in Parliament, in the press, and from the pulpits claimed disaster for Protestant England. Fueling these fears was the mass immigration of poor Irish that followed declining conditions in Ireland, the influx of foreign clergy seeking exile from political turmoil in Europe, and a growing Protestant obsession with Catholic life and ritual.

In the second half of the century, the Catholic Church assumed a far more Roman character than had previously been the case—a trend that became known as Ultramontanism.[8] The power of Ultramontanism was in its heightened sense of ritual, its opulent European aestheticism, and its pursuit of exterior manifestations of the sacred. Rome was in a belligerent and defensive mood, its increasingly intransigent position made clear with the papal declaration on infallibility in 1870.[9]

Roman Seductions

In England the reestablished Catholic Church cut its path through a swath of controversies. Its most disturbing power to Protestants was its ability to attract, unsettle, and "seduce" pious Protestants—taking them over to Rome.[10] In this climate of Gothic obsessions, private religious scruples, evangelical revivals, and nonconformist resistance to the established church, defections to Catholicism questioned not only the English Reformation but English sovereignty and national identity. As Florence Nightingale put it,

I have always thought that the great theological fight has yet to be fought out in England between Catholicism and Protestantism. In Germany it was fought three hundred years ago. They know why they are Protestants. I never knew an Englishman who did and if he inquires he becomes a Catholic.[11]

There was an element of scandal attached to conversion. By mid-century it became something of a fashion — a daring act to be overcome by religious compulsion and "turn" to Rome. Catholicism's most famous Protestant scalps were the Oxford scholars and leading Anglican clergymen John Henry Newman (1845) and Henry Manning (1851), both of whom eventually became cardinals in the Roman Catholic Church.[12]

Irish Catholicism

In Ireland Catholics endured the persecution of the Penal Codes with Celtic stoicism and stubbornness. Stripped of their hierarchy, oppressed by onerous tithes that had to be paid to the hated Church of Ireland (Anglican), the people clung to their faith. The church relied heavily on France for the Catholic education of its moneyed classes and the training of priests (no priest was permitted to be ordained in Ireland).[13] But there were few priests, few churches, and millions of souls to care for. In those years of persecution the Catholicism of the common people became blended with local customs. Celtic festivals and celebrations merged into a world of holy water, saints' relics, and miracles. The Irish church had survived the Reformation, but it was a Catholic Church unlike any other, full of a medieval love of festival and magic, ignorant of doctrine.[14]

Prior to the Reformation ordinary people (from Italy to England) knew little of religious doctrine, nor were they expected to. Such matters were left to a pious, highborn elite. One of the effects of the Reformation was what Jean Delumeau described as the "confessionalization of Europe."[15] Over the course of the sixteenth, seventeenth, and eighteenth centuries, through religious wars and intense conflict between the confessions, the common peasant became the object of evangelism. All citizens came under scrutiny from the priest, pastor, or community of elders. In the Protestant world they became Puritans, Anabaptists, Lutherans, Calvinists, and so forth. They fought and felt religion, argued over scripture, and for the first time developed a personal relationship with God. In Catholic districts the parish was energized by lay societies, by a new breed of better-educated clergy, by close surveillance of sacrament attendance (particularly confession), and by the large numbers of religious vocations to the priesthood, brotherhoods, and, overwhelmingly, the sisterhoods.[16]

The Irish had not been subject to this process. The English-ordered Reformation in Ireland had been a spectacular failure. It was the English who made so many Irish militant Catholics and, in Irish eyes, made conversion to Protestantism a traitorous act.[17] With Emancipation in 1829, the major tasks facing the newly established Irish Church were to rebuild Catholic institutions in Ireland, evangelize among the poor, and bring them back into the fold. The pressures on existing services in the first half of the century were massive. In Ireland under the Penal Code, poor relief had been tied to membership of the (Protestant) Church of Ireland. Following the repeal of the Penal Code in 1829, Catholic institutions for the care of the poor and infirm were established, but they were swamped even before the Famine of 1845 drove millions out of the countryside to relief centers in the cities and all over Britain (and in the United States and Canada).[18] Ireland needed workers for the Church, it needed priests, brothers and nuns, and it needed them in their thousands.

Catholicism in England

> *The rapid expansion of British industry could not have taken place had there not been available a reserve of labour among the poverty-stricken people of Ireland. . . . Nearly all of them settle in the big cities of the industrial areas, where they form the lowest stratus of the community.*
>
> —*Friedrich Engels, 1845*[19]

Well before the first potato crop failure in 1845, the Irish, Protestant and Catholic, had been steadily coming to England to work as both skilled and unskilled workers.[20] There was great poverty among the Irish immigrants, and they became much loathed as "drains" on the poor relief of a community.[21] More than this, their poverty and appalling living conditions led to poor health. When cholera and typhoid epidemics struck, they struck hardest on the Irish quarter of each British city.[22] The Irish mortality in epidemics became so evident that the Irish began to be considered the cause of these epidemics — including the so-called "Irish fever" or dysentery.[23]

Once Ireland's successive potato crop failures set in (which began "the Great Hunger" or "the Famine"), the numbers of poor Irish in British cities swelled. This rapid influx of desperate Irish only served to increase the British community's abhorrence for the dirty, ignorant "Paddy."[24] In mainland Britain (as in Canada, the United States, and Australia) panic arose over the implications for civilized society if all was to be overwhelmed by peasant Irish.[25] In the eugenics-dominated nineteenth-century world, fear led to hysteria over racial contamination by the Irish — widely considered the "missing link" between the Negro and the Anglo Saxon.[26]

In this hostile English world, the struggling Catholic Church became the center of solace and refuge for hundreds of thousands of Irish poor.[27]

The small, elite English Catholic community was forced to accommodate Irish weavers in the north, dock workers in the seaports, and mill workers in the Midlands. Its aristocratic churches with their private pews for the wealthy were bursting with standing Irish poor.[28]

For the English church, the Irish came to be its greatest challenge. For some it was considered God's great work to which they had been called as a consequence of Catholic Emancipation. A ministry to the poor Irish was both their duty and their destiny. But as the church reestablished itself in Britain, despite its Irish congregations, it carefully avoided the appointment of an Irish hierarchy and stayed well beyond the reach of the internationally powerful archbishop of Dublin. So the Irish congregations of the English Church were served by a mixture of Irish, convert English, and Continental priests.[29] But unlike every other English-speaking Catholic Church in the world, it did not become dominated by Irishmen in the nineteenth century.[30]

Sisters of Mercy, Bermondsey

Some would rather pray than dress a cancer

— *Catherine McAuley*

It was to one of these overwhelmed poor London parishes that a request came to Mother McAuley in Dublin, foundress of the Sisters of Mercy, to establish the first convent in England since the Reformation.[31] In 1838 Bishop Griffiths, vicar apostolic of the London District, requested permission from Archbishop Murray of Dublin to send two ladies from England to be instructed in the religious life of the Sisters of Mercy.[32] According to the Annals, it was decided that the Cork house was appropriate for these ladies, both of whom were converts and members of prominent English families.[33] Late the following year these two women, joined by four women from Cork and Mother McAuley, "quietly took possession" of their partly completed convent in Bermondsey,[34] designed by the fashionable architect of the period (and Catholic convert) A. W. Pugin.[35]

The English newspapers were obsessed with the story of these women and the establishment of a Catholic foundation, and enchanted by the prominent role the aristocracy was playing in this sensation. A group of six women had been living piously under the guidance of Bishop Griffiths waiting for the house to be established. This group included Lady Barbara Eyre, daughter of an earl. Barely had the community been established, under the formal administration of the young but experienced Mother Mary Clare Moore,[36] than the first English reception of nuns (the taking of vows) in three hundred years took place. It was by all accounts an astonishing event, Lady Barbara in silk and diamonds, her hair dressed by Her Majesty's hairdresser.[37] It was featured (with illustration) in the *Illustrated London News* on 12 December 1839.

Perhaps in deference to the families of the novices, or for maximum impact in Protestant England, the presentation ceremony was more like a society wedding than a religious ceremony.[38] Witnessed by over five thousand people, it caused a sensation. At least one woman, who would later convert to Catholicism and become a Sister of Mercy, heard about the ceremony as a schoolgirl in Yorkshire and determined to become a nun.[39] For the Church, anxiously reestablishing itself in England, it was of tremendous benefit to be able to attract, instruct, and admit women of birth and influence to a religious order. Thus the parlor at Bermondsey was said to be always brimming with those seeking instruction.[40]

There was a great deal of work for the sisters to perform among the poor of London, and the death toll from nursing the ill was high during the first few years.[41] The sisters established twenty-two foundations in England:[42] schools, a hospital, a creche for working mothers, a night shelter for the homeless, a hostel for women.[43] Over this period the would continue to nurse the sick poor in their houses, provide nursing care to members of the wealthy classes and ailing clergy,[44] and, most notably, respond to the call for nurses in the Crimea.[45]

It appears that relations between the sisters and Bishop Griffiths, and later Bishop Grant and Cardinal Wiseman, were most cordial. Mother Moore was an intelligent and diplomatic leader and there is no hint of the personality clashes and power struggles that dominate the early years of other communities. Most remarkably, the community was not starved for funds. Benefactors were plentiful and dowries were substantial. Thus the more usual tale of poverty and exploitation does not apply to the Bermondsey community.

Nonetheless, there were difficulties. The most notable problem that dogged the Sisters of Mercy in their early years was the tension between the English Catholic Church, its converts and supporters, and the spirituality and rule of the Irish nuns. There was little choice of vocational approach for the eager English convert. There was, too, ignorance of the differences between communities and the divergent religious rules that existed within the church. The Sisters of Mercy were (and remain) a working community. A product of the revitalized Irish church, the community existed to help the poor, not for the spiritual aspirations of its members. Mother McAuley declared that "God blesses labour, not ritualized asceticism." In fact, she considered "love of labour the rock upon which so much false spirituality is wrecked."[46] Work, she felt, "offers the holy grail of martyrdom."[47] Mother McAuley was derisive of the fact that "some would rather wear a hairshirt than scrub a grate; rather pray than dress a cancer. . . . works of mercy are generally more mortifying than other penances — bad smells, loathsome diseases, more disagreeable than the discipline."[48]

But "love of labour" was not the prime virtue of the English converts left to conduct the Bermondsey convent once Mother Moore returned to Cork. Without Irish leadership, the community began to drift from their rule, and new provisions were made for those who wished to live a more traditional religious life — the enclosed life of prayer and asceticism as opposed to work among the poor. Manias of religious devotion began to emerge and, finally, bizarre experiments in rule and religious life led to the recall of Mother Moore after an absence of only six months.[49]

The idea of work as a means to self-mortification was a central tenet to the religious life of this Irish order. This view did not meet with the Gothic and romanticized notion of Catholicism, popular in nineteenth-century England, a view that was reinforced by the aristocratic and medieval sentiments of the English church. The vow of poverty was also one that concerned the families of well-born recruits. The hard frugal life of the Sisters of Mercy was considered far more extreme than their asceticism (their acts of pious self-denial), and it was felt to be inappropriate for such genteel women.[50] The challenge, then, for this Irish foundation was to absorb its English entrants yet retain the rule and the spirit of the vocation as Catherine McAuley had intended. After its uncertain beginning, the English foundation of Sisters of Mercy was led by Mother Moore for thirty-three years, thus successfully avoiding fashionable manias and rule by poorly trained convert religious. The proof of their success, and of Moore's adaptability, came with the invitation to nurse soldiers in the Crimean War.

The Crimea

Mother Moore had become acclimatized to dealing with the English, calming anti-Catholic anxieties, and building bridges between the two communities. After all, she had had to deal with English clergymen, English aristocrats, and English converts. Her nuns had included members of the royal family, daughters of Protestant ministers, and daughters of members of the British High Command.[51] Moore was experienced at guiding the manias of convert women into a disciplined and useful religious life, and accustomed to dealing with the elite of English society. Florence Nightingale, therefore, was perhaps not such an unfamiliar creature for Moore to deal with on the highly sensitive political mission to the Crimea.

The Sisters of Mercy set off to the Crimea as soon as the call for nurses was made. The opportunity to further the Catholic hand in Britain was a prime one. Mother Moore led her party of sisters to France even before Nightingale had agreed to go. After some frantic letter writing, the Catholic contingent waited for Nightingale's group and joined her party in France, diplomatically accepting her leadership.[52] The larger goal of the expedition was for Catholics to be seen to serve the British military cause, assisting, without favor, the poor British soldier. The public relations impact of this exercise made it possible for Catholics to counter the continuing opposition to their presence in Britain, and to provide their friends with a case for tolerance and support. It was, therefore, necessary for Moore to cope with Nightingale, to avoid sectarianism and Irish/ English disputes, to work well and hard, and in so doing make friends for the church in high places.

The church hierarchy in England was overjoyed at the outcome of the Crimea — notwithstanding a rebuke from Ireland and Rome for allowing the English nuns to be placed under the leadership of a Protestant woman.[53] At the very time that the Irish sisters were on the verge of being recalled (due to unsatisfactory arrangements over their chaplaincy and tensions with Nightingale),[54] Mr. Newdegate, a member of Parliament who had made his entire parliamentary career into a single-issue campaign to rid England of convents, was speaking to his Convent Inspection Bill.[55] Its fate in the House of Commons was a matter of great anxiety for the church in England, especially for Moore. Bishop Grant wrote to Mother Moore on 12 August 1855 to apprize her of its progress:

Bless the sisters for me, and tell them that during this last session of Parliament no one dared say a single word against convents or religion, although the bigots have been otherwise very active. This silence is attributed, through the divine blessing, to the Sisters.[56]

The Bermondsey Sisters of Mercy, then, were key actors both in the establishment of Catholicism in those early decades after Catholic Emancipation and in nursing's great nineteenth-century saga — the Crimean War. There they won the admiration and lifelong friendship of Florence Nightingale (although her relationship with the Irish contingent of Sisters of Mercy never warmed). They later worked in the first Catholic hospital to be established in post-Reformation England, supporting the high profile campaign of Cardinal Wiseman. Before they even returned from the war, the Catholic hierarchy was of the view that the popularity and support of the sisters would be usefully turned to establish a Catholic hospital for incurables.[57] As Dr. Whitty, vicar general of Westminster, put it, "we ought not to lose the opening now made for your sisters."[58] Again it was to be a first such institute since the Reformation and was therefore subject to enthusiasm, ceremony, and opposition.

Like the convent, the first Catholic hospital in England was the object of aristocratic patronage. Officially it came under the Knights of Jerusalem, a lay order of wealthy Catholics. The hospital was the bishop's showpiece, with the sisters almost props in his display of Catholic skills and success. The patients, incurable children, were well endowed with toys and books. The hospital was visited by the royal family; vestments in the hospital chapel were presented by Pope Pius IX.

In nursing terms, however, the direct impact of the Sisters of Mercy was limited. The sisters' most memorable nursing came with the call to the Crimea. They served the church's purposes both there and with the Hospital of St. John and St. Elizabeth, and nursed wealthy patrons and clergy in their homes.[59] They did not establish a hospital of their own and did not engage in the professionalization of nursing in England. Nursing remained one of many activities they pursued when called.[60]

In fact, the sisters were campaigners — a shining Catholic light for all to see. They were campaigners for Catholicism, exemplars of the power and utility of vowed women. Nursing, thanks to the Crimean War and Florence Nightingale, was an asset to that campaign. But most important of all, they were there, walking the streets of England in habits,[61] calmly going about their business, tending the sick and poor, singing their prayers. Through their piety, devotion, and even death, the sisters raised the profile of Catholicism, offering an English path to a Catholic vocation. They led by inspiration, bringing an English presence to the iconographic Soeur de Charité who fascinated so many English visitors to the Continent. And it is to the impact of this image and its emblematic power on the nineteenth-century pious imagination that we now turn.

The Protestant Response

> . . . *with all the devotion of Sister of Mercy but with none of the mistakes of her creed*
>
> — *T. Bowman Stephenson, 1890*[62]

The tensions that erupted in nineteenth-century Protestantism can be seen in the conflict over religious nursing. To have nuns abroad in England crystallized Protestant England's quandary of what to do with its pious women. The Sister of Mercy, or Soeur de Charité, was well known as the generic, if inaccurate, term for a nursing nun.[63] Visitors to the continent witnessed their labors and on occasion directly experienced their care. The cult of St. Vincent de Paul and the work of the Soeurs de Charité greatly appealed to civic-minded and virtuous people concerned to find solutions to the overwhelming social problems caused by industrialization.[64] These problems of crime, poverty, child labor, and civic disorder were understood by both Catholics and Protestants in evangelizing terms. The aim of the numerous groups who worked and proselytized among the poorer classes throughout the nineteenth century was that Christian practice might civilize the dangerous and unruly mass of the poor.[65] Through prayer, literacy for Bible reading, meditation, and regular sober living, the unruly and raucous working classes were to be transformed into model citizens.

For well-born members of English society, their regular visits to the Continent provided opportunity to study Catholic methods of charitable relief. More specific "fact-finding" missions also took place early in the nineteenth century. For instance, in the 1830s, prior to the establishment of Anglican sisterhoods, Edward Bouverie Pusey (influential leader of the Oxford Movement) visited Dublin and was given permission by Mary Aikenhead to attend the profession of Sisters of Charity.[66] Nightingale was specific in her research: she described her Roman holiday as "a course on convents and hospitals."[67] By the mid-nineteenth century the notion of a female institute had become the common topic of sermons and pamphlets.[68] As Augustus Muhlenberg stated in 1872 in his *Thoughts on Evangelical Sisterhoods*, "The question no longer is, Shall we have sisterhoods? But of what kind shall be their form, their organization, et cetera, in order to conformity [sic] with the genius of our Protestant religion."[69]

Protestant Models of Female Religious Life

EVANGELICAL PATHS

In 1833 an Anglican clergyman, John Keble, gave the Assize Sermon at Oxford that was later published under the title of "National Apostasy."[70] It is difficult to read this sermon today and grasp just what caused such controversy and led to a radical movement that dominated nineteenth-century religious life in Britain. The position statement implicit in Keble's seemingly innocuous sermon was that Anglicanism is a divinely ordained religion of ritual, sacraments, and apostolic authority. It was a defensive position, one that was responding to a fundamentalist revival in Anglicanism that, along with the Great Awakening revivals in the United States, made the Bible the sole tool for Christian practice.

The debate that erupted around the emergence of Protestant communities of women religious in England was colored by the controversies within Anglicanism and inflamed by continuing high profile conversions of Anglicans to Catholicism.[71] There was great controversy, debate, and acrimony over the appropriate religious life for women, and there existed wide variation in approach. For those of an evangelical temper the essential elements of any organized activity by women were, first, that it be supervised and superintended by a pastor. Second, the pastor was only a substitute father. The woman's own father retained full authority over her and could recall her to home duties as required. This was the key issue according to the bishop of Lincoln, Charles Wordsworth: "No vow of obedience to a superior of a sisterhood can be defended which militates against any clear duty to God or to Parents."[72]

Early efforts at nursing came as evangelical philanthropists responded to epidemics. In 1829 Quaker Joshua Hornby established a home visiting service for the poor in Liverpool. In the cholera epidemic of 1831 the care of the sick was the work of pious individuals. The first formal training of nurses in nineteenth-century England occurred as a result of the efforts of Quaker Elizabeth Fry. Following a visit to the center of the revival of the female diaconate, at Kaiserswerth, Germany, Fry founded the Protestant Sisters of Mercy in London, in 1840, in order to train women to care for the sick in their own homes. The name was changed to Institute for Nursing Sisters in deference to concerns over popish tendencies. The Fry nurses were Protestants of good character who had received training at Guy's Hospital, London. The cost of the Institute was borne by donations from paid patients, which subsidized care of the poor.

Fry's broadly Protestant Institute was ahead of its time. It also garnered the skill and energy of working women. For the better class of woman, two paths gradually emerged for those who wished to dedicate their lives to God's work — the deaconess and the nun.[73] Within this evangelical framework, espoused principally by "low" elements of the Anglican Church, Quakers (such as Fry), and Methodists, there were variations to the model. For instance, Mildmay Park, founded in 1861 by the Rev. William Pennefather and his wife Catherine, was run along the lines of Pastor Fleidner's Kaiserswerth. Pennefather also welcomed Presbyterians, and the women who completed training were not in general Anglican deaconesses. By 1884 there were 200 deaconesses and 1500 associates. The deaconesses took no vows, wore a distinctive uniform, and lived at Mildmay Park, superintended by Mrs. Pennefather.[74] Mr. Pennefather's enthusiasm for the contribution of women was tempered by the wish to prevent them from getting "above" themselves. He wished "to make the ministry of Christian women as efficient as possible, without tempting them out of the lowly sphere assigned to them by God."[75]

The North London Deaconesses Institution, established in 1862 by Elizabeth Ferard, the first Anglican deaconess to be "set apart" (the deaconess version of profession or vow taking), was also modeled on Kaiserswerth.[76] As "it is exceedingly desirable that a Deaconess should be, to a great or less extent, a practical nurse," this community assumed responsibility for nursing at the Great Northern Hospital, London, in 1863.[77] They were assisted in this task by an experienced nursing deaconess sent over from Kaiserswerth for that purpose.[78]

A different model was that of the Rochester Deaconess Institution, which offered a two-year training program for women in preparation for parish work. These women resided in their parishes, not in a community house. They gained nursing, home visiting, and scripture class training to equip them to "most fully fulfil their roles as man's help-mate." The Methodist and Anglican deaconess institutes in England did not attract moneyed or high-born women to the same extent as did the Anglican sisterhoods. But neither were they for the lowly. For instance, the Methodist Deaconess Institute at Mewburn House, London required candidates to be "women of good education and address."[79] The deaconess role was not necessarily a lifelong state, though it could be. It was assumed to be the domain of single women or widows. The women were expected to have the permission and support of their families and, unlike Kaiserswerth, to be provided for by them as required.[80]

ANGLICAN SISTERHOODS

> *Newman and I have separately come to think it necessary to have some* Soeurs de Charité *in the Anglo-Catholic church. . . . My notion was that it might begin by regular employment as nurses, in hospitals and lunatic asylums, in which last Christian nursing is sadly missed.*
>
> —E. B. Pusey[81]

A second initiative in the development of modern nursing occurred as part of the Oxford Movement within the Anglican church. In 1845 an Anglican religious order, the Order of the Holy Cross, or the Park Village Sisters, was established to minister to the sick poor. This group, founded by Pusey, underwent no training. The sisters cared for the sick poor in their homes. A second group, the Sisters of Mercy, was established in Devonport in 1848 by Miss Priscilla Sellon. In 1855 the Park Village Sisters were absorbed into the Devonport Sisters of Mercy, under Miss Sellon's leadership.

The model commonly adopted by Anglican women was that of dowry requirement for choir sisters and the option of lay sister status for poor women. The life of the women was generally ordered around liturgical observances and set prayers. Sellon was a key figure in nineteenth-century Anglicanism. In her organization there were three levels of participation. Each group had a distinct habit, identity, and rule. The tertiary group was composed of women who lived at home, took a modified vow, and maintained regular prayer observances. These women would perhaps come together at retreat time. The second group lived within the convent but went abroad performing charitable works such as nursing and home visitation. The third group adhered to a severe rule of prayer, discipline, and fasting. They were enclosed, went barefoot, and rose at night for prayers. In this community all domestic work was performed by the sisters, and the many critics of Sellon were concerned at the severity of the rule.

One of Sellon's most widely read critics was a Miss Margaret Goodman, who wrote a best-selling book following her experiences as a member of the community. Goodman portrays Sellon as unstable and cruel.[82] This perception of women dominated nineteenth-century fears of female communities. It was thought that women lacked the stability and reasoned nature of men and therefore required the moderating influence of the pastor to prevent them from succumbing to religious mania. There are those for whom Sellon personified these traits, and her administration, by more than one account, was quixotic and tyrannical.[83]

Mumm argues that the Anglican sisterhoods were in fact quite autonomous and conducted under the authority of the mother superior. She claims that the role of the pastor was to provide a place for them to do their work, as opposed to wielding power within the community.[84] As with the Catholic sisterhoods, the impetus for the foundation of Anglican communities involved the women themselves.[85] With a sympathetic pastor, informal parish associations of women became formalized into communities. Officially the sisterhoods had little place in the Anglican polity until the twentieth century, but if they existed within a sympathetic diocese there was little their opponents could do about them. Likewise, if they felt the need to find a more sympathetic bishop they were free to move.[86]

The role of the pastor in gaining recognition and acceptance of the community—for mounting its defense—has led to the notion that the community itself was the product of clerical initiative. It is the names of the male founders or cofounders that are often best known beyond the community. Pusey's encouragement of sisterhoods is better known than the identities of the women who founded the communities (with the exception of Priscilla Sellon). In East Grinstead the Sisters of St. Margaret were the inspiration of John Mason Neale, who made the formation of the sisterhood an important part of his life's work.[87]

The story of a member of the Sisters of St. Margaret, Emily Scobell, well illustrates the tensions between "high" and "low" elements of the Anglican Church and the way the sisterhood epitomized this division. Emily Scobell was the daughter of an evangelical Anglican pastor. Her father had opposed her "high" tendencies, forbidding her to go to confession or visit the poor. His opposition is instructive. When she joined the community (against his wishes), he wrote demanding of the mother superior by what "right" she had invaded his home and stolen his child.[88] His resistance to auricular confession goes to the heart of Protestant anxieties over the intimate relationship that was thought to occur between a confessor (a priest) and a woman — another man's wife or daughter. According to Bishop Wilberforce, the confessional superseded "God's appointment of intimacy between husband and wife, father and children."[89]

Soon after joining the community, Scobell died of scarlet fever contracted through nursing. She left a generous bequest of £400 to the community (and the larger part of her inheritance to her brother). There was a riot at her funeral. The sisters had their habits torn and Neale was attacked by a large mob incensed that Scobell's property had been "stolen" by the church, and that Neale and the sisters had assumed the role of chief mourners at the funeral.[90]

The issue of inheritance and the disposal of fortune was a sensitive one. According to Mumm, most communities gave the women time to make a will and organize their funds before taking vows. Mumm claims that the record on such financial transactions demonstrates a surprising degree of financial autonomy for Victorian women. There was certainly a great deal of money involved. Inheritances of diamonds for chalices, railway stock, full funding of convent buildings, and so forth came from wealthy entrants.[91] The dowry paid by choir sisters averaged around £500, but in a great many instances it was much more than this. Like the Bermondsey Convent of Mercy, these affluent and well-bred institutes were something of an English phenomenon — Catholic and Anglican. In some cases a woman could even enter, as in medieval times, with her servant as a lay sister (though she did not retain her servant's services in the nineteenth-century convent).[92] Lay sisters were part of nearly all communities in the nineteenth century, and these entrants and the novices generally preformed all the manual work — something that required great training for aristocratic novices.[93]

Nonetheless, the work ethic that distinguished the Catholic communities inspired by Vincent de Paul was strongly manifest in these Anglican sisterhoods too. The rules of the Sisters of Charity (Anglican) required the sister to make service to the poor her first devotion. Both the Sisters of the Holy Church and the Sisters of the Holy Rood decried burdensome prayers and offices that would interfere with their work. One prospective candidate to the Community of All Saints recalled the first question asked by the mother superior: "What can you do?"[94]

Perhaps not surprisingly, a habitual peril for these communities was the defection of its members to Catholicism.[95] Mass defections occurred at the time of the Gorham Judgment.[96] In fact, Mumm reports that 36 percent of the women who left Anglican communities did so to become

Catholic. Not only did such dramatic changes of side undermine the confidence and stability of the fledgling communities, they reinforced popular prejudice that the sisterhoods were all crypto-Catholic in the first place.

Thus Protestant nurses were produced from a range of innovative and experimental religious and practical trainings. There were deaconess programs where women remained at home for their training, wore no uniform, experienced no community, right through to vowed women who punctuated their nursing work with regular periods of prayer. All these women, from Methodist deaconess to Anglican nun, had to fight for their place in the sun, and that place was far from stable. But of all the varied tasks they undertook, their nursing impulses had often prompted calls for their establishment, developed loyal followings for them, and profoundly influenced the subsequent course of professional nursing in Britain, and thereby the world.

Protestant Nurses

The spontaneous philanthropy of pious women in the nineteenth century was given direction by the establishment of female religious communities. At the same time, the magnetic pull the Catholic Church appeared to exert over these women was lessened by the provision of acceptable (though still debated) Protestant alternatives. Although teaching, orphanage work, and care of penitents assumed great importance, particularly into the twentieth century, in the nineteenth century it was the nursing work of the sisterhoods that provided maximum impact. It was also highly relevant to subsequent professional developments in secular nursing.

The earliest groups of religious women in England, Catholic and Protestant, were all primarily engaged in nursing. The epidemics of the first half of the nineteenth century, the swollen ranks of paupers due to the Irish famine, and the lack of any suitable institutional provision for their care, called the pious and compassionate to their aid. The precise training each sisterhood offered its members was highly variable. Most received some rudimentary nursing training, and they generally received broad practical experience in home nursing, epidemic nursing, and hospital nursing. Deaconesses received about two years training to equip them for Bible reading, health mission work, management of parish charity work, teaching, and care of the sick. In addition to home visiting and epidemic nursing performed on occasion by all the sisterhoods, the Anglican communities offered England skilled clinical nurses with experience in hospital administration, war nursing, and medical and surgical care. From as early as 1851 the All Saints Sisterhood, one of the leading

Anglican nursing communities, received formal training at Westminster Hospital, London.[97] By the 1860s and 1870s the nurses of St. John's House, All Saints, the Holy Rood, and the Community of St. Margaret provided the most experienced and best-trained nurses in the country.[98]

Anne Summers has shown how remarkably effective these sisterhoods were in raising the standards of organization and care in the teaching hospitals.[99] These women were professionally competent; they demanded better provisions (from bandages to diet) for patients. They also supervised and trained the nurses working with them and insisted that cleaning work be performed by cleaners and not nurses. In practical terms, these groups of nurses performed important work, establishing the moral integrity of nursing as a pious vocation, and furthering the cause of trained nurses. Even before the Crimea, the Fry nurses and St. John's House sisters worked in the homes of the poor and rich alike, in hospitals and in poorhouse infirmaries. Their success engendered debates about the ability of hospitals to afford trained nurses, and of the role of nurses in the management of epidemics and other public health measures. It was they who pioneered the field as an area of virtuous activity, as well as a focus of emergent expertise — moral and scientific.

St. John's House

The most influential of all communities in this respect, and in relation to its impact on Florence Nightingale's thinking and experience of nursing, was St. John's House, formally the Order of St. John the Evangelist. This community was founded in 1848 as a "Training Institution for Nurses in Hospitals, Families and for the Poor." The nursing focus of St. John's House (named after its parish location), its subsequent impact on London teaching hospitals, and its atypical organization and rule distinguish it from the other sisterhoods and deaconess foundations, and link its history more vitally with the emergence of secular nursing following the Crimean War.

As Carol Helmstadter points out in a series of papers, St. John's House owed its foundation to a pious medical reformer, Robert Bentley Todd, a far-sighted individual who achieved prominence as a medical innovator and teacher.[100] He was aware that his goal for hospital reform required a new type of nurse. St. John's House was to provide and train these nurses. Their nursing successes were impressive. In 1856 they assumed control of King's College Hospital, London, in 1866 Charing Cross Hospital, London, and in 1867 the Hospital for Sick Children in Nottingham.[101] Over this period they frequently rejected proposals to take over other hospitals due to lack of resources.[102]

Unlike other religious communities of women, St. John's House sisters were administered by a council of twenty-four men. St. John's House was an experiment—a model nursing community, established to reform patient care and aid the development of scientific medicine. Under sympathetic patronage it succeeded in these tasks, controlling the hospital environment, training nursing staff and providing a stable environment for patient recovery. The sisterhood provided women with an opportunity to unite professional, spiritual, and philanthropic goals within an Anglican context. This was an innovative approach to complex practical problems and a pragmatic meld of models that at first appeared the solution to hospital needs and the vocational desires of women.

Difficulties soon emerged. The first superior of the community was a low church woman, Elizabeth Ferard. She acquiesced in a structure that gave the House Master primary control over the sisterhood. This structure swiftly proved a major obstacle when a high church woman, Mary Jones, close friend and mentor of Florence Nightingale, took over the community. In 1868 Jones led a defection from St. John's House, leaving it bereft of sisters. She declared: "I am by the voice of the Sisters the Superior of my Sisterhood, and as such I must diligently care for the needs and jealously guard the rights of my Sisters. A constitution of our own is essential, and we must claim the right to regulate our own inner life."[103] Jones and her sisters formed a new community, the Sisterhood of St. Mary and St. John, and achieved self-governance and spiritual freedom. For its part, the council little understood how problematic these structural issues were for the sisters and simply began again, perceiving the issue as a symptom of incipient Romanism among the sisters.

A decade later St. John's House was managing two major London teaching hospitals, King's College Hospital and Charing Cross Hospital, with thirty-five sisters overseeing 219 nurses.[104] The sisterhood withdrew yet again due to continued dissatisfaction with the controlling role of an increasingly unsympathetic council. Problems also rose directly through clinical and professional conflicts with medical men. For instance, at King's College Hospital, the famous Lord Lister's impromptu on-ward surgery would take over the entire ward for long hours (full troop of medical students observing, loud and terrifying explanations, blood on the floor, and so forth), making the care, even the feeding, of other patients impossible. Other difficulties involved the abusive and insulting treatment of women by one attending obstetrician, Dr. Hayes, which led to a formal complaint by the sister in charge. The absence of acknowledgment of Sister Aimee, the Sister Superintendent, in the annual reports of King's College Hospital served as the last straw.[105] The second rift ended in a nasty press war and the sisters being unable to reclaim £15,000 of their funds from St. John's House. The Anglican *Guardian* was the sole support for the sisters. The *Times* and medical journals claimed that the issue was one of ignorant and overbearing women standing in the way of medical progress.[106]

This second defection effectively caused the demise of St. John's House, although it did continue in an attenuated form until World War I. Meanwhile, the community that had seceded continued its work and remained in great demand internationally.[107] The successive failures of St. John's House highlighted the failure of the hybrid model where well-born pious women trained and regulated nursing in a major teaching hospital, superintended by a combination of male religious and medical men. The model foundered on the need for the women to establish a realm of independent spiritual and temporal authority within the hospital and within their community. Both the lack of recognition of their spiritual needs and the refusal of the council to recognize that their expertise and experience demanded a corresponding area of power and authority led to a collapse in relations between the hospitals and the sisters, and the council and the sisters.

The movement for religious women in Protestant England, then, achieved a great deal of success in the second half of the nineteenth century. It was the Anglican sisterhoods in the south of England and evangelical Anglican and Methodist deaconesses throughout the country that achieved the most formal and prominent communities of women. They achieved recognition and visibility for women, forming the critical mass of active women who participated in a host of community activities, such as Bible and mission groups, overseas missions, and temperance societies. It was in this manner that the political and social landscape of nineteenth-century society came to include women. Women, for their part, colonized more and more territory as belonging to the "the female sphere." Education, orphan care, prison reform, rescue work, home nursing, and higher education formed the locus of such activities. Institutional nursing by religious women, with its organizational and infrastructure demands, was left to the Anglican sisterhoods.

Unlike the Lutheran deaconess movement, the deaconesses in Protestant England largely remained part of the pastoral machinery of the parish. Under the authority of the pastor, safe within the patriarchal home, their range and professionalism were limited. In England trained and professional nursing activity demanded a more centralized and autonomous organizational base than was generally allowed in the deaconess movement. Through a separate organizational structure, women such as Elizabeth Fry, Mary Jones, and Sister Aimee were able to set up skilled nursing organizations for pious women. Over the period from the 1840s to the 1870s, these women were able to offer good care from respectable women to private patients and to hospitals on a contract basis. Anne Summers charts the remarkable yet largely unobserved impact of these groups.[108] In the first instance they offered a high standard of postsurgical care. This was in an era when surgical innovations were being developed and private surgery by the country's leading surgeons took place in the homes of the wealthy. Postoperative recovery then as now relied on skilled aftercare. These English "Soeurs de Charité" developed these skills and became highly sought after. Second, as contract nurses to major hospitals, they brought these skills and a high standard of practice to the teaching hospitals. The records of the Boards of Governors meetings complain about the cost of the sisters, and the heavy costs in improved patient diet, bandaging materials, and so on that they insisted were necessary for proper care.[109] Moreover, they refused to perform domestic work, so the hospital had to fund "scrubbers" in addition to nurses. It is, therefore, from this group of predominantly Anglican women that the awareness of the possibility of reform and its uses and benefits permeated medical and hospital practice in the years leading up to the Crimean War. Following the Crimea, the enthusiasm for trained nursing raised the sisters' own stakes even higher, as they were the only group to provide trained nurses for almost another twenty years.

However, despite their success and clear viability, the limits of their approach for England had become clear. The Anglican affiliation of these communities was intolerable to both the nonconformist elements of English Protestantism and the evangelical elements of Anglicanism. Moreover, this occurred in a more general climate of secularization and democratization. The sectarian tensions evident in the upheavals within Anglicanism, between Anglicanism and the nonconformist sects, and between Protestantism and Catholicism strengthened the case of "liberals" who held that the secularization of state and civic institutions was the only sane and peaceful response to religious division. The liberal-democratic framework strove to prevent the extremities of revolution that dominated continental politics, and at the same time to limit the official role of the Anglican church and the capacity of the Catholic church to influence British politics. Franchise debates, the rights of women, attitudes to immigrants, and colonial responsibilities were all issues that expressed religious, patriotic, and civic turmoil.

In this climate it was not possible for Catholic women to take over the administration of English hospitals, nor was it desirable for Anglican women to reinforce the ascendancy of the established church. The deaconess groups did not address the issue of institutional care of the sick to any great measure, and therefore the reform and secularization of nursing required an English solution.

Religious nursing was, then, a force for reform and a doorway for respectable women to the public domain. However, for Protestant England it was a movement with clear limitations. Neither Catholic nor Anglican sisterhoods were able to make significant inroads into the well-established hospital system. Unlike the situation in New South Wales and North America, the nineteenth century in England was a period not so much of hospital foundation as of reform.[110] The established hospitals in England operated within preexisting governing structures. Boards of governors, who generally represented respectable Protestant England, would have considered it their charter to preserve English institutions from the hands of Catholics. The heritage of the English Reformation could not be squandered by the restoration of hospitals to the hands of nuns. For the Anglican sisterhoods much of the same thinking applied. Medical support for the sisterhoods had waned by the 1880s. Moreover, the sharp distinction between "high" and "low" church and the presence of nonconformists on hospital boards would have made the wholesale appointment of Anglican sisterhoods to the management of hospitals extremely controversial. For nonconformist churchmen, keeping public and private resources out of the control of the "official" but resented Anglican church would have underlain much resistance to the sisterhoods.

As opposed to continental Europe, where the nursing communities were commonly exempt from anticlerical decrees,[111] in England the divisions within Protestantism and virulent anti-Catholicism meant that there was not to be an English religious solution to the problem of nursing. This was despite the brave and innovative Protestant modifications to the Catholic model engineered over the course of the century. In England, the model of a modern, scientific, and democratic nation, a view developed that it was desirable to move beyond religion in the fields of education and government and scientifically to shape its citizenry in civic, nondenominational Christian virtue. It was in this context that the Nightingale response to the problem of religious nursing provided such a powerful and resonant solution.

The Nightingale Solution

Despite her singular qualities and achievements, Florence Nightingale was a woman of her era. Like other serious-minded and pious Victorian women, she felt called to a useful life and thwarted by the constraints of the role of daughter.[112] As an adolescent during the controversies of the Oxford Movement, she was well aware of the religious life that a good many of her peers would choose. She must have followed the scandals caused by conversions and the love affair the English upper class conducted with the trappings of Catholicism, if not Catholicism itself. She had her own struggle, too, in this respect. In her correspondence with Henry Manning, whom she had met in Italy, she expressed the urge to become a Catholic and envied the life and training of nuns.

In 1852 Nightingale wrote to Manning, now a Catholic priest,

> If you knew what a home the Catholic Church would be to me. All that I want I should find in her. All my difficulties would be removed. I have laboriously to pick up, here and there, crumbs by which to live. She would give me my daily bread. The daughters of Saint Vincent would open their arms to me. They have already done so; and what should I find there? My work already laid out for me instead of seeking it to and fro and finding none; my home, sympathy, human and divine. . . . Why cannot I enter the Catholic Church at once as the best form of truth I have every known and as cutting the Gordian knot I cannot untie.[113]

Nightingale continued to observe the nursing work of Catholic nuns. She educated herself on the difference between Daughters of Charity (whom she always praised) and communities where the sisters did little hands-on nursing and made their own spiritual life, not care of the sick, their essential work (such as communities she observed in Rome).[114] In addition to her efforts to secure time at a hospital run by religious women, she visited Pastor Theodur Fleidner at Kaiserswerth. There she was able to study the organization and training of the deaconesses. But it was the nuns who really fascinated her. First she followed their work from afar, envying their training, utility, and purpose. It was this training that was such a problem for her. She understood that efficient nursing and hospital reform entirely relied upon the effective training of women. She even temporarily entered a convent to learn more about that training.[115]

When the call to the Crimean War came, Florence Nightingale was well researched but not well experienced. The war proved a battle for Nightingale on a number of fronts: she had to maintain the support of the War Office, the army, army medical men, and her heterogeneous group of nurses—including her adversary, Irish Sister of Mercy Mother Francis Bridgeman. Two things we can say emerged clearly from this experience. First, Nightingale hated the sectarianism and controversy that dogged every issue when it was clouded by religious conflict.[116] Second, she developed a close and highly spiritual relationship with Mother Moore, the leader of the Sisters of Mercy from Bermondsey, London. Not only did these two women correspond for many years following the war, but Nightingale's attachment for Moore is evident from the fact that on her return to London she immediately went to the Bermondsey convent, and, finding the sisters about to commence a spiritual retreat, remained with them for a few days before announcing her return from the war.

Although Nightingale was the undoubted heroine of the war, the nursing sisterhoods, too, grew in popular confidence and stature. Other Crimean lady nurses published their own accounts of the war, many of which were critical of Miss Nightingale and lauded the Catholic nuns.[117] As we have seen, Catholic sisterhoods, for their part, took advantage of public enthusiasm to open a hospital in London in 1856. Nightingale was particularly concerned to discover a plan in the Army Medical Department to introduce (Catholic) Sisters of Mercy as female nurses at the Victoria Hospital at Southampton. Apparently this lobby came from a Catholic convert, Dr. Andrew Smith.[118] The Protestant sisterhoods also had friends in high places, with Deputy Inspector General Mouat putting their case: "women, as a rule, can only make good and useful nurses when led to the adoption of this most trying and disagreeable of occupations from strong moral feelings . . . and Protestant sisters must form an integral portion of the community."[119]

As a woman of her generation, Nightingale had begun as something of a Catholic fellow traveler, inspired by the life and work of the nuns with a vocational sense that God had called her to forge her own path and lead others along it. But, as Bolster puts it, "Her attractions are for the organization rather than the doctrines of the Catholic Church."[120] The religious order constituted the spiritual/ethical "space" from which, when pressed by the Nightingale Fund, she formulated a nonsectarian form of nursing suitable for English society. Her European research, the Crimean experience, and the advice and inspiration of Mary Jones, formerly of St. John's House, and Mother Moore, Bermondsey Sister of Mercy, provided the accumulated wisdom from which the "Nightingale System" was to emerge.

The Nightingale System

> But two thoughts which God has given me my whole life have been, first to infuse the mystical religion to the forms of the other . . . especially among women to make them "handmaidens of the Lord." Secondly — to give them an organization for their activity in which they could be trained to be "handmaidens of the Lord."
>
> —Florence Nightingale, 1889[121]

During the patriotic fervor of the Crimean War, the grateful British public (including loyal citizens from New South Wales) contributed generously to a fund to establish a system of trained nursing. This was not Nightingale's initiative; she was far too busy examining army sanitation, the water supply of India, and a thousand other pressing questions to focus on nursing.[122] Nonetheless, the Nightingale Fund demanded her response. Taking copious advice from Mary Jones (a frequent, privileged visitor to Nightingale's sickbed), studying the rules and contracts of St. John's House, and drawing on her own encyclopedic knowledge of hospitals following decades of research, she began to develop her own system.[123] The sisterhoods provided the model for hierarchical organization, with the Nightingale sister responsible for ensuring decorum and respectability, supervising the conduct of patients, nurses, and doctors. The invention of the nurses' home was another "cloistered" element of critical importance. In addition to the improvement in hygiene and health the homes facilitated, they provided the crucial opportunity for the training in "character" that Nightingale considered so essential to improve nursing.[124] The homes, too, made it possible for respectable girls to train as nurses, reassuring their families that a safe and chaperoned environment was provided for their nonworking time. The nurses' home was "A place of moral, religious, and practical training of character, habits, intelligence, a place to acquire knowledge, both technical and practical. . . . It is there that order, discipline and method . . . must be first taught, or they will not be amenable to ward discipline."[125]

What was later to become known as the "Nightingale system" of training and hospital reform involves a number of key aspects: matron in authority, nursing probationers in residence, instruction from the ward sister, and supplementary lectures on hygiene. Monica Baly's thorough examination of the historical record points out that this "system" was not the result of a thought-out master plan. Nightingale did not, in fact, have control over St. Thomas's, where the system was introduced. Mrs. Wardroper, the matron, was not a lady, and Nightingale frequently despaired of the entire business.[126] Nonetheless, as a result of Nightingale's profile and the Fund's effective publicity machine, the St. Thomas's experimental model became nursing scripture. In fact, Nightingale became synonymous with nursing.[127] Her influence extended from military nursing to all matters concerning nursing, poorhouse nursing, home visiting, and midwifery.

The failure of Catholic nursing to make an impact on Victorian nursing reform in England is indicative of the fact that hospital reform remained a Protestant concern in Britain. However, disunity within the Protestant confessions, in the context of the Oxford Movement and nonconformist anger, left the highly successful Anglican nursing sisterhoods without the broad popular support enjoyed by Catholic sisterhoods elsewhere. The success of Florence Nightingale, like the success of the active orders of religious nurses that preceded her, was that she provided a solution to the problem of religious tensions in Britain. Vocational nursing led by godly women could achieve a miracle among the old hospital nurses.

The Anglican sisterhoods, like the Catholic sisterhoods in Catholic countries, had shown what could be done. The improved management of hospitals, better clinical skill, and improved care were undisputed. But there had to be a way to provide this care without fueling the religious tensions that dominated Victorian Britain. As Baly has well demonstrated, St. Thomas's training was not very successful, and Nightingale privately did not think much of it. Its success was that it offered much of what the sisters had proven to work, without the religious intrigue to upset the board or the secret sisterhood to upset medicine. But most important of all, it successfully harnessed the vocational wave of women in a way that removed religious tensions yet maintained its pious energy—Victorians loved it.

Chapter 5
At the Margins of the Empire
Religious Wars in the Hospital Wards of Colonial Sydney

Despite its position at the very margins of the British Empire, colonial New South Wales played its part in the Nightingale movement for the reform of nursing.[1] As patriotic members of the British Empire, colonials contributed generously to the Nightingale Fund set up during the Crimean War by an enthusiastic British public. Miss Nightingale honored this contribution in 1868 by providing a team of women to bring her distinctive style of trained nurse to Australia. However, long before the Nightingale sisters disembarked at Sydney Cove, a group of French-trained Irish nursing sisters had been busy caring for the people of Sydney at St. Vincent's Hospital. Sydney's St. Vincent's was an excellent hospital, led through the century by distinguished and educated women.[2] It was funded by subscriptions and supported by a wide section of the Sydney community.[3] St. Vincent's became the hospital of choice for all private patients, foreign visitors, and embassy staff, and even boasted a suite for the Royal Navy.

Yet despite the achievements of the Sisters of Charity, professional nursing in Australia is commonly considered to have begun in 1868, when Miss Nightingale's distant relative and protégée Miss Lucy Osburn and her team of five newly trained sisters arrived in Sydney. Their task was to reform nursing at the Sydney Infirmary, the oldest hospital in Australia.

The story of the English Nightingales and the Irish nursing nuns in nineteenth-century Sydney's two hospitals continues the Victorian story of Catholic Emancipation, Irish politics, Anglican tensions, and the emerging terrain of women's work into the colonial world of New South Wales.[4] In Sydney, at the boundaries of Empire, the juxtaposition of these two communities of nursing women provides a case study that addresses the issues of competence and professionalism, religion and sectarianism, and church and colonial politics as they shaped the emergence of professional nursing.

The Tyranny of Distance

The Colony of New South Wales was only fifty years old when five Irish Sisters of Charity disembarked at Sydney Cove, in early summer, on the last day of 1838.[5] The voyage had taken four months. The sisters were accompanied on their outward voyage by an English Benedictine priest, Father William Ullathorne. It was his responsibility to ensure that arrangements were made for the sisters that befitted their holy and unworldly status, and that they avoided the unseemly task of communicating directly with crew and fellow passengers.

In 1838 Sydney was the administrative center for the entire continent and for New Zealand. At that time the total population of the continent was 152,000. In New South Wales there were 77,000 Europeans.[6] New Holland and Van Diemen's Land,[7] as Australia was then known, were settled in 1788 when the British finally accepted the loss of America and needed somewhere other than Virginia to transport their convict ships. The European community of Sydney consisted of the military presence required of a garrison outpost of the British Empire, plus administrators, convicts and former convicts, guards and their families, and a handful of free settlers. Half the population was English, a quarter Irish, with Scottish and sundry other nationalities making up the remaining quarter. The English were in charge, the Scots worked hard and prospered, and the Irish were a thorn in everyone else's side. It was thus a microcosm of British society.[8]

Irish Versus English: Sisters of Charity and Dr. Polding

But there was one major difference between "Home" and the colony: in Sydney there were few women.[9] The shortage of women meant that the domestic and sexual services of convict women were at a premium. On arrival the women were placed in the homes of the colonial leadership and settlers. Women who committed a further offense or became pregnant (a common occurrence) were put to work (accompanied by their babies) in an institution known as the Female Factory at Parramatta — a half-day journey by ship inland from Sydney. The Female Factory was first established in 1801 for about fifty women, who were occupied weaving linen and wool. It was rebuilt by Governor Macquarie in 1818 and by 1842 accommodated 1,203 women.[10]

It was here that the Sisters of Charity were first put to work, among a thousand women and children, two-thirds of whom were Catholic.[11] The niceties of their chaperoned journey to Australia were somewhat at odds with the brutal reality of the Female Factory, the lack of suitable accommodation or financial support available on arrival, and the way they were left to fend for themselves in the hostile society of New South Wales. Despite these difficulties, the sisters took to the work with energy. Even accounting for the enthusiasms of insider historians, the sisters must have been a welcome change to at least some of the inmates of the Female Factory and their children.[12] The concentration of Irish among convict women in Sydney was high.[13] Before 1815–21 nearly 55 percent of convict women were Irish; overall in 1788–1828 40 percent were.[14] For homesick Irish women, the sisters brought the consolation of the church and taught the children. Their success in moderating the mood of the Factory was enough to be mentioned in dispatches to Rome by the vicar general of the colony, Dr. John Bede Polding. Characteristically, the sisters are invisible in this clerical correspondence. Their achievements were attributed to the genius of their confessor, Ullathorne, who according to Polding "goes to Parramatta once a week . . . he has formed the house of the Sisters of Charity, . . . his labours have made the Factory the abode of penitence."[15]

Relations with the vicar general began badly and were to deteriorate. In a decision that showed a startling innocence of the colonial situation, Sister Mary Cahill declined a government stipend for the sisters.[16] Meanwhile, Polding (also an English Benedictine) did not provide for them. Polding received a government stipend of £800 per year. He also had possession of the £2000 Ullathorne had brought out with the sisters in 1838. Polding had assured Mary Aikenhead, foundress of the Irish Sisters of Charity, that he would provide for the sisters, However, once in Sydney he instructed the sisters to write to Dublin for their dowries. Unknown to the sisters, Mary Aikenhead forwarded the dowries to the Benedictine agent in London, the Reverend Thomas Heptonstall. So while Polding mustered the resources to give property to Benedictine nuns and other property purchases, the substantial dowries the sisters had brought to the order were at Polding's disposal and never made available to them, and the sisters struggled in desperate poverty and actual hunger.[17]

The confusion over dowries was part of a more general confusion over the nature of the Sisters of Charity, how they were supposed to live, and where they fitted into the Catholic Church in Sydney. The Irish Sisters of Charity had only begun in 1815. Mother Mary Aikenhead, their foundress, was still alive in 1838. In 1841 the total number of women religious in Ireland was only 987 — of a population of eight million.[18] The rule by which the community lived was formed under Jesuit influence that emphasized a worldly mission requiring flexibility and adaptability and a strong spiritual interiority.[19] It was founded as a centralized institute under the motherhouse system, which stipulated direct rule within the community as opposed to rule by a bishop.[20] This was new territory for women both in Ireland and in Australia, and Polding's understanding of or interest in issues may have been limited.

Mother Aikenhead's Sisters of Charity

Mother Aikenhead was the daughter of an apothecary, and her religious vocation to the poor gave special emphasis to care for the sick. Aikenhead was also a convert to Catholicism, and from the beginning her mission was one of outreach with hospitals open to all. She determined that she would find a means to provide the poor with care that could match anything money could buy. This was not simple philanthropy but a philosophy that encompassed material goals and expectations for the community. The foundation of St. Vincent's Hospital in Dublin expressed this pragmatic merger of clinical and philanthropic goals. One of Aikenhead's early problems had been the death rate among the sisters involved in sick visitation. Moreover, not only was home visiting a personal health risk to the sisters, but Aikenhead was concerned that the sisters were themselves a source of contagion as they traveled from house to house. Her only solution was to bring the poor to the sisters, where their wants could be supplied and the sisters could care more efficiently for greater numbers of poor. It was this "logistical" consideration that led Mother Aikenhead to the possibility of a hospital.[21] Once the money was found to commence the institution, she sent three sisters to Paris to the Hôpital de Notre Dame de la Pitié, conducted by the Sisters of St. Thomas of Villanova. There the sisters were sent to the different departments to gain a broad experience. St. Vincent's, Dublin was opened in 1834, and run by nurses with the only training available at the time,[22] offering medical support from Dublin's best. St. Vincent's medical care was given by men such as Joseph O'Farrell (1790–1877), one of the founders of, and keen contributors to, the Dublin Pathological Society, forerunner to the Royal Academy of Medicine, and O'Bryen Bellingham (1800–1867), an Edinburgh-trained Protestant aristocrat who developed the "Dublin Method" for aneurysm surgery.[23] The group that was sent to Sydney in 1838 included Sister Francis de Sales O'Brien, who had received her nursing training in Paris, and Sister John Baptist de Lacy, who had trained at St. Vincent's in Dublin.[24]

It was also in 1834 that Dr. Polding, as the new vicar apostolic of New Holland and Van Diemen's Land, approached Mother Aikenhead for Sisters of Charity for the Colony of New South Wales. The Sisters of Charity were focused on their service to the Irish poor, and they did not establish overseas missions as readily as did other communities. However, Polding's tale of the plight of the Irish convicts in Australia moved

Mother Aikenhead. In the first years of convict settlement Catholicism was proscribed, and the Catholic community had to rely on Irish convict priests (who were flogged for performing their calling).[25] The convict women were in a particularly vulnerable position, at the mercy of all, with no provision for their care or guidance. Aikenhead agreed to supply Polding with a group of five sisters for the mission to "work a change in at least the female part of the convict population."[26]

Finding a Place for the Sisters in Sydney

As for so many other nineteenth-century female religious foundations, from Chile to Newfoundland, the sisters endured remarkable hardships. The death rate among the Sydney sisters was high, and the small community was stretched to the limit of its human and financial resources.[27] The sisters taught children and adults, cared for orphans, and visited the sick. They moved from Parramatta to Sydney at the bishop's command, were shifted from house to house, and on one occasion were almost dispossessed by him.[28] Even though Polding had begged Mary Aikenhead to spare him some Sisters of Charity, whom he knew to be skilled nurses and teachers, he made no effort to provide them with their own schools or hospital. Instead he put them to work walking all over the town to visit six schools and the Sydney Infirmary, where no trained nursing was carried out and the nursing work (such as it was) performed by unskilled servants. The sisters' lack of permanent housing hampered their ability to train novices, hold religious services, and stabilize their religious and professional lives.[29]

Most important, Bishop Polding and his vicar general, Father Gregory, interfered with the rule of the sisters, appointing and dismissing leaders, accepting and rejecting novices, and so forth.[30] The acrimony in relations between the church hierarchy and the sisters is clear in the abusive tone of the letter extract below.

The character of the Church in this Colony must indeed be very low in the estimation of some of its members, when the conduct of its highest Official is considered such that even women deem it their duty to subject it to investigation. Truly this is a new Era in ecclesiastical discipline when those whom St. Paul says may not open their mouths in the Church of God, fearlessly ascend the Tribunal of Justice, undertake an office involving responsibility from which Men of the highest standing of the Church distinguished by their piety and learning shrink with a God-inspired dread, privately to sit in judgment upon the actions of one whom they are bound by vow to obey.[31]

Sydney was a very small community, however, and the trials of the Irish Sisters of Charity imposed by their English bishop and vicar general did not go unnoticed by the Catholic community and friends of the sisters. In

1853 the attorney general of New South Wales, John Hubert Plunkett, initiated a public appeal to enable the Sisters of Charity to procure a permanent residence in Sydney. In an anonymous pamphlet entitled *A Brief Sketch of the Pious Congregation of Sisters of Charity, carefully selected from authentic sources*, he referred to them as "the Australian Sisters of Charity," emphasized the recent deaths of three sisters from influenza, and called on those who "proudly call themselves the daughters and sons of Australia" to assist the sisters.[32]

At a second public appeal in 1855, this time launched by Henry Parkes, Plunkett asked the crowd whether "Miss de Lacy, a Sister of Charity, who had devoted her whole life to the relief of the sick and comfort of the poor, were not equally entitled to the gratitude shown to Miss Nightingale."[33]

Meanwhile, European settlement in Australia expanded rapidly. Other Australian colonies had begun to be settled and the basis of the future six states laid down with settlements at Hobart, Melbourne, Adelaide, Perth, and Brisbane. This expansion occurred through survey and exploration, land grants for farming, and a steady increase in free settlers. However, this gradual pace was to change when, in 1851, the gold rush began.

It had been noted by crown surveyors that the mountains, river valleys, and plateaus of southeastern Australia contained gold. What was missing was the experience to recognize good gold country and the simple portable technology to extract it from wild country. When the Australian veterans of the Californian gold rush came home in 1851, they brought with them the technology and American knowhow to find and exploit the rich gold deposits of Victoria and New South Wales.[34] As in California, the gold rush was to change the landscape forever. It was the beginning of the new settler-society Australia and the end of Australia as a penal settlement.[35]

Despite the rush of migration of free settlers to the gold fields, the Catholic community of Sydney remained overwhelmingly Irish. Throughout this period the Irish nationalist movement was becoming increasingly vocal as Ireland moved slowly toward separation from Britain and the establishment of Home Rule. In general, the political passions of the Irish were seldom supported by the Church.[36] The Catholic Church had its own political agenda in the nineteenth century, and the British Empire provided the newly reestablished Irish church with the perfect infrastructure on which to build its own English-speaking Catholic empire.

Interestingly, the Sisters of Charity was one community that did not remain avowedly Irish. While it did attract Irish women and the daughters of Irish immigrants and convicts, the Sydney community of the Sisters of Charity actively welcomed Australian women and did not reinforce its Irishness through direct recruitment drives in Ireland (as did the

Mercy sisters and a good many others).[37] The Sisters of Charity saw themselves as Australian, proud of their place as the foundation order for this new society.[38] Not only were they not so "Irish" in their outlook, their brief was charitable care and service to the entire community — not simply the care of Catholics. Their "place" in Sydney was not in the Irish community or in the bosom of the Church — as mere "hands and feet" for the bishop. The sisters had their own vision, their own mission. By 1857 the sisters in Sydney had been nursing the sick in their homes for nineteen years. They had also been "homeless" themselves for many years. So when the opportunity arose to obtain the land and buildings suitable for a hospital and a convent, the sisters seized the moment.

Battle Lines: Clergy Versus Sisters

> *I was never a very sanguine advocate for the advancement of the hospital.*
> — *Archbishop Polding, 20 June 1859*[39]

Through the generosity of Sir Charles Nicholson (a non-Catholic) and their friends in the community, the sisters were able to obtain the property Tarmons for a hospital and convent.[40] On Nicholson's return to England, his parting gesture to the colony was to sell his house to the sisters, for the purpose of a hospital, at an extraordinarily generous price, and to donate one thousand pounds toward the cost of purchase.[41] To the sisters, Sir Charles Nicholson had undoubtedly been sent by God. The sisters were particularly delighted with the position of the building. It was in a beautiful spot on a hill overlooking the harbor with floor to ceiling windows that allowed for maximum ventilation by sea breezes. Friends rapidly raised eight thousand pounds, which left a debt of only two thousand pounds.[42] Sir Charles, along with Mr. Plunkett, the treasurer, Father McEncroe, and Sister de Lacy were established as hospital trustees — one priest, one Catholic layman, one Protestant man, and one woman.[43] The hospital came about through a community effort that combined wealthy philanthropy, Catholic support, and a broad subscriber base that included everyone from the governor of New South Wales and Colonial Secretary Henry Parkes to Protestant ministers and Jewish shopkeepers. The sisters, flushed with success at having raised such a large amount of money, marshaled the broad community behind the effort as subscribers, and attracted the leading medical men in Sydney to work (gratis) for the poor in their hospital, as honorary medical staff. It was a mutually beneficial arrangement, as St. Vincent's also provided them with the first good avenue for private surgical and medical care in Sydney.

The celebrations were short-lived. Dr. Polding had been absent during these developments. When he returned to Sydney he did not take the news well. He was furious, not only viewing the entire venture as a challenge to his authority, but also because such a large charitable initiative would take continuing resources to sustain. And despite the fact that so many of the fundraising committee and the subscribers to the hospital were non-Catholic, Polding insisted that the hospital would be a "drain" on the diocese.[44] There were schools and orphanages to build, fallen women and children to protect. All this work, as he saw it, would be significantly affected by a Catholic hospital.

Other issues about the hospital also bothered Polding. He did not like the Protestant doctor, Dr. Robertson, who was the sisters' medical officer; he did not care for the fact that the governor and all the Protestant establishment had appeared on the subscription list.[45] The archbishop's personal donation of five pounds, published in the first annual report, was well eclipsed by the ten-pound donations of a Protestant clergyman, Reverend Wolfrey, and M. Sentis, the French consul.[46] In the years to come Polding did not shift from the view that the hospital was a thorn in his side and a "burden" to Sydney.[47]

On his return in 1857 Polding moved to reassert his authority over the Sisters of Charity. He demoted and promoted sisters, transferred women from one house to another, and generally repaid them for their insolence. He established his own community that year, the Good Samaritan Sisters, to do diocesan work. He insisted on a Charity nun, Sister Scholastica, becoming their head and training the novices.[48] Matters drew to a head in a Bible scandal. The Sisters of Charity had accepted a donation of Protestant Bibles for the use of Protestant patients. In 1859 a zealous chaplain, Father Kenyon, seized these texts and removed them. Immediately all the Protestant doctors and the treasurer resigned, and the more ablebodied Protestant patients left too. After something of a standoff the case was mounted in legalistic terms to the bishop that subscriptions were raised on the basis that St. Vincent's welcomed patients of all religions. Should it be determined that Protestant patients were discriminated against, the money might have to be repaid.[49] The bishop backed down and the Bibles were returned.

The hospital continued as a battleground. The authority to command the institution was denied the woman who had the experience to do so. In 1859 Sister de Lacy, along with a postulant, left the Sydney community, and the chief medical consultant also resigned. Sister de Lacy returned to Dublin against the orders of Polding. By virtue of her vow of poverty, de Lacy owned nothing and was forbidden by the archbishop to take anything (even her clothes) with her. Outrage at her treatment led to a public fund, with over 130 subscribers, set up to provide funds for Sydney's own "Florence Nightingale" on her voyage home.[50] Both the *Free-*

man's Journal and the *Sydney Morning Herald* lamented her parting. The latter proclaimed: "We are not the less strongly attached to the distinguished principles of Protestantism, because we cherish toward these virtues [nursing] a feeling of the highest veneration, whether a Fry, a Nightingale or a de Lacy."[51]

On her return to Ireland she was given the opportunity to explain herself to the Directress of the Sisters of Charity and was sent as superior at Kilkenny.[52] The matter, however, did not end there. Polding was determined to have de Lacy returned or excommunicated for disobeying her bishop. He wrote to Archbishop Cullen in Dublin demanding that she be sent back to Sydney. Meanwhile her supporters in Sydney wrote to Rome demanding that Polding be prevented from persecuting the Sisters of Charity. Cullen in Dublin also referred the issue to Rome. Cullen's eventual response to Polding was that Sister de Lacy was "doing much good here in Dublin, and besides is rather advanced in age, whence it would be perhaps expedient to let her finish her days here in peace."[53] Rome began an investigation of Polding in which he was called to account for his lack of respect for the rule and autonomy of the sisters. It was an astonishing defeat, the more so since it had been completely unexpected by Polding. He responded: "It was extremely bitter to me to learn from your eminence's letter that the most illustrious and Most Reverend Archbishop of Dublin is a promoter of Sister de Lacy's idle tale."[54] He felt crushed, the victim of an Irish conspiracy.[55]

It is the strength in community that shows up in this tale. For even though every individual sister who came out to Australia and struggled under Polding had left or died, St. Vincent's, as a mission and priority of the Sydney sisterhood, remained on track.[56] In fact, aside from the difficulties with the church hierarchy, the story is one of steady progress. The people of Sydney, of all religious persuasions, supported St. Vincent's through the subscription system. Protestant ministers shared the right with Catholic priests to send poor patients to the hospital. The religious background of the patients was published by St. Vincent's in each annual report to disabuse the government of any notion that it was a Catholic hospital for Catholics. The sisters insisted that they served the entire community, without favor, and were thus entitled to government subsidy, although they were singularly unsuccessful in this campaign.[57]

The lack of government assistance forced the sisters to rely on their commercial talents. In 1870 the new extended hospital was finally opened. This hospital included a private wing. Here the sisters began to gain ground. Sydney had no private hospital facilities, nor was there a cadre of experienced nurses available to care for the well-off in their homes. Sydney had wealthy (increasingly so) as well as poor residents; it also housed numerous embassy staff and was a British naval base and port of call for many foreign vessels, military and civilian.[58] It was unthinkable that a person with a modicum of self-respect would be cared for at the only other hospital in the colony, the Sydney Infirmary, and thus St. Vincent's was in constant demand as a private hospital. It provided a clean and orderly environment, well-fitted private suites, good private surgeons and physicians, and well-educated and well-born nurses (described by the Nightingale nurses' champion, Henry Parkes, as "the cultured ladies of religious sisterhoods").[59] It was a successful combination. Official anti-Catholicism notwithstanding, St. Vincent's had a public ward for the Royal Navy, with officers treated in private rooms.

In fact, St. Vincent's became something of a favorite for sailors, caring for 448 merchant sailors in 1862–82 and 187 men of the Royal Navy in 1872–75, as well as men of the French and German navies. In 1881 Rear Admiral Tyron, the senior medical officer for the Royal Navy fleet, was appointed to St. Vincent's.[60] St. Vincent's and the Charities were also praised by members of the medical profession. In 1871, at the height of tensions between the Sydney Infirmary nursing and medical staff, representatives of the medical profession commented that the infection rate at St. Vincent's was much lower than at the Sydney Infirmary.[61] A veiled comparison was also made of the nursing in the respective hospitals. The comparison could not have cheered the embattled Nightingale incumbent, Miss Osburn: "They (the Sisters of Charity) attend upon the sick with a degree of care and kindness which could be expected of no person who nurses for hire."[62]

There is no doubt that throughout the course of the nineteenth century the Sisters of Charity had a prickly relationship with diocesan clergy, who continually attempted to interfere with their internal management. Nonetheless, the troubles of the sisters cannot simply be put down to acrimony between themselves and the Englishman Polding — bitter though that battle had been. The Irish clergy, too, were nervous at the intimacy of the Sisters of Charity with the Protestant community. They considered it improper for them to work so closely with Protestant doctors and to take money from Protestant subscribers, but, worst of all, the sisters were even on friendly terms with visiting Protestant clergymen who sent patients to the hospital. The church was sure that women — as weak-minded creatures — were in danger of falling under the influence of those men. This is despite the fact that the diocese had found the Sisters of Charity singularly impossible to influence.

English Versus Irish

The struggles of the Sisters of Charity did not pertain only to the place of women within the nineteenth-century Catholic Church. A second group of nursing women, over this same period, also found themselves at the center of a storm in colonial Sydney. These were the Nightingale nurses who were sent from Britain in 1868 to reform the Sydney Infirmary and establish professional nursing in Australia.

The scheme to bring a team of Florence Nightingale's nurses to New South Wales was the result of the efforts of the exuberant Henry Parkes, colonial secretary for New South Wales, 1866–68. Parkes had been so moved by Nightingale's achievements in the Crimea that he orchestrated Australia's contribution to the Nightingale Fund and was keen to involve New South Wales in the Nightingale vision for the future of nursing. When, a decade after the Crimea, he inspected Sydney Infirmary after receiving complaints, he knew exactly what to do.[63] Nightingale responded to Mr. Parkes's pleas and promised to send a cohort of sisters as soon as possible, declaring that "I would fain repay my heavy debt to Australia according to my powers."[64]

The Sydney Infirmary had begun as a convict hospital. Its inglorious beginnings were enhanced in 1816, when rebuilding was financed through the rum monopoly (whereby it became known as the Rum Hospital), and nurses continued to be drawn from the ranks of convicts well into the nineteenth century.[65] There was no provision for private work and when a free settler's wife was admitted in obstructed labor doctors refused attendance as they were not entitled to charge a fee. There was community outrage when the woman died.[66] The vermin infestation at the hospital was a consistent source of complaints. When a young sailor died in 1866 at the Sydney Infirmary after the master of his ship had found him in a "filthy state and swarming with vermin," St. Vincent's took over the care of merchant and Royal Navy seamen and officers.[67]

Lucy Osburn arrived in Sydney with a group of five trained nurses in 1868. No sooner had they arrived than an Irishman attempted to assassinate the visiting Prince Alfred, son of Queen Victoria. It was some compensation for the shame of the attack that Sydney was able to offer the prince an English Nightingale to nurse him back to recovery. "Our fair Sisters of Charity," clamored the newspapers and the grateful public.[68] The attempted assassination of Prince Alfred stirred a hornet's nest of anti-Irish feeling. The assailant, O'Farrell, was hanged following a confession in which he allegedly claimed to be part of an Irish Fenian organization.[69] It was in this climate of passionate pro-British feeling that the Nightingale nurses commenced their campaign to reform the Sydney Infirmary, and to usher in the new age of nursing.

Despite the rhetoric and the red carpet, the Nightingale mission was certainly not a runaway success. When Osburn led her team of Nightingale sisters to the Sydney Infirmary in 1868, she was aware that a challenge awaited her. Her goal was to transform the colony's only public hospital into a respectable, ordered environment where, according to the sanitarian view of the universe espoused by Miss Nightingale, the patient would find the resources to heal himself. Osburn quickly made an enemy of Dr. Alfred Roberts, the hospital superintendent and chief surgeon, who had been a prime mover in the plan to introduce trained nurses. In Roberts's view the reform of nursing did not involve the control of the hospital, which remained firmly in the hands of the medical superintendent.[70] The limit of Osburn's authority rested with her sex. She had no authority over male nurses, orderlies, kitchen staff, and so forth. As a leading member of the colonial medical profession, Roberts kept a close eye on developments in Britain. His private war with Lucy Osburn kept pace with the territorial struggles between trained nurses and the newly empowered medical profession in London teaching hospitals, such as Mr. Guy's (his own training hospital) and King's College.[71]

Nightingale Sisters and Irish Nurses

Notwithstanding the somewhat predictable opposition of the medical superintendent, what confronted the English sisters at the Sydney Infirmary was far worse than they could have imagined. The prime difficulty was not the filth and disorder of the institution but the caliber of the nurses. According to Sister Mary Barker in her letter to Miss Nightingale, 30 May 1868: "I think the scrubbers at St. Thomas's Hospital were a respectable class of women in comparison with what we found as day nurses at the Sydney Infirmary's."[72] Osburn describes them as "rough raw nurses brought up in huffer muffer Irish ways without a clear or systemic idea in their heads."[73] According to Sister Miller, "the climate is horrid and the people all Irish and bad."[74] The servants, the management of whom is always key to running the hospital, "are all Irish Roman Catholics."[75]

Osburn recounted to Nightingale that she sought the immediate resignation of the worst of the nurses. She confessed to great relief at the fact that she was able to do so without occasioning violence. For the remainder of these rough Irish women, she immediately ordered "four-posted iron bedsteads and looking glasses."[76] Once these arrived, she instructed the English sisters to teach the nurses to put up their hair.[77] The Irish women's uncovered heads with "luxuriant hair fuzzy as oakham" (rope), to use Mayhew's description, were evidently Osburn's prime concern.[78] Thus the reform of Australian nursing was launched, not with training or a recruitment drive, but with hairdressing lessons and twice-daily prayers on the wards.[79]

The paradox of nineteenth-century nursing was that only women who did not need to work (i.e., they worked from vocational fervor) were able to command enough respect to reform nursing into respectable work — a profession. This is clear from Osburn's experience when in 1873 she was called before the Commission of Inquiry to Inquire into a Report on the Workings and Management of the Public Charities. Who and what she was seemed to perplex the committee. Their questions revolved around not the hospital, but Miss Osburn's background and status. "May I," interrogated the chairman of the committee, "if it is not an impertinent question, ask you whether your taking such a position as you now hold was a necessity, or did you come from the love of the work?"[80] Osburn goes on to explain the distinction between sisters and nurses, how they live quite separately, and an entirely different standard of etiquette is expected of them: "they [the sisters] are quiet steady people as we can get. The nurses are of course a merry set, and like music and dancing and that kind of thing; and that I could not allow with the sisters."[81]

Australian women, it appears, were altogether too much of a merry set for the speedy reform of the Sydney Infirmary. They were entirely lacking in the skills in personal grooming and domestic management considered necessary for professional nursing. This is hardly surprising. As Beverley Kingston notes, domestic help was sorely lacking in the colony and ladies were poorly served compared to their European counterparts.[82] The general shortage of women in Australia, too, seemed to militate against a good supply of nurses. Despite the emblematic significance of Florence Nightingale, few nurses came from the higher classes. The professionalization of nursing required the inculcation of these supposedly feminine middle class virtues into common women. It was not an easy task.

The first register of nurses at the Sydney Infirmary records Osburn's opinion of her recruits to nursing and follows their progress through life. The register opened with Ann Branagan, 23, in the colony two and a half years, in hospital first as servant and then as night nurse. Described by Osburn as "Simple. Roman Catholic," she commenced at £26 per annum, and then was moved to be in charge of day ward at £48. In 1876 she married Henry Macguire and they opened a small hotel in Bourke Street. In 1880 she came asking for work. In 1881 she was admitted to the hospital after "a couple of nights drinking and fighting with husband."[83]

The register is full of such stories. "Wesleyan Irishwoman" Jane Morrow moved to Newcastle Hospital in 1870 and then "took to the drink and neglect of the place." Elizabeth Morror was involved in a lawsuit with a Maitland doctor about "some dreadful scandal." A good many nurses, it seems, "took to the drink" or "went mad." A few revealed a religious vocation. One high church Anglican woman from Victoria, Gertrude Moule, entered the Convent of the Holy Trinity, Oxford when she completed her training. Another, Lucy Millard, died at the Institute for English Nurses in Paris in 1884.

English Sisters and the "Colonial Air"

Osburn's problems began with her nurses but soon moved to her sisters. Twelve months into their three-year contract, one married. Worse still, there were rumors about the precipitous nature of the marriage — rumors spread by other sisters. Osburn described it to Nightingale as "Another vexation. Sister Haldane is propagating, even in my presence, all through the establishment that Sister Bessie was confined three months after she left here . . . I have no means of ascertaining if it is true or false."[84]

This was the same Sister Bessie Chant, who was caught making love with a patient (she kissed him in the ward and they afterward exchanged letters).[85] Sister Annie Miller flirted with a resident physician years younger than herself and had to be removed from him — love sick.[86] Sister Eliza Blundall flirted with patients and wardsmen. Osburn began to wonder if there were something in the air of the colony that led her sisters to behave so outrageously. Her astonishment at the lack of propriety and decorum of her own sisters caused her to doubt herself. She opened her heart to an increasingly unsympathetic Nightingale:

Imagine one of them [the nurses] telling at their dinner for the general amusement something which she overheard when waiting for the steward. It was a warm evening and after dusk Bennett [the porter and messenger] — who is married and lives here with his wife and children — was sitting on the balcony with the male cooks and Sister Eliza, the latter was explaining how she could marry any moment as she had five or six beaux waiting for her. "I believe it," says Bennett with a sigh, "for I have often wished myself a bachelor for your sake." This pretty speech was greatly applauded by the cooks. Now none of them were as bad as this when they came, what has altered them?[87]

Amazingly, despite such blatant husband-seeking and total lack of "nunlike" behavior among the sisters,[88] there was still something "Popish" about the English nurses that disconcerted many in Sydney.

Battle Lines: Clergy Versus Nightingales

> *I am your humble servant ready to go to the world's end at an hour's notice.*
> — *Lucy Osburn to Florence Nightingale*[89]

The general perception that the Nightingale sisters were crypto-Catholic may have been due to the fact that, according to Osburn, Florence Nightingale was commonly considered a Catholic by people in New South Wales. In her letter to Nightingale of 16 June 1869 Osburn informs her of this:

Do you know that both here and in London almost everyone thinks you to be a Roman Catholic and sometimes they shut me up by saying point blank Miss Nightingale is a Roman Catholic, is she not? I feel there is a certain amount of impertinence in sucy [sic] enquiries. I get off always now by saying — I have always believed Miss N to be ch of England but I should never think of asking.[90]

Apparently Nightingale was not so bemused, because four months later Lucy Osburn writes: "In future I shall take the liberty to contradict my friends when they assert so confidently that you belong to them hitherto I have just raised my eyebrows and said oh."[91]

But the whiffs of papism were not only confined to Nightingale. A series of trivial events led to suspicions of Catholic conspiracies. To begin with there were difficulties with the term "sister," and Osburn's official title. "Lady superintendent" was unacceptable as this intimated the wife or partner of the male superintendent, Mr. Blackstone — not an uncommon arrangement for institution management in this period. "Lady Superior" was too ecclesiastical for Sydney, and Osburn was advised that "matron" had very vulgar associations in the colony. Osburn's solution was to simply call herself "the nurse from England."[92]

During the inquiry, the commissioners wished, too, for clarification of the usage of the term "sister." "Is it not on religious grounds or from sentimental feeling that you were called 'sisters'?" Osburn strongly denied the accusation.[93]

In fact, the controversy over the title of Osburn and her sisters had major ramifications for the hospital. Once Osburn had been decreed by the hospital board to be "head nurse" and the sisters simply "nurse," prospective trainees withdrew their applications and the hospital was unable to attract applicants for nursing training over the period 1868–73.[94]

As if to feed Catholic rumors and Protestant phobias, Osburn received a set of statuettes of Nightingale by Hilary Bonham-Carter. Osburn set them up on the walls. She thanked Nightingale, remarking how she "looks as if you were pointing the way to the heavenly kingdom. The Roman Catholics look upon it with great reverence, I suppose they think you have been canonised."[95] Osburn even referred to her graduation from St. Thomas's as her "vows," declaring: "I completed the six years I took my vows last 10 September and I should value very much if it were only an official statement that I had been in connection with your school or any certificate the Council might have deemed me to have deserved."[96]

Lucy Osburn, the lady superintendent, found every step of her path to reform nursing and the hospital blocked by a coalition of medical men and evangelical members (male) of the governing body of the hospital.

Miss Osburn was High Anglican while the Church of England in Sydney was very evangelical.[97] She was no novice to these difficulties; according to Freda McDowell, there is a possibly apocryphal story that Osburn's devoutly evangelical father turned her portrait to the wall when she disobeyed him and commenced nursing.[98] Like her father, these Sydney men were singularly unimpressed with Osburn's role and the entire idea of female nurses assuming responsibility for the management of the hospital (laundry, kitchen, orderlies as well as nurses). In fact, they found the whole enterprise deeply suspect. Aspects of Osburn's behavior caused additional concern. Her custom of attending early morning service attracted suspicion;[99] she had demanded the title of "Lady Superior" and called her nurses "sisters"; she had even been spotted slipping into St. Mary's (Catholic) Cathedral (apparently to listen to music).

Finally, Osburn did the unthinkable: in her frustration over not being able to have the hospital cleaned (she was always thwarted in her attempts to have men do work for her), she ordered a pile of cockroach-infested rubbish burned, unaware that somewhere in the rubbish was a pile of old Bibles. The next thing she knew she was in the eye of a storm. Questions were raised in Parliament and the press. In October 1870 the hospital governing board undertook a formal inquiry to examine allegations made in the *Protestant Standard* over the management of the institution and review accusations of sectarian bias relating to the conduct and suitability of the lady superintendent. At this stage, an exasperated Florence Nightingale considered the whole enterprise a failure, despite the fact Osburn was completely exonerated by the committee.[100]

A second inquiry, by the Public Charities Commission in 1863, was another victory for Osburn. Here she argued her case with more success. The commissioners recommended that full management of the wards, patients, nursing, and cooking and control of all workers in these departments should be under the command of the lady superintendent. It was recommended that the title "sister" be reinstated; the committee observed that its change to "nurse" had been "injudicious," as the title "gives the head nurse a moral power."[101] Finally, after a five-year war, the Nightingale system finally arrived at the Sydney Infirmary.[102]

Lucy Osburn was the victim of Protestant sectarianism. She bore the brunt of a powerful faction in Sydney that was unhappy with women assuming a role in the world without the direct supervision of men. A combination of medical resentment and evangelical suspicion worked against her — despite her friends in high places (such as Henry Parkes and the governor). Evangelical Sydney was unhappy about Osburn's lack of deference to male authority and outraged by the recognizably Catholic trimmings of the new secular nurse.

The Place of Women, God's Men, and Good Nursing

> *I love you women, but I hate your religion!*
> *Thank God, my child, in all the bad things we ever did we didn't marry!*
> *— Mary Aikenhead*[103]

To implement reformed nursing successfully, virtuous and vocationally motivated women needed to uplift the nursing staff, manage the wards and departments of the hospital, and support medical practice. This meant strong female leadership, religious discipline, and medical cooperation. The sisterhoods excelled in this, especially where, as in Sydney, the hospitals belonged to the sisters. The secular nurses, on the other hand, had to negotiate every inch of progress. Thus, in nineteenth-century Sydney we have a microcosm of the revolution that was occurring for women in the religious context and in work, in the parallel stories of these two communities of women.

What was it about the Sisters of Charity that made them so successful in establishing and conducting a modern hospital? It certainly was not the unqualified support of a well-endowed church, for the Church had little money and resented every penny that went to the hospital. Despite this opposition and the great human cost among the sisters caused by opposition from the bishop, the community succeeded in creating a fine clinical institution with very high standards.[104] The sisters achieved an institution with good doctors, good facilities, and skilled nurses. St. Vincent's was the only respectable hospital in the entire country for some decades.

Sydney also lacked any respectable, reliable nurses for home care. Doctors had many private patients who were more than willing to pay to be in such a well-run hospital. So there was a need for the sisters' hospital and a market to pay for it. Yet the sisters lacked support from both church and state. To survive, the sisters had to move beyond devotion to the poor and also provide care for those who could pay. This shift to service provision, as opposed to simple charity, was a trial for the sisters. They felt they required dispensation from the pope to obtain income from their hospital work, which they considered contrary to their vow of poverty.[105]

In overcoming these scruples the sisters were then firmly in the commercial domain. They had the best doctors, medical training, private patients, and always a waiting list for the poor of the city. In order to gain support from the government they constantly strove to highlight their achievements, their nonsectarian community service, and their professionalism. By continuing to present themselves as a high quality service to the Sydney community, they distanced themselves from Catholic politics and found some protection from episcopal interference.

For instance, in 1884 Bishop Vaughan promised employment to a Belgian (Catholic) doctor at St. Vincent's. The medical staff resigned at the appointment of one they considered unqualified. The rectress did not "obey"; she called her lawyers. St. Vincent's had received a small grant of land for the hospital that was decreed for the use of a hospital solely conducted by the Sisters of Charity. Diocesan interference challenged this autonomy and placed the donation at risk. When the archbishop backed down, a hiring process was initiated. All medical positions had to be advertised and applicants interviewed by the medical staff. Recommendations were then to be made to the rectress. She retained the right of veto, which she did in fact exercise.[106] This control, astonishingly, even applied to teaching appointments with the University of Sydney.[107] It was always the sisters' hospital, and this independent position was critical to their financial security. As neither the state nor the diocese committed support to the hospital, the sisters relied on their network of supporters. This community was not the same as the "Catholic community" and, in fact, included some who despised the church.

The sisters' vow of service to the poor was also subject to some redefinition. There were poor in New South Wales, but this poverty could not compare with that in Europe. In fact, the pioneer pride of many citizens led them to insist on the right to pay for the education of their children, or for hospital care. It was the emerging respectable working class, more than the poor, that the sisters served in Sydney. As they explained to Rome, "in this country the poor are comparatively few . . . and because the people in this country, in general, not liking to appear poor, refuse gratuitous services, despise even those who offer them, and often end by turning to Protestants and paying them."[108]

Finally, the mission of the sisters was always ecumenical. One of the radical features of Mary Aikenhead's apostolate was outreach and community service. It had not been popular with the church from the start. When the rule of the community was ratified by Rome, its ecumenical flavor was distinctly watered down and the word "Christian" was changed to "Catholic."[109] The sisters were perfectly comfortable working with Protestant doctors, and with Protestant clergymen, who not only referred patients but were also welcome to minister to them in the hospital. In 1867 the sisters refused to place an altar in the front room of the hospital, unwilling to claim it solely as a Catholic space. They considered the altar in the chapel quite sufficient.[110] They accepted donations of Protestant Bibles[111] and appeared not to exploit the opportunity that sickness provided to proselytize among Protestant patients.[112]

Pragmatism remained dominant. For instance, they did not consider cleaning part of nursing training but a simple issue of resources. When one early student nurse offered to pay for a charwoman to relieve her and her fellow students of this work, the sisters agreed, and after this student had completed the course the sisters continued the practice by demanding a subsidy from the students.[113]

The Nightingales also had a vision of a clean, efficient hospital. What they lacked was power. They had no authority over the male staff or domestic, maintenance, or kitchen staff until the Commission of Inquiry recommended that this be so. It was simply not possible for them to reform the hospital under such constraints. Another great challenge to Lucy Osburn was the quality of her nursing staff. Whether it was the English Nightingale sisters, the Irish nurses, or the new recruits, Osburn found it impossible to muster the feminine moral authority from nurses of less than desirable backgrounds. She was forced into a campaign to "uplift" her nurses, to teach them to dress, to walk, and behave in a way that desexualized nursing and provided the women with authority over their working class patients and shared administrative and clinical power with medical men.[114]

But pious women's work had another difficulty. The entire project was deeply suspect to evangelical Christians. It empowered women in an unseemly way — by mimicking the style and manner of nuns. For sections of the Sydney Protestant community, including members of the Sydney Infirmary hospital board, it represented a radical and unwelcome challenge to the position of women and to the authority of men. From medicine and the churches, Lucy Osburn suffered continuous innuendo and slander.

The differences between the two communities of women are perhaps less surprising than the similarities. Among the Sisters of Charity dissent and conflict were the result of their precarious situation and the constant interference of clergy. However, the mission of the hospital succeeded in overriding their problems. The establishment of St. Vincent's was the women's impulse, their vocation, and it was achieved in opposition to the church hierarchy. Because the Sisters of Charity formed a community, they were able to succeed even where individuals failed. As each woman left or was replaced, St. Vincent's remained at the core of the sisters' mission, a legacy of the two trained nurses who arrived to establish the Sisters of Charity in Australia.

The Nightingale system too allowed for this chain of continuity in the secular world. Lucy Osburn came to Sydney in the spirit of a sacred vocation, willing to be Nightingale's instrument to the "ends of the world." Osburn had limited authority over an undisciplined group of women. She left Sydney in 1884 after sixteen years, largely unrewarded — in fact rebuffed in not being offered the position of matron at the model hospital opened in 1882. Nevertheless, her training system was established under Nightingale principles. It did survive, and did produce graduates who went on to train Australian nurses.[115] It was thus the implementation of a system, not the work of an individual, that succeeded.

Resistance to the Nightingales indicated the extent to which the very notion of pious women organizing themselves to perform work in the world was a radical one. In common with their vowed Catholic sisters, it was only the utility of the Nightingale nurses that eventually broke through this resistance. But what is shown here in both stories is the way in which care of the sick by hospital nurses struggled and strained against the limitations of female influence and authority. On both sides of the confessional divide, men in authority sensed a transgression — they were troubled by the directions of such behavior and struggled to reassert their authority over it.

Care of the sick by pious skilled women was moving beyond the sphere of influence of male religious leaders, and over the course of the century, as delicate coalitions with medicine and government were negotiated, women (secular or vowed) who could run good hospitals became indispensable. Catholic piety may have led the nuns to establish the field, allowing for the entrance of women into professional practice, but they left the door open behind them. The men who ran the churches in nineteenth-century Sydney were right to worry.

Chapter 6

Frontier: "The Means to Begin Are None"

We had to struggle against fanatical Protestantism here; against unbelief, atheism, impiety and, unhappily, not a single notable Catholic here to encourage works of charity.

— Mother Joseph of the Sacred Heart, Sisters of Providence, Washington Territory, 1878.[1]

Despite the vast number of immigrants crowding into the industrial north of the United States, changing forever the ethnic composition of the country, the Catholic sisterhoods did not restrict their efforts to the needy poor of the cities. Part of the extraordinary force that nineteenth-century America exerted upon the European imagination was the pull of the frontier. There were other frontiers, such as the wild penal settlements of what was to become Australia or Britain's dominions of India and the Far East, where Protestant and Catholic missionary women nursed and taught to extend the borders of the Christian world. South America, with its poverty and wealth, needed sisters too, and the turmoil in Europe provided many refugee sisterhoods. Nonetheless, in the European imagination the American frontier stood alone, dauntingly full of danger, beauty, and possibility.[2]

In this respect the sisters were no different from other American settlers, immigrant or native born. The great drama of nineteenth-century expansionism and nation building provided the same irresistible urge to the Catholic Church and its sisters as it did to other travelers. The risks and possible gains the open territories offered were seized with both hands. In the frontier they found that almost anything became possible. The role of vowed women in this green field for pioneers was shaped as they went—by exigencies and adaptation. In common with other pioneers, the Catholic Church was stretched to the maximum extent of its resources. The Protestant ascendancy that had proved such an obstacle to Catholic acceptance in the East, and fostered the leadership style of men such as New York's Bishop John Hughes, was not as much in evidence out West. Not that there was an absence of opposition to the sisters or of anti-Catholic sentiment, far from it; simply the hardships of pioneering life made it less possible to maintain such divisions between groups within the community.[3]

Pioneers needed hospitals. Doctors needed hospitals. The companies that opened the west — railroad companies, logging mills, and mining ventures — needed hospitals, too. Bishops, for their part, were keen for the sisters to come to their dioceses. Through the sisters the Church provided much-needed services, and the sisters, with great labor and perhaps a benefactor or two, were able to become self-supporting. This was essential. As in the east, there was no money for the sisters. They were invited, pleas were made for them to come, but once they disembarked from ship, riverboat, stagecoach, or train they were expected to support themselves and to establish and nurture an expanding foundation of social and educational institutions for the church. As Mother Saint Pierre Cinquin so aptly put it, for the sisters arriving west to build their foundations, "the means to begin are none."[4]

Two Communities at the Frontier

In this chapter we examine the hospital foundation work of two very different communities of sisters in the west. In San Antonio, Texas we find the extraordinary development of the Sisters of the Incarnate Word. Here a vicarious mission for an enclosed community in Lyons, France, was established to recruit women for nursing work in Texas. The Sisters of the Incarnate Word embody the international nature of this missionary work for Catholic women — a French mission, realized principally through Irish and German women, was acted out in the landscape of the American west. The second is the French Canadian missionary community, the Sisters of Providence, pioneers of the Pacific northwest in Alaska, British Columbia, and the northwest states of the United States.

These two communities have been selected from the dozens of possibilities because they embody a number of characteristics important to this discussion of vowed women, hospital foundation, and frontier. The Sisters of the Incarnate Word personify more clearly than any other community of women the particular confluence of international Catholic forces that led women to work in hospitals in the American west. This group was founded specifically for this endeavor, and it used French traditions for female religious life and Irish and German (and finally, Mexican) womanpower to carve itself a place in the history of the West. The Sisters of the Incarnate Word are also of interest because they emerged from an enclosed community. The religious traditions they embodied were therefore distinct from those of the Vincentian movement for women that takes up such a large part of this story so far.

Although a separate community from the French Daughters, the Sisters of Providence studied the Conferences of Vincent de Paul, practiced his spiritual exercises, and honored Monsieur Vincent along with their own foundress, the Venerable Emilie Gamelin, a Montreal widow who died of cholera while nursing during an epidemic in 1851.[5] In this sense the Sisters of Providence perfectly embody the tradition of religious vocation that inspired women to enter nursing and hospital work in the name of God. But this community is atypical in other ways. The Sisters of Providence attracted few Irish women (or daughters of Irish immigrants) for their American mission in the nineteenth century. It was not simply a case of language (as with the German communities), for many French communities were overwhelmed by Irish women — the Sisters of the Incarnate Word for one. It was the fact that the Sisters of Providence in the northwest were a missionary branch of a Montreal community. Nurtured by their motherhouse in Montreal and sustained by plentiful vocations among Quebec women, the community was able to maintain its French-Canadian identity until well into the twentieth century.[6]

Sisters of the Incarnate Word

> *Be perfectly dead to yourself; make interior acts of abnegation to your tastes and aversions and that will make it possible for you to live in a manner befitting the title you have of Spouse of the Incarnate Word. . . . we no longer belong to ourselves; we have given ourselves to Him.*
>
> *— Mother Saint Pierre, 19 January 1878.*[7]

The Sisters of the Incarnate Word were formed as a missionary branch of the French community, the Order of the Incarnate Word and Blessed Sacrament. The mother community was founded in 1627, at Lyons, France, by Jeanne Chézard de Matel as an enclosed community of women vowed to "the ministry of Christian education." Following their suppression by the Revolution, the Order of the Incarnate Word and Blessed Sacrament was restored in Lyons in 1832. In 1866 the French-born bishop of Texas, Claude Dubuis, was able to convince Lyons to send him sisters to nurse epidemic victims in Galveston and San Antonio. This group of women were formed as "Hospitallers" of the Incarnate Word and became known as the Sisters of Charity of the Incarnate Word.[8]

In Texas the Sisters of Charity of the Incarnate Word were sustained by immigrant recruits. In fact, it was not until 1972 that the general chapter elected its first American-born superior, Sister Eleanor Cohen.[9] For the first fifty years French-born women dominated the leadership of the community (with the exception of one Prussian), and in 1918 the first of five successive Irish leaders was elected.[10] Over the nineteenth and twentieth centuries the ethnic composition of the entrants changed, reflecting changing immigration patterns and European politics. The mother-house in Lyons was closed and the sisters expelled to Switzerland by the Third Republic in 1906. World War I and then World War II affected immigration from Europe; and Irish immigration continued to climb through this period. Ties with Mexico strengthened, too, with increasing numbers of Mexican foundations and entrants.[11]

During the nineteenth century, however, the Sisters of Charity of the Incarnate Word retained their French identity and strong ties to Lyons. Although the community was diocesan and Bishop Dubuis is recognized by the sisters as the founder of their San Antonio foundation, the links to Lyons were vital in the spiritual development of the community and in sustaining their clear sense of an American apostolate. For instance, the one non-French leader in the nineteenth century, Prussian Sister Ignatius Saar, who led the community from 1884 to 1897, had been trained in San Antonio. However, as part of her preparation for leader-ship, she had made three trips to Europe over the years to spend time in the Lyons monastery in order, according to Sister Madeleine Chollet, to "imbibe from our saintly mothers of Lyons much of her knowledge of the spirit that should animate the daughters of the Incarnate Word."[12] This "spirit" was grounded in hospital work.

"We Have Nothing But That Which Is the Result of Our Industry"

The impetus for the formation of the Sisters of Charity of the Incarnate Word of San Antonio was the pleas to Bishop Dubuis from San Antonio's Dr. Ferdinand von Herff and civic leaders for sisters to establish a hospital.[13] Lyons responded, sending women for both the Galveston and San Antonio foundations. The San Antonio group, comprising the illiterate Mother Madeleine Chollet, the charismatic Sister Saint Pierre, and Sister Agnes Buisson, arrived to open the city's first hospital — open to all, doctors and patients, private and public alike.[14]

The sisters announced their new institution, the Santa Rosa Hospital, in 1869, in the local newspaper in the following unambiguous terms:

No regular physician is excluded from our institutions. Every one has a right to send in his patients, whether they be paying or charity patients. He will have entire control over them in the hospital; and his prescriptions with regard to food, nursing, and medicines, will be strictly followed.

We beg leave to remark, however, that the number of charity patients must be proportioned to the number of paying patients, or else we should be in a state of bankruptcy at the very beginning; since we have no revenue, no resources, no other income, but that which is the result of our industry.[15]

The Remark Book of the Santa Rosa Hospital records the wonderful mix of evangelistic business and clinical concerns that dominated the day-to-day life of the hospital.

Thursday 20 January 1898. Operation on Mrs. Sophie Bulter the colored lady, by Dr. A. Herff assisted by Dr Oldham and the sisters. They removed a large tumor from her bowels. — Dr. Razor went home on the 9.30 am train. Mrs. Varnell's daughter arrived today. She will remain with her mother for some time. Mr. R. H. Billingslea received his First Holy Communion this morning in our chapel. Professor Whitehouse gave another lesson on massage [to the sisters]. Mr. Hubbard left this morning for Tampico, Mexico.
Rev Mother went to Boerne.
Saturday 5 February 1898. Mr Moran's sister left today — George Hamel the Aransas Pass Engineer died this evening about 8.30 pm with spasms caused from neuralgia of the stomach or rheumatism. Paid Theodur & men. Gave a note to Mr. S. W. Johnson for $800.00 with interest at 4% for one year. George Hamel's remains were removed immediately to the office of Sloan & Shelley the undertaker. He died a free mason.[16]

Demand for the sisters as "nurses-for-hire" was high. In 1885 they were contracted to staff the Missouri Pacific Railroad Hospital at Fort Worth, Texas. This particular contract had been pressed on the sisters by Bishop Dubuis and the company doctors. Mother Saint Pierre needed persuading that the mission was worth the spiritual risk for the sisters. Not even the prospect of a regular monthly income from the sisters' salary ($15 per sister, $20 for the superior) convinced her. It was only the realization that the sisters would be able to engage in missionary work as they cared for the injured and dying railroad workers, many of whom were Irish and lapsed Catholics, that clinched the deal.[17]

This was the heart of their American mission. As Mother Saint Pierre boasted to Lyons in 1884:

In the hospital [Santa Rosa] we did good work with souls this year. I think that's why the devil torments us so much in our works; he is losing some fine fish under the roof of the Incarnate word. We have had several conversions; baptism has regenerated many a good thief who has gone straight to heaven after having received the grace of reconciliation.[18]

In 1887, ten years after the Santa Rosa Hospital opened, the first county hospital of San Antonio was completed and the sisters agreed to manage it. So for a while the Sisters of the Incarnate Word ran both the Catholic and the county hospitals in San Antonio.[19] In addition to dominating hospital provision in San Antonio, the sisters extended their operations in railroad hospitals, which provided them with an entry to new regions and new opportunities.[20] Typically these hospitals were established in response to persistent pleas from medical practitioners in towns without a hospital, through railroad company offers and invitations from bishops.[21] By the time of their silver jubilee in 1894, membership of the Sisters of the Incarnate Word, San Antonio had increased from 3 to 197. They owned and operated two hospitals, Santa Rosa, San Antonio and St. Joseph's, Fort Worth, and they operated seven railroad hospitals across four states — Palestine and Tyler, Texas; Las Vegas, New Mexico; Fort Madison, Iowa; and St. Louis, Sedalia, and Kansas City, Missouri. They ran more than a dozen schools in the United States and Mexico, two orphanages in San Antonio, and a home for the aged in Monterrey, Mexico.[22] Spurred on by increasing demand for their hospitals and improvements in medicine and nursing training, the Santa Rosa Hospital began its Training School for Nurses in 1903. Their immediate priority was the professional training of their own members, and the first cohort of thirteen students was made up entirely of Sisters of the Incarnate Word.[23]

Recruitment Drives

This rapid expansion required sisters. In 1878 Mother Saint Pierre returned to France and visited Germany to find recruits for the San Antonio mission. She brought back ten women. In 1881 she included Ireland on her recruitment tour and returned with four women from the Continent and fifteen Irish women. In 1895 a recruitment tour yielded twenty-one candidates from Ireland, seventeen from Germany, and three from France. In 1900 the touring sisters brought back six from France, twenty from Germany, and forty from Ireland.[24]

Mother Saint Pierre made moves to establish a house in Europe to prepare women for the Texan mission.[25] The recruitment house was to gain English-speaking recruits from the "Island of Saints," as they could not be attracted in the United States. Second, it was to prevent the possibility of women using the novitiate to escape from their homeland. Mother Saint Pierre complained that they had "to pay the travelling expenses of close to forty postulants . . . several of these creatures came under false pretext and we had to send them home."[26] In order to avoid these difficulties, she negotiated with a Presentation house in Ireland to found a receiving center.[27] Her correspondence with Lyons pushed for this initiative and requested Lyons's blessing. However, the receiving house idea did not come to fruition in Mother Saint Pierre's lifetime, and her successors met obstacles in Germany and France when attempting to establish recruitment houses.[28] The problem of recruitment and preparation of suitable candidates for the Texas mission continued to occupy their energies well into the twentieth century.

Sisters of Providence: Missionary Nurses

Another French-speaking community (this time French Canadian) that responded to the call for missionaries to the western United States was the Sisters of Providence in Montreal, Quebec. Following gold strikes in the Pacific northwest, European settlement expanded rapidly. This part of the United States was the home of many Native American communities, and French missionary priests of the Society of Jesus had long been involved with this fur-trading society. The Sisters of Providence shared the Jesuits' Francophone mission and moved west not only to serve European settlers, but to work among and bring into the church the Native American communities of the northwest. In 1856 Mother Joseph of the Sacred Heart (Esther Pariseau, 1823–1902) led four women from Montreal to Fort Vancouver, in the Washington Territory. These women were pioneers and missionaries. Later, in response to repeated pleas by Chief Seltice of the Coeur d'Alenes people for "women blackrobes" to come to care for and teach their girls, they became the first white women to cross the Bitterroot Mountains into Montana.[29]

These French Canadian women embraced the challenges of frontier life under the leadership of Mother Joseph to build a remarkable network of thirty charitable institutions (hospitals, orphanages, academies, and Indian schools) between 1856 and 1902 (see Table 2).[30] For this group of women the term "build" held literal meaning. Mother Joseph was a carpenter, builder, and architect; she is today recognized as one of the first architects in the northwest and by the West Coast Lumbermen's Association as the first artist to work in the medium of wood. In 1980 a statue of Mother Joseph was installed in the National Statuary Hall in Washington, D.C. as a pioneer leader in Washington State.[31]

When she first entered the motherhouse in Montreal her father told Mother Gamelin, foundress of the community:

I bring you my daughter Esther, who wishes to dedicate herself to the religious life. She is twenty years old, and for some time she has prayed with her family for enlightenment. It is a great sacrifice for me to part with Esther, but if you will accept her into the Sisters of Providence, you will find her able to give you valuable assistance.

She has had what education her mother and I could give her at home and at school. She can read and write and figure accurately. She can cook and sew and spin and do all manner of housework as well. She has learned carpentry from me and can handle tools as well as I can.

Moreover she can plan and supervise the work of others, and I assure you Madam, she will someday make a very good superior.[32]

On arrival in Fort Vancouver, Mother Joseph knocked together the altar for their cabin. On 7 June 1858 she opened an extension of the

TABLE 2. SISTERS OF PROVIDENCE INSTITUTIONS ESTABLISHED UNDER THE LEADERSHIP OF MOTHER JOSEPH

1856	Providence Academy, Vancouver, Washington
1858	St. Joseph Hospital, Vancouver, Washington
1863	St. Joseph School, Steilacoom, Washington
1864	St. Vincent Academy, Walla Walla, Washington
1864	Holy Family Hospital, St. Ignatius, Montana
1868	Our Lady of Seven Dolors School, Tulalip, Washington
1873	Sacred Heart School, Colville, Washington
1873	St. Patrick Hospital, Missoula, Montana
1874	St. James Residence, Vancouver, Washington
1875	St. Joseph Academy, Yakima, Washington
1875	St. Vincent Hospital, Portland, Oregon
1876	Our Lady of the Sacred Heart School, Cowlitz, Washington
1877	Providence Hospital, Seattle, Washington
1878	Providence Mary Immaculate School, DeSmet, Idaho
1880	St. Mary Hospital, Walla Walla, Washington
1880	St. Mary Hospital, Astoria, Washington
1881	St. Michael School, Olympia, Washington
1881	St. Martin School, Frenchtown, Montana
1885	Sacred Heart Academy, Missoula, Montana
1886	Sacred Heart Hospital, Spokane, Washington
1886	St. Clare Hospital, Fort Benton, Montana
1886	St. Joseph Academy, Sprague, Washington
1887	St. Peter Hospital, Olympia, Washington
1890	St. John Hospital, Port Townsend, Washington
1890	St. Eugene School, Kootenay, British Columbia
1891	Providence Hospital, Wallace, Idaho
1891	St. Elizabeth Hospital, Yakima, Washington
1892	Columbus Hospital, Great Falls, Montana
1893	St. Ignatius Hospital, Colfax, Washington
1900	St. Genevieve Orphanage, New Westminster, British Columbia

laundry and bakery building with a few adjustments as St. Joseph Hospital, Fort Vancouver.[33] Throughout her life she worked as both leader and property manager for the Sisters of Providence. Her correspondence appears to deal, in equal measure, with spiritual concerns and with renovations. It is peppered with quotes from builders, compliments on an altar she built, or requests for her opinion on building repairs or elevator design.[34] The sisters' first foundation was in Fort Vancouver, but, according to the Chronicles and correspondence, they were desperate for an opening that would allow them to extend their operations into Seattle. They had to wait from 1856 until 1877 for this opportunity. As is so often the case in the annals of religious women, the intercession of a saint caused a reversal of circumstances for the community. In this case, a special devotion to St. Joseph produced an invitation to apply for the contract to care for county patients in Seattle.[35]

Hospital Foundation

The first patient register for Providence Hospital, Seattle, makes clear the sisters' primary goal in their hospital work. The conversions and baptisms are recorded as a great honor: "We admitted a pregnant mother. When the baby was delivered it already had been dead several days. We were grieved to not be able to baptize the child, as that was our purpose in receiving the mother. She, however, returned to the sacraments before leaving us."[36]

In fact it appears to have been impossible for a member of the local Native American tribes to die in their hospitals outside the Catholic fold. For instance, in the first register of St. Joseph's Hospital, Fort Vancouver, in 1858, the six "Indian" patients were all claimed as converts (four died).[37] As each death was an opportunity for redemption, the sisters tried hard with everyone — regretfully declaring Freemasons the most unconvertible of all.[38]

This is not to say, however, that the sisters' spiritual goals of hospital work contravened their clinical aims. The sisters not only were pleased by their many conversions and secret baptisms, and the various forms of subterfuge they inventively used to bring prodigal souls back to God, they were also very proud of their nursing and of the regard and affection of their patients. They were extraordinarily aware of the power of their work to impress the unbeliever and the opportune nature of pending death to turn even the hardened sinner back to God. As Mother Joseph put it in her "begging" letters to the faithful back in Quebec:

The Sisters of Providence were happy to respond to the invitation of the Bishop of Nesqualy, to come to his assistance, *and to follow him in the apostolate of charity which, in the eyes of our separated brethren, holds so much prestige and accomplishes so many conversions.* (emphasis added)[39]

The evangelistic nature of their work was something the sisters were fervent and open about. The deathbed conversions in particular were claimed by the sisters to "excite our ardor."[40] The Chronicler of Providence Hospital, Seattle records:

More temporal prosperity blessed this year than formerly, but the salvation of souls is still our most important blessing. In coming to us seeking cure of the body, our patients usually also find cure of the soul. To achieve this we spare no means to let our patients see their illness as a blessing — a mark of the love of God, who wants to win their souls.[41]

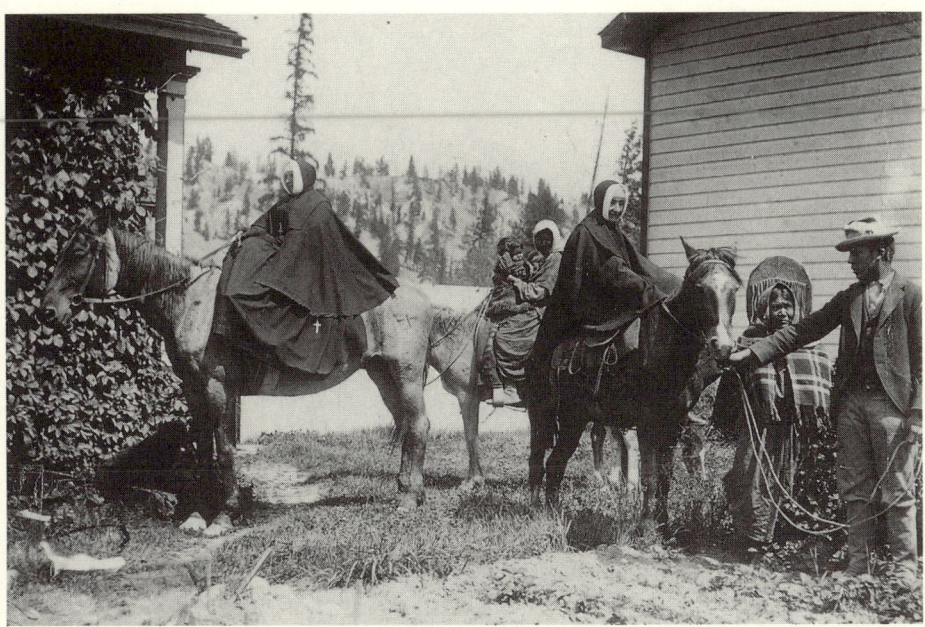

Figure 5. Fund raising, St. Eugene Mission, Kotenay, British Columbia, 1880s. The Sisters of Providence conducted rugged begging tours to the mining camps of eastern Oregon, Idaho, and Montana, where they collected thousands of dollars in gold and coin. Reprinted with permission of the Sisters of Providence Archives, Seattle, Washington.

In fact, the object of a good death for all led them to consider only those who died without grace as failures — "lost." It was a failure that caused them to reproach themselves. They took to heart Vincent de Paul's admonition to the original Daughters of Charity that they were responsible for souls who died without God's grace.[42] Barbra Mann Wall argues that closeness to death was the real interest for the sisters in nursing. It was an evangelical opportunity that belonged to them alone, and as such the sisters were able to participate in "man's work" of saving souls without overstepping their place.[43]

To the sisters, the conversion of patients to Catholicism was evidence of the continued intercession of the saints. A firm belief in the miraculous was a sustaining and enabling force and guided their lives and their work. They interpreted all events as evidence of the hand of God and His saints — particularly property deals, the subject of much prayer. Burying medals of St. Joseph in the lots adjoining the hospital was a favored approach to property investment. St. Joseph was "appointed" the spiritual president and financial patron of the sisters' corporation at incor-

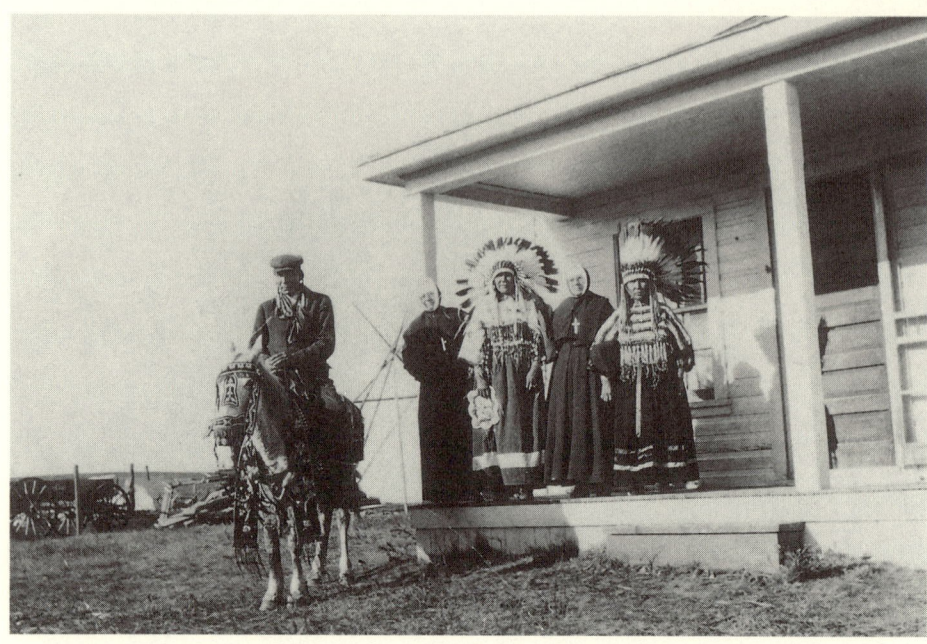

Figure 6. Sisters of Providence Sister John of God and Sister Jeanne de Chantal with Chief Corlo and his companions, St. Ignatius Mission, Flathead Indian Reservation (Jocko Reservation), Montana, late 1880s. Reprinted with permission of the Sisters of Providence Archives, Seattle, Washington.

poration in 1859. In the Articles of Incorporation found in the Corporation Ledger book St. Joseph's role is formalized:

St. Joseph chosen to be the protector of the Sisters of Charity, March 19, 1859. The Corporation of the Sisters of Charity of the House of Providence in the Territory of Washington wishing to testify its confidence in the protection of St. Joseph most humbly request him to be the protector and guardian of all the works, property and affairs connected with it, and declare that it holds him as its good Father and its spiritual President. . . . Made and passed at the House of Providence at Vancouver on the 19th of March 1859, Sister Blandine, Secretary, Sister Joseph of the Sacred Heart, President.[44]

As a consequence, St. Joseph was actively involved in all property decisions. For instance,

St. Joseph chose the property on his feast day as we had asked him to. It had been impossible to get it before without paying a huge price; even then the owner would not sell. Then, a few days later, Mr. Massey just decided to sell. Mother Praxedes and Sister Joseph came and found the place so beautiful and so advantageous that they bought it.[45]

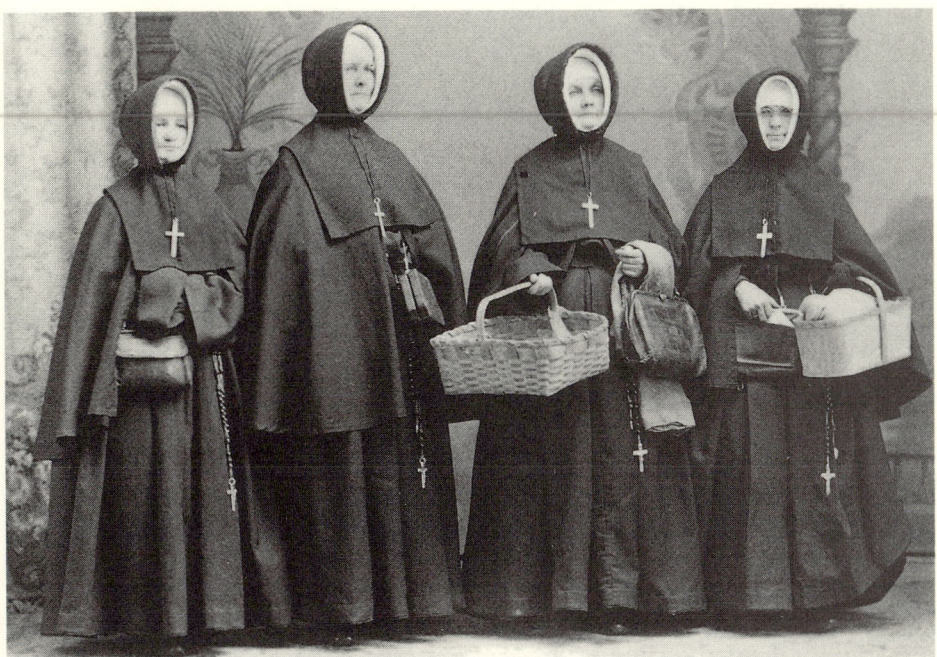

Figure 7. Sisters of Providence dressed to go begging, Montreal, 1900. Reprinted with permission of the Sisters of Providence Archives, Seattle, Washington.

St. Joseph was also relied on — sometimes impatiently — to put food on the table. At one stage, in 1878, the Providence Hospital was in debt for $1,452 and there was only twenty-five cents in the house.

In extreme difficulty one uses extreme measures. After having knelt before the Lord many times, first asking his love and then money, and seemingly getting no money and seeing our need so great, the *Economie* went right to the tabernacle door and knocked three times and continued to knock when she got no answer. "I bring you my purse with the twenty-five cents in it," she said. "I am leaving it here until tomorrow." The next evening she went to get her purse, sure that God had heard her. Then the next day two private patients arrived, one bringing $123 and the other $84 . . . a sufficient sum to satisfy our creditors.[46]

This faith in the miraculous and belief in the real presence of saints was essential for the sisters to sustain their courage and their confidence that they could rise to fulfill God's demands. It also placed their work outside the realm of the ordinary or the individual, and reinforced the view that it was God who was to be honored in their successes. The sisters were only His instruments and remained unworthy of praise or recognition. In fact, Mother Joseph was gently criticized, in a pastoral letter from Canon Alfred Archambeault, their confessor, for not "fostering a calm and perfect confidence in Divine Providence" in her houses. Canon Archambeault had observed much concern with temporal problems, and insufficient faith and confidence among her sisters.[47] He blamed Mother Joseph for this worldly preoccupation and excessive concern with debt. Total faith, then, was clearly something to work on, to perfect in oneself. Its successful inculcation resulted in a freedom from worldly concerns that endowed women with the courage and confidence to succeed in the material world.

Skilled Nurses

For the early sisters, hospital work was central to their mission. *The Traité élémentaire de matière médicale* was published in 1869 as a medical guide for the Sisters of Providence. Translated in 1889 to become the *Materia Medica* and edited by Sister Peter Claver, the text came with glowing testimonials from the medical faculty of McGill University in Montreal. Sister Peter Claver traveled from hospital to hospital throughout the northwest, establishing the dispensaries and training the sisters and nurses.[48] The text provided an extended pharmacy section (plus herbs of North America); it included anatomy and symptomatology, pathology and disease; there was a section on insanity that included mania, monomania, dementia, and idiocy with the nursing treatment listed as "rest of mind, attend to functional derangement."[49] It also included an "Advice to nurses" section that detailed observation of ventilation, light, cleanliness, noise, temperature and warmth, sleep, and diet. It decreed that a nurse should have knowledge of dressings, poultices, fomentations, leeches, cupping, enemas, hypodermic injections, suppositories, gargles, nasal bougies, nasal douches, inhalations, and baths. There was also an extensive dictionary.[50] In all, it was a sophisticated and comprehensive modern text that provided the sisters with information on treatment regimes equal to any available to nurses at the time.

The sisters understood the value of skill and dedication in care of the sick. The Chronicles of Providence Hospital cite the time that none had any rest for four weeks while nursing two patients, a typhoid and a sawmill accident victim, "not leaving them for five minutes alone. The odor from the wounded patient was very bad."[51] Both men survived. In 1885 the same Chronicles regretfully declared that "after eight years of existence, we lost our first case of typhoid fever — and that after only a week's illness."[52] At St. Joseph's, Vancouver, Washington, Sister Mary Faith was said to have "exhausted her strength caring for Mrs. Pulski, who had cancer of the stomach. She was with us for six months. She demanded constant care and later, towards the end, she was delirious day and night."[53]

This is not to overstate the "clinical" dimension to the sisters' nursing. Rather, the point is that there was no division for the sisters between devoted and attentive nursing and evangelical work. These were one and the same. It was actually *through* good nursing that hearts were opened to God and souls on the way to hell were rescued. The Catholic sisters did not avoid direct patient care, and the Sisters of Providence did full "body work" when required. For instance, the Chronicles of Providence Hospital tell of "one paralytic man suffering for ten years . . . [who] became horribly afflicted, full of sores so that no nurse would take care of him. Sister Eugene and Sister Annunciation took full care of him then. Their charity touched him and he asked for instruction and baptism."[54] In the interests of propriety, however, the sisters did employ male nurses for the intimate care of male patients in "so corrupt a country" — as was usual practice in all hospitals at this time.[55]

Thus through their practice and determination sisters became skilled nurses, worked closely with doctors, and were extremely sensitive to anti-Catholic criticism of their hospitals and their nurses. They were openly competitive with other hospitals, county or private Protestant institutions, which they considered very inferior to their own. They relished the opportunity, when it arose, of caring for someone who had opposed them and proudly chronicled many tales of the transformation of former foes into firm friends (with or without conversion).[56] There were, then, strong motivations for them to succeed as nurses, to run efficient hospitals, to work well with good doctors, and to show a world that would have delighted in their failure that they were the best possible nurses.[57] For their part, the sisters too delighted in the failure of opponents and were not above malice — such as when in 1900 the Chronicles of Providence Hospital accused the deaconesses at the competing Methodist Hospital of "going back to the fleshpots of Egypt" at the slightest opportunity![58]

The community's reputation for hospital foundation grew through success. In 1897 Sister Blandine of the Holy Angels wrote to Mother Joseph of the Sacred Heart, putting the case for hospital work very pragmatically:

hospitals are what should be most dear to our hearts, since this is where we can carry out all the works of mercy, whether spiritual or corporeal. For me, this seems to be the useful effort, from all standpoints. It is true that we must act wisely. However, if we do not accept this, others will step in ahead of us, and there will be nothing left for us. We are short of subjects who are familiar with English for our Schools, and our novitiate regularly admits each year enough members who are willing to work in hospitals. This is the Providence for our Western Missions and the best approach to the harvest which lies before us. Other works are decreasing bit by bit, but hospitals are growing day by day.[59]

The best approach to reap the "harvest" that lay before them, the sisters decided, was through prayer, determination, and a realistic appraisal of how best to utilize their increasing recruits (vocations). In a remarkable document, the *Régistre des missions démandées à la Province du Sacre Coeur*, the sisters faithfully recorded all invitations to work and their acceptance or refusal. Although they responded positively to many, most requests were signed off with the phrase: "remercié faute de sujets" (refused due to a lack of sisters). Requests for schools, hospitals, orphanages, and Indian schools were repeatedly refused for this reason.[60]

The invitations were presented in both religious and entrepreneurial terms. For instance, on 5 March 1884 a Jesuit, Father A. Parodi, wrote to the sisters from Ellensburg, Washington. His letter was followed shortly by a second from another Jesuit, Father Kusters. The priests outlined an attractive proposition for the sisters to set up a hospital at a logging camp at nearby Roslyn. The proposition detailed how the coal company dispute had resolved that the men would take care of their own sick and injured and sought to employ "some Sisters of Charity" to take care of their hospital. Single men would pay $1.00 per month and married men $1.50. They would also undertake to provide the sisters with a school for 200 children, plus additional land. They requested five sisters, two for the hospital and three for the school. As an added incentive it was mentioned that there were "many more logging camps and sawmills with whom the same monthly agreement or else ticket system could be made." The sisters had to decline.[61] Another request came in December 1896 from Father William Judge (another Jesuit) in Dawson City, Northwest Territories. He wanted the sisters to come and open a hospital for miners. He urged them to come and to make sure they brought printed tickets (as there were no printing presses in Dawson City). His plea was strengthened by the information that during the previous summer Episcopalians had purchased the supplies to establish a hospital, but had been unable to organize delivery — so the sisters still had a chance to get in first! They declined.[62] A Father Hartleib of Moscow, Idaho began his request with the claim that this offer should override all others. Moscow, he declared, offered everything: two railroads; timber, water, and no canyons; 5,000 people; good Catholic families (some of whom were principal businessmen). The county had agreed to provide a bonus plus pay for county sick, and citizens had promised to also give a bonus to the sisters. They accepted.[63] Having so few sisters made it necessary to pick and choose. Persistence on the part of the priest, good relationships, and the potential for growth were the key indices for the sisters' decisions. They chose well, too; their hospitals lasted.

The sisters' well-thought-out sense of their place in the "marketplace" also led them to take a professional approach to nursing training, something they implemented "for the renown and the growth of the hospital."[64] In 1890 Miss Theresa Cox, a graduate of the training program at Bellevue Hospital, New York, began instructing the sisters at St. Vincent Hospital, Portland, Oregon in new nursing procedures and surgical techniques. She used her first edition textbook of Clara Weeks along with the sisters' own *Materia Medica*, while medical staff taught the sisters in their specialty areas.[65] At the end of twelve months the sisters completed examinations, but no diplomas were awarded as Cox considered them unnecessary for sisters.[66] Sister Andrew was then sent to the Presbyterian Hospital, New York to observe teaching and practice there. She recalled the warmth and kindness shown to her there and returned to establish St. Vincent Hospital's own training school in Portland, Oregon in 1892. Sister Andrew also apparently disagreed with Cox's view on diplomas for sisters and made sure she was awarded her diploma when she became superintendent of nurses in 1890.

The success of the sisters' foundations was linked to their nursing abilities and their preparedness to move with the increasing professional demands of hospital administration and nursing training. However, this is only part of the story. These women in the remote north and southwest required not only administrative ability, nursing skill, and piety, but an adventurous and entrepreneurial spirit.

Beggars and Businesswomen: Adventures in the Wilds

We sat upright in the wagon, with rosary beads in hand; frightened at the howling of the coyotes, wolves and panthers, and by noises of various kinds, real or imaginary, that tended to excite fear. Sister Mary Jesus, alone, was fearless, and would even laugh at our apprehensions. After tying the horses to the wagon, she would spread her blankets on the ground, then say her night prayers, take out her pistols, and placing one of them at each side of her, at a convenient distance, she would lie down and sleep as peacefully as if she were in her bed.[67]

The Wild West was larger than life. Somehow the sisters' communities all seem to have found characters to fill the boots of western legends. In Minnesota a six-foot, 200-pound Sister Amata Mackett toured the cowboy camps and lumberjack mills by train, handcart, ox, or snowshoe to raise revenue for St. Mary's Hospital, conducted by the Benedictine Sisters of St. Joseph.[68] Sister Blandina Segale, Sister of Charity of Cincinnati, heroine of the Santa Fe Trail, was protected by the outlaw Billy the Kid for the care she gave his wounded men. The Sisters of Charity of the Incarnate Word played their own part in the larger-than-life legends of the West with Sister Mary of Jesus Noirry, one of the founding group from Lyons, who went out into the wilds, armed with a brace of pistols, dressed in an oversize man's coat, boots, and straw hat (to disguise her habit). She begged money, provisions, and hay for her horses on begging missions lasting five or six weeks.[69] For her part, Mother Joseph of the Sacred Heart, Sister of Providence, was an accomplished saleswomen and intrepid beggar who faced wolves, bears, and Indians in the mountains of the northwest.

It is difficult not to romanticize such adventures; however, Sister Catherine Mallon, who accompanied Sister Blandina and wrote a journal in order to assist Blandina's recollections, recalled the hardships somewhat bitterly.[70] She admitted many years later that she found it hard to bear the lack of appreciation from new sisters of the difficulties that had been faced by their community's pioneers.[71] Nevertheless, adventure or lonely drudgery, begging was a particular feature of frontier missions. Begging was degrading and humbling, a traditional religious practice of mortification since at least the time of St. Francis of Assisi. It was thus perfect as a spiritual practice to induce humility. The sisters were able to turn a traditional practice, to erase pride and self, into an effective means to raise funds for their work. There was much opportunity for self-abasement, such as the time Sister Stephen from San Antonio, after being spat upon, persisted, "Thank-you sir, that was for me. Now would you give me something for the orphans."[72]

In 1880 one begging mission of the Sisters of Providence even went to Chile (where a sister foundation existed). Despite the trip's difficulties, the sisters returned to the northwest with $10,000.[73] In the two communities under examination here, begging involved long trips into the wilderness, among working men in camps, to cavalry outposts and isolated settlements, searching for the "kind generous Irish heart."[74] The Sisters of Providence sent begging missions over the mountains to the mines of Idaho, Montana, and the Caribou Country in British Columbia. The camps were often a wonderful source of revenue. Mother Joseph commented that she found the miners especially generous:

They [the sisters] were largely rewarded by the excellent reception they encountered from the miners, who were very respectful at all times, and more generous than one would have expected of people who subject themselves to such hard labor and privations to earn a small fortune.[75]

Over the decades of her work in the northwest Mother Joseph personally crossed the northern states many times, living hard and fearless. As in

Texas, begging missions required toughened frontier women. Sisters of Providence journeys involved riding some 400 miles on horseback in infamously wet country.[76] Special waterproof riding habits were made, and watching the travelers undergoing their riding and "sleeping rough" training was the cause of much amusement for those staying at home.[77] Mother Joseph, always the intrepid leader on these dangerous excursions, recorded one brush with an Indian war party:

As we were preparing to decamp, we heard the trampling of horses and saw a troop of Indians in the war paint surround our caravan. When they recognized our pectoral crosses, they immediately gave a sign of friendship and respect, our fears were dispelled. We treated them to a meal, but cringed at their scalping knives which they kept ready to carry off scalps of whatever Americans they would encounter. How happy we were to see them depart peaceably. God be praised.[78]

Business Initiatives

The move from begging to the ticket (*billet*) system, where for two, five, or ten dollars per year the workers bought the right to care at the sisters' hospitals, was an important shift in the commercial relationship between the sisters, their patients, medicine, and business. As we have seen, the sisters were on occasion directly contracted by companies to run small camp hospitals or hospitals in the cities to care for workers. In 1885 a Seattle doctor, Dr. Carmel, set up a small hospital, "luxuriously furnished with Turkish carpets," furniture with marble tops, and so forth, in competition with the sisters at Providence Hospital. This doctor's agents began selling admission tickets for $5 or $10 a year as a form of insurance voucher to individual workers at the many mining and logging camps in the region. These tickets "authorized the purchaser, in case of illness, to come to the hospital free and receive the ordinary and extraordinary care of doctors and nurses, get board and so forth, without any further cost."[79] It was a move that caused the sisters great consternation.

Our opponent is meeting with success with the workmen. We regretfully see ourselves losing this class of workmen, who are usually poor even in this country where wages are high. It is this class of people who are our bread and butter. What to do? They forced us to send out tickets too . . . [but] our opponent has been in the field for four months.[80]

In an effort to hold onto their custom from these sites, the sisters too began to sell tickets that entitled bearers to free care in the hospital with a choice of their own doctor. They were surprised at their own success, able to compete with the doctor even in areas where his custom was firmly established. By 1887 Dr. Carmel's hospital was bankrupt and the sisters' revenue from tickets was $5,700.[81]

In Washington the company whose workers took so many of these tickets was the Port Blakely Mill. This powerful company ran the largest milling operation in the world during this period.[82] Logging, of course, was dangerous work, and it was not possible for men to look after themselves when away from home and family. Under the ticket scheme, the only cost incurred by the company for the health and welfare of its workers was the administrative burden of pay deductions. So useful was the role of tickets in health care that it apparently became customary for companies to deduct the payment from the men's pay with or without their permission — something that put casual workers at a disadvantage. In fact, patients were at times admitted from the logging camps concerned about payment for hospitalization, only to discover that they had been paying health insurance all along.[83] There is no evidence that the sisters colluded with the company managers and pay officers to deduct payment without permission for hospital insurance. However, as the universal health provider for such an enormous and high-risk employer, the beneficiaries of this "compulsory" coverage were clearly the sisters and their acute hospitals.[84]

A further element of significance to the billet system was the provision in the contract for choice of medical practitioner, which promoted the development of private medical practice within the sisters' hospitals without any necessity for medicine to develop or support the institution. Here again the sisters' efforts to stave off financial ruin supported the development and extension of private medical practice in their hospitals.

The tight business management practices of the Sisters of Providence (and the fact that they incorporated as soon as they possibly could) are evident in the records of transactions, property lists, and "Deliberations of the Corporations." All property decisions were carefully minuted and accounting records maintained. Board meetings were conducted, as demanded by the by-laws, and the provincial superior was president of the corporation — only Sisters of Providence were members of the board. Accounting records distinguished between *balance en caisée* (money in hand) and *billets abonnements* (agreements). The latter term included all contracts for patients, whether with logging camps, sawmills, railroads, or counties, and specifications were listed such as whether the agreement included cost of physicians (*salaire et honoraire*).[85]

The well-maintained records, fostered by the need to report all their dealings to Montreal, extended to property registers.[86] The best illustration of this tradition can be found in the book of architectural drawings and land survey documents, *Inventaires des immeubles de la Province du Sacre*

Coeur[87] This document was meticulously executed by Sister Anatolie (evidently a talented draftswoman) in 1919 when she was sent from Montreal to undertake an inventory of all properties. But despite this level of corporate pragmatism, what determined the way the sisters lived and worked, their relation to the surrounding society, and the connections between their various houses was their motherhouse, their training, and their rule.

The Sisters' Bill of Rights: The Rule

The Sisters of Charity of the Incarnate Word, San Antonio

The Sisters of Charity of the Incarnate Word were established as a tertiary or third order community of the Order of the Incarnate Word and Blessed Sacrament. Their rule, what Mary Ewens has referred to as a sisterhood's "Bill of Rights,"[88] was within the Augustinian tradition and was a modified form of the motherhouse's rule to accommodate sisters living an uncloistered life of active work, in regular contact with the laity. This rule had been something of a generic rule for nursing communities since the time of the Hospitallers from the Crusades. When the first group of sisters arrived in Galveston, however, there had barely been time to prepare them for the mission: they had responded swiftly to the yellow fever epidemic then raging and arrived without any written rules.[89] In fact, the three women in the first party had only received six days preparation in Lyons. This defect was remedied in the second group sent to Galveston, in 1866. These women had been rigorously prepared and given strict instructions to make sure the foundation was conducted according to the rule of the Sisters of Charity of the Incarnate Word. It appeared that the concern of the superior in Lyons, Mother Angélique, that the sisters were insufficiently prepared to establish a religious community so far from the motherhouse, was warranted. When the second party arrived in Galveston they found the Sisters of the Incarnate Word wearing four variations of habit or dress.[90]

The simple rule of 1869 referred to the sisters as hospitalers. It made clear provisions for their conduct as religious in the company of the sick, extolling the sisters to "keep a continual watch over themselves."[91] The "great vigilance" required also forbade them from being "employed" nursing in the home. They were, however, allowed to visit the sick in their homes. This rule provided a detailed schedule for prayer and exhortation from first thoughts on rising to invocations to say if awakened in the middle of the night.[92]

A second, more developed rule, devised by Bishop Dubuis in 1872, specified spiritual exercises, specifically mentioned the vows of chastity and obedience, and discussed modesty, elections, and the "life, dress and lodging of the sisters."[93] This rule included issues of dowry (not a requirement), fasting (not allowed), travel by sisters, and detailed instructions for the care of sick and behavior of nurses (they were never to joke with patients of "a different sex," never to "familiarize themselves with doctors").[94] Dubuis falls back on the words of Vincent de Paul, "postponing God for God," in his description of their work and the sisters' relationship to their work, affirming that care of the sick had priority over their daily regimen.[95]

Insight into the spiritual formation of Sisters of the Incarnate Word is offered through the extensive writings of Mother Saint Pierre, community leader from 1872 to 1891. Attention to the rule and to each sister's spiritual formation was a constant theme in her writings. Mother Saint Pierre's awareness of her role as pastoral guide to her foundations and her strong links with the French motherhouse illuminate her letters to both her superiors in Lyons and her "children" in Texas. Correspondence between Lyons and San Antonio remained affectionate and close. The women in Lyons shared the trials and sufferings of the sisters and gave them heart. When Mother Saint Pierre felt overwhelmed by the work, the foreignness, and the responsibility, she would write to Lyons "how we should like to have you with us in these sufferings and struggles."[96] The motherhouse in France was her confidante and spiritual advisor, and for the enclosed Lyons community the Irish, French, and German women of the San Antonio foundation provided a vicarious mission in the world.

One such struggle occurred when the sisters had agreed to supply a group of sisters to help form a community in Chicago. Mother Saint Pierre developed second thoughts at the way the party was being organized. The Polish priest from Chicago had taken a high-handed approach to the endeavor, overruling Mother Saint Pierre's selection of women and then whimsically changing arrangements, demanding sisters of Polish extraction.

It was the rule of the sisters that empowered Mother Saint Pierre to take a dramatic stand against this priest, withdrawing the women until her terms were met. She described her turmoil and difficulty in frank correspondence back to Lyons. Mother Saint Pierre was away in Eagle Pass and was telegraphed that the priest had arrived and had changed his mind again about which sisters he did and did not want.

So praying and asking God to help me, I set out in spite of the danger in case Sr. Assistant might yield to the entreaties and so lose our right to judge which

Sisters are suitable to do the work of God. The train left at 7.40 pm and I travelled all night praying, praying. I arrived home at 6.50 am. The carriages were there to take the Sisters; Sr. Assistant had thought it best to yield to this good father who preferred to take only three sisters rather than four since the fourth was not to his liking. Having comprehended this spirit my Mother's heart suffered from the injustice done to some of my children [Sisters] and my authority as Superior and guardian of the spirit of our community was being sacrificed to caprice. Then I was clearly strengthened by the thought that it was better not to allow the beginning of a house of the Incarnate Word than to allow it to be begun contrary to the principle of universal charity of His adorable heart. Not being able to consult all our sisters and let them know my reasons — for the carriages were there — I called all the sisters in the house and the priest and said to him in their presence, "Father I am angry that you have come so far for our Sisters but, as we understood and believed that you wanted Sisters of the Incarnate Word but instead it is 'such and such a person' you want, we cannot continue with what we promised you. Our sisters will not go." The struggling and the wrangling would take too much to relate here. I was as calm as calmness itself and it was extraordinary. I allowed no excuse, no reasoning. "They are all equally human," I told him. . . .

The good priest then lost his equilibrium; he began to cry like a child. To my own great astonishment, the good God sustained me so strongly that I wasn't even moved. . . . then he yielded, said he was wrong and asked for mercy. . . . The storm was great, my good mother, and the struggle painful but I must say that grace surpassed the pain. I felt myself enlightened and urged on by a surprising firmness to yield to nothing in what seemed to me so evidently contrary to the holy will of God and to the spirit of the Incarnate Word.[97]

For even though the rule of the Sisters of the Incarnate Word of San Antonio had been developed in part by Bishop Dubuis, it had been approved by Lyons, and the sense of connection and continuity with the spiritual tradition of the Order of the Incarnate Word and the Blessed Sacrament was vital to the identity of the order in America. Over the years, the sisters voted to retain their experienced French leaders, despite the dominance of Irish recruits. In fact, the election of the first Irish superior in 1918 spelled the decline of the French connection. The election result was conveyed to the motherhouse in a reassuring tone, and Lyons was consoled about the new superior: "Rev. Mother Mary John is really a true daughter of the Incarnate Word from Lyons. She loves you very much. . . . I am sure she will always remain submissive and affectionate towards you."[98]

Pius X granted papal approbation for formal separation from Lyons in 1910.[99] With this the work of both foundresses, Mother Madeleine and Mother Saint Pierre, was completed. They had led the new foundation from France to the United States, shaping it to the demands of Texas and the southwest, and shaping recruits from many nations, through strict adherence to their inner life sustained by their rule.

SISTERS OF PROVIDENCE: "OUR STRENGTH COMES FROM OUR MOTHERHOUSE"

The rule was the lifeblood of the Sisters of Providence, too. Nonetheless, the sisters appear to have been given some latitude to accommodate the needs of a new country. For instance, Mother Joseph dispensed with the rule of silence at meal times, arguing that frontier life was grim and lonely and the sisters needed to socialize and sustain each other. Montreal reinforced this change in tradition and urged the sisters to use the normally silent meal times to practice English.[100] Emphasis was also placed on never missing meals — to keep their health and spirits strong. Prohibitions on the care of women in labor, too, were somewhat relaxed for missionary hospitals.[101] As a self-conscious missionary community, the Sisters of Providence were sustained in their isolation by the formal connection that their rule maintained with their motherhouse home in Montreal.[102] Their Chronicles express great joy at observing their foundress's day (23 September) in the awareness that all their houses, from Montreal to Chile, were united in this observance. The union of prayer and ritual reinforced their special identity as Sisters of Providence and sustained them in their challenges as foreigners in an anti-Catholic place.[103]

On a less profound but equally powerful level, their vow of obedience to rule and superiors gave the sisters a line of command independent of local clergy. At the same time, Montreal appeared to actively administer the missionary outpost, with frequent visits from their superior general, a steady supply of new recruits, and visits back to Montreal by members of the community. This connection with Montreal, however, could be invoked or not as circumstances dictated. The superior appears to have had a great level of discretionary power. For instance, when the offer to take county patients in Seattle first came to the sisters, they declared it impossible to make a hasty decision as the invitation would have to be considered by Montreal. Furthermore, their immediate superior, Father Prefontaine, was away, so the issue simply could not be resolved under these circumstances. Nonetheless, rather than forsake the offer, the sisters agreed to the deal. Their reasoning justified this independent action thus:

Mother Praxedes, Vicar, had prayers upon prayers said [to extend their mission]. Then one day she placed at the feet of St. Joseph's statue a letter pressuring him to make known the will of God. The next day, February 1877, we received the following telegram:

"Do you wish to take the county patients? Respond immediately." Father Kauten

This unexpected request of the assistant priest put us in a quandary, for we feared the disapproval of the pastor, who was away. But, we thought, this absence in so difficult an occasion was a true act of Providence.[104]

The combination of obedience to their rule and utter faith that they were instruments of God's will was capable, on occasion, of empowering these women to use their initiative and exercise their judgment. Paradoxically, these actions occurred wholly within a framework of submission, obedience, and indifference.

Mother Saint Pierre: "Remain Hidden"

The paradox of power and submission underscores the tension between temporal achievements and the spiritual formation of the sisters as vowed members of a religious community. Mother Saint Pierre counseled Sister Alphonse in February 1889:

Remain hidden, Alphonse. I cannot recommend this as much as I would like to, and beg you to give this spirit to our sisters. It is better that people take us for imbeciles, in no matter what, than to consider us clever and intelligent, agreeable to popular or worldly opinion.[105]

In the nineteenth century the promotion of self was considered anathema in religious life. As members of a religious community the sisters considered that the idea of the "self" belonged to the temporal world and was to be "eradicated" through religious practice, submission, and obedience. Thus the desire to avoid "singularity," or distinction, by women religious was integral to their religious identity and their efforts to achieve spiritual perfection. Despite this emphasis on modesty, humility, and submission, God's work, especially on the frontier, demanded courage, initiative, and resourcefulness. It was never the sisters' intention to build an empire for the themselves; they were agents of God's empire. But despite their need to shun the limelight, God's work deserved illumination. Their institutions were a beacon for Catholicism and they were proud that God had allowed so much to be accomplished through them.

Foundations at the Frontier

In the west the great hardship was that of poverty. The Catholic businesses of successful immigrants in the east and midwest were few and far between, and out west the sisters' work embraced a motley community of miners, immigrant workers in camps, Native Americans, and freed slaves. The opportunities for a well-endowed community were scarce. In the new towns only the local business people and pious congregation members could be approached for alms; therefore the sisters were soon forced to look further afield. Given that railroad work teams and miners had money and, not infrequently, the need for acute hospital care and nursing, the sisters devised an entrepreneurial solution for their cash need. First, they rode among the men, in railroad, mining, and logging camps, begging from the workers. Then they moved to collaboration with industry to provide care for workers. In this way the sisters worked in a contractual relation with mining and railroad companies, setting up hospitals with beds allocated to private companies, and also setting up mobile hospitals at the campsites. Eventually the sisters worked the camps to sell vouchers/tickets/billets, what we could today call insurance vouchers. Buried in the pious language of beggars, the significance of this step from begging donations to purchasing possible services can easily be overlooked. Nonetheless, their entrepreneurial activities, their need to seize anything that worked to keep their foundations alive and growing, meant that in a thoroughly contingent manner the sisters worked to establish a system where the support of a private hospital (even support of the major provider of health care services for an entire city or region) came through insurance subscriptions.

The two communities under discussion in this chapter, the Sisters of the Incarnate Word of San Antonio and the Sisters of Providence, were both motivated by missionary zeal to work in the west of the United States. As foreign women who relied on material and moral support from their far away motherhouses, they also provided a means for women back home to participate vicariously with women at both locations, sharing prayers and offerings, sharing successes and failures at conversion. On the frontier the sisters drew courage from the demand for their nursing skills to move further and further into the commercial realm of company hospitals, nursing contracts, and insurance schemes. These efforts funded their mission, brought them close to lapsed Catholic souls, and gave them the opportunity to inspire Protestants with their piety and self-sacrifice. The sisters knew that their nursing work was the potent brew that could "accomplish so many conversions."

At the same time, however, the sisters had detractors. Against these detractors there was only one defense — the sisters' hospitals had to be better than any others. This meant they had to facilitate modern medicine and provide skilled nursing. It was the combination of these factors: evangelism, financial difficulties, developments in medical and nursing training, and anti-Catholic forces, that led the sisters continually to improve their skills, their services, and their institutions to be leaders in their field. At the same time their religious training made them eschew, in principle, the notion of profession or businesswoman.

In both the Sisters of the Incarnate Word and the Sisters of Providence we find frontier women — intrepid and entrepreneurial. But these classic hallmarks of individualism were achieved through a complex religious shaping that eradicated self and extolled simplicity and group identity. Thus, through an ancient path of religious perfection acted out at the frontier of a foreign land, these women moved with confidence and competence, building institutions and creating health services both for themselves and for their sisters back home.

Chapter 7

Crossing the Confessional Divide
German Catholic and Protestant Nurses

Immigration is a tale of the movement not only of peoples, but of social practices. Religious nursing could be understood as one such social practice, one that many German peoples sought to reestablish in the New World. The German experience brings together a number of critical themes to this study of nursing work by pious women in the nineteenth-century Protestant English-speaking world. First, there is the revival of Catholicism in Catholic regions of Germany in the mid-nineteenth century. Central to the German experience was the establishment of Daughter of Charity motherhouses, and the proliferation of new communities of vowed women dedicated to work among the increasingly desperate poor. This phenomenon corresponded closely with the Irish and French experience, where a multitude of religious communities and lay societies were generated in the flowering of Ultramontane Catholicism.[1]

A second theme is the entry of Protestant women into this territory of active, public work in the community. The German story is critical here because Pastor Theodur Fliedner's Kaiserswerth deaconesses were the first non-Catholic attempt to harness the evangelical energy of women in a public role. The deaconess movement was created by Fliedner (1800–1864) in 1836, as a revival of the biblical female diaconate outlined in Romans 16:1, 2.[2] The deaconesses thus are of immense significance to the opening out of nursing work to Lutheran women, then to various evangelical and Methodist groups, and finally to secular women. The deaconesses are also important for the attention they received from the Protestant world outside Germany. The model not only spread through Scandinavia, but interested great numbers of British women (including Elizabeth Fry and Florence Nightingale) and pastors who subsequently introduced deaconesses to their parishes. But equally significant is the fact that deaconesses were imported directly to the United States by Pastor Fliedner himself in 1849, transplanting the German Lutheran model for a working female diaconate directly into the German community of mid-century Pittsburgh. It is these multiple strands, Protestant,

Catholic, German, and Scandinavian, as they intercept with both the Vincentian Daughters of Charity and the Nightingale reformers that this chapter sets out to explore.

Finally, this chapter discusses particular elements of religious communities of nursing women. Both the Catholic and Protestant German examples appear to share certain characteristics less evident in non-German communities. The role of the pastor is highlighted for German communities, and the independence of the women, perhaps in line with the position of German women more generally, appears circumscribed. A further issue that provides a consistent undercurrent to the work of these women in the United States is the tension between assimilationist moves to integrate immigrant institutions into mainstream American society, and the powerful forces that pulled German communities toward cultural and linguistic distinctiveness.

Religious Revival in Nineteenth-Century Germany

One of the great errors in the everyday understanding of religious nursing is the notion that Catholic nursing represents an unchanging two-thousand-year tradition. The power of such rhetoric is obvious, stamping nursing, charity, and care as Catholic practice. But such a view underplays the achievements and innovations of the nineteenth-century Catholic nurses, and disguises the fact the vital and innovative nursing communities, which it has been argued had such an impact on the modernization and secularization of nursing, were for the most part formed in the nineteenth century.[3]

German Catholicism had been severely battered by the Reformation and its ensuing wars, the subsequent decline of the Holy Roman Empire, the Napoleonic Wars and French occupation, liberation and the Treaty of Vienna (1815) (which broke up Catholic states into minority regions in new Protestant states),[4] and, finally, revolution (1848) and the rise of socialism and liberalism. The net result of this turmoil and devastation in the first half of the nineteenth century was a rise in illegitimacy rates, secularism, and anticlericalism. In the new Germany, bourgeois Catholics joined Masonic lodges and read liberal and left-wing papers, and working class Catholics filled the taverns on Sundays. Those who did come to church commonly formed "tobacco collegia and conversation circles" during the sermon. There were even complaints of congregation members climbing the rafters from the choir gallery or mounting the organ to mock the priest — even assaults on priests were reported.[5]

The revival of Catholicism over the two decades 1850–70 was energized by Swiss and Alsatian priests who, through massive mission gatherings, activated a resurgence of pilgrimages and lay societies or sodalities.[6] This resurgence resulted in a dramatic shift in the social and demographic profile of Rhenish and Westphalian Catholics, so that by 1870 late marriage, low illegitimacy, and high lifetime celibacy rates became the distinguishing features of a generally churchgoing and sober population.

But the successes of Catholic revival were to become the cause of its trials under Chancellor Bismarck. Coupled with the increase in clerical authority over the lives of Catholic Germans was an increase in the political influence of the pulpit — ever the enemy of both Prussian militarism and liberal forces. The dissenting role of the Catholic Church, and its spectacular ability to mobilize masses of Catholics against the Prussian government, resulted in the declaration of open war between church and state under the political program known as Kulturkampf.[7] As relations between church and state deteriorated, Catholic clergy were expelled, church property seized, and Catholic religious communities persecuted.

It was, then, a politically experienced and effectively organized form of Catholicism that traveled in the form of one million immigrants to the United States during the peak decade of German immigration, 1870–80. These immigrants brought with them a deep suspicion of secular government, a cherished sense of the glory of German Catholicism, and a hard-wrought determination to keep that flame alive.[8]

The Sisters of St. Mary: "We Feel Inclined to Cross the Ocean"

Dear Mr. Wegman
The present state of affairs with regard to religious, and convents especially, is so discouraging that we feel inclined to cross the ocean; therefore I would ask you to try to make the acquaintance of some priests, Jesuits or Franciscans if possible and inquire of them whether or not it would be advisable for five sisters who devote themselves to the care of the sick to come to America. We do not want to travel without knowing our destination and, therefore, would ask the guidance of some religious authorities to whose guidance we would gladly submit, without, however, expecting any material aid from them. (Mother Odilia, 1872)[9]

This chapter on German nurses begins with the story of the Sisters of St. Mary of St. Louis. Like millions of immigrants before her (and millions more to come), Mother Odilia Berger wrote in desperation to a sympathetic contact and, receiving an encouraging response, headed off to the New World. It was unusual for German women to go to the United States unchaperoned by brother or father (religious or familial). Throughout the century Irish women immigrated in larger numbers than their brothers, but for Germans the reverse was the case.[10] German women, too, had the added barrier of language, and for this group as obvious religious women there was the additional risk of sectarian harassment. It is worth examining, then, what led Mother Odilia to overcome such obstacles and take a desperate step into the unknown.

Gustave Wegman, a German immigrant to St. Louis, presumably responded to this plea for assistance, because in 1872 Mother Odilia and her four companions arrived in the United States. These women were refugees of the Kulturkampf. But Mother Odilia had been a refugee on many occasions before this most recent and severe spate of persecution, and her peripatetic attempts to establish a community of women are illustrative of both the difficulties of the time and the opportunities for determined women on God's mission in the nineteenth century.

Mother Odilia Berger, founder of the Servants of the Sacred Heart and subsequently of the Sisters of St. Mary of St. Louis, began her religious life when she joined the newly established Congregation of the Poor Franciscans in 1857 in Pirmasenz, Germany. It was an impoverished community. After years of suppression under Napoleon and religious and political upheaval following liberation, the Catholic Church had neither wealth nor community support as the powerful movements of liberalism and socialism seemed to be moving Germany toward complete secularism.[11] In these desperate times, Mother Odilia's novitiate had consisted entirely of begging for her religious community. In pursuit of funds she found herself in Paris in 1864, where she came under the influence of the German-speaking pastor of the area, Vincentian Father Victor Braun. At his urging she established a home for poor German factory women. Unable to do this work under the blessing of her motherhouse in Pirmasenz, she obtained a dispensation to quit the community and began a new community in Paris, the Servants of the Sacred Heart of Jesus.[12] Apparently these women wore a uniform dress and called themselves "sister," but retained their baptismal names.[13] Father Braun wrote the rule for the group, but after two years he accused Mother Odilia of "attempting to destroy the filial respect which the sisters owed to him as their founder" and the community split.[14] Supported by Monseigneur George Darboy, archbishop of Paris, Mother Odilia remained in Paris providing shelter for the working girls.[15] However, the outbreak of hostilities between France and Germany in 1871 meant that all Germans had to leave the area, and Mother Odilia and a companion returned to Elberfeld, in the German Rhineland, where they had to take work in a garment factory in order to survive as itinerant religious woman.

The war, of course, brought casualties, and the women, now known as sisters of the Third Order of St. Francis, soon began to work as nurses to Prussian soldiers at the city Society Hospital in Elberfeld. Following the war, their expanding group nursed smallpox victims in their homes.[16]

Once Germany had been declared victor over France, Bismarck moved to consolidate his power domestically with Kulturkampf. Although Bismarck's expulsion order specifically excluded nursing communities, Mother Odilia's nurses were members of a new order and were therefore banned. Their only possibility for a future as women religious was through emigration.

Mother Odilia, then, was an experienced, committed woman with many years of active work and religious life behind her, with experience in founding communities and dealing with pastors and bishops. She had, however, no formal affiliation or religious training and was therefore not a "religious." Her goals for America were to formalize the establishment and regulation of a religious life for women who nursed the sick.

She was welcomed in Missouri, the home of many Catholic and Protestant Germans. The community was quickly set up, as the Sisters of St. Mary, under a sympathetic German bishop, Monsignor Henry Meuhlsiepen, vicar general for the German-speaking people of St. Louis, and a German pastor, Father William Faerber. For the rest of her life Mother Odilia ensured that all further developments of this community occurred with the German parish boundaries, and so remained under the jurisdiction of German clergy she trusted.

> *Greetings from all your companion Sisters who are continually praying and weeping for you.*
> — *Mother Odilia*

Within the first year of their foundation the sisters worked again as smallpox nurses, and thereafter they nursed during cholera outbreaks. In 1878 they were among those who responded to an appeal for nurses to assist victims of yellow fever in Memphis.[17] The small community sent thirteen of its thirty-one sisters to tend the victims. All the sisters became infected; five died.[18] When the entire group of sisters contracted yellow fever, they were instructed by Sister Mary Mechtildis to have their habits within reach and to put them on when they felt death approaching, for there would be no one to prepare them for burial.[19] It was both a tragic and a glorious public beginning to their work in the United States. German-American women joined the community, and Mother Odilia chose to pattern her order on the rule of Franciscan communities she had been part of in Germany, striving, like all foundresses, to make the novitiate a solid foundation to religious life. Sisters were sent to Cincinnati to a Franciscan community to undergo training, and they returned to establish further novitiates along this model.[20] Mother Odilia personally held conferences (religious training sessions) for her sisters in addition to those given by Father Faerber and Monsignor Meuhlsiepen.[21]

Hospital Foundation

The Sisters of St. Mary were a nursing community, and the need for a hospital was obvious to them from their extensive home nursing work. Nursing the sick poor in unsanitary homes without water, food, or medical help was becoming increasingly unsatisfactory.[22] In 1877 they purchased a property that was to become St. Mary's Infirmary, St. Louis. The hospital patient lists of the 1890s are dominated by American-born patients, followed by Irish- and then German-born. Overall, charity patients represented approximately 50 percent of patients at St. Mary's.[23]

When the smallpox epidemic of 1883 broke out, the city forced patients to use the quarantine hospital. They handed the management of this hospital over to the sisters, who nursed 1400–1500 patients there that year.[24] In 1886 the sisters again nursed at the quarantine hospital, this time during a diphtheria epidemic. In addition to the quarantine work, in 1884 the sisters were called on by the chief surgeon of the Missouri Pacific Railroad, German countryman Dr. W. B. Outten, to take charge of a large railroad hospital. In 1885 they were invited by the same company to run its hospital in Sedalia.

Following their success in managing their own institutions, St. Mary's in St. Louis (1877), St. Joseph's in St. Charles (1887), St. Mary's in Chillicothe (1888), the Quarantine Hospital in St. Louis, and railroad hospitals in St. Louis and Sedalia (all in Missouri), the Sisters of St. Mary were invited to replace Franciscan sisters from Illinois and take over nursing at the German Hospital in Kansas City, Missouri.[25] This hospital was nonsectarian, with strict decrees on the role of ministers and priests. Nonetheless, the board's inability to secure skilled and useful secular nurses led them to contract with the Catholic Sisters of St. Mary until 1900. At this time the board felt confident that it would be possible to staff the hospital with trained nurses and conduct a training school. The sisters were then persuaded to open their own hospital in Kansas City, Missouri.[26]

The Sisters of St. Mary continued to operate hospitals, independently and under contract. Members of this community developed their skills in a variety of hospital contexts. For instance, Sister Clara Harbers was superior of the motherhouse, St. Mary's Convent, St. Louis, 1876–77; superior at St. Mary's Infirmary, St. Louis, 1877–78, 1880–82; superior at Quarantine Hospital, St. Louis, 1883–85; superior at Missouri Kansas, Texas Railroad Hospital at Sedalia; superior at St. Joseph's Hospital, St. Charles, 1890–94; and superior at St. Mary's Home, St. Louis.[27]

Over the last decade of the nineteenth century and into the twentieth, new developments in hospital management, changes in the role of medicine, and the professionalization of nursing were shaping hospitals throughout the United States. As was the norm for Catholic hospitals, the Sisters of St. Mary conducted their hospital business as an in-house affair, and the sisters were signatories of their original articles of incorporation.[28] The Sisters comprised the total membership of their hospital boards, and the role of medicine was that of welcome visitor. Nonetheless, the impression given by the annual reports, anniversary publications, and pamphlets emphasized the role of medical practitioners within the hospital and the "guiding hand" they gave to the sisters to assist them to adapt to the changing demands of the American health care system.[29] In fact, it was not until the period following World War I, in anticipation of the hospital standards movement, that a more professional approach to administration, patient records, and formal collation of patient histories and review of medical staff qualifications became usual practice.[30]

Throughout the first decades of the twentieth century, the Sisters of St. Mary were sustained by recruits from Germany. The amount of English spoken within the community was limited; evidence of a concerted effort to become American and to speak English, as occurred with the Sisters of Providence in Washington and the Sisters of the Incarnate Word in San Antonio, does not appear until the 1920s, when the prayer book was translated into English and the non-American sisters naturalized.[31] In fact the efforts to improve the English of new recruits seem paltry—one new word a day was a goal for sisters in 1903.[32]

Second, the general level of education for German women was something of a limitation for a community needing to professionalize its qualifications. In 1909 the State Licensure Board Committee contacted the superior of St. Mary's, Kansas City, Missouri, Sister Mary Eulalia Steinkrueger, and asked her to obtain registration papers for her sister nurses.[33] They commenced intensive training with the hospital doctors, and eventually four sisters received diplomas, while others went to St. Louis to attend the Sisters of St. Mary training school.[34]

The registration movement and the professionalization of nursing proved a challenge for the Sisters of St. Mary in those first decades of the twentieth century. The nurse-sisters at St. Mary's Hospital, St. Louis had been undertaking a course of lectures from medical staff and studying nursing textbooks in English since 1900, but this did not translate to diplomas or licensure. The first formal sister training school opened in 1907, but the sister diplomates were not awarded licensure until 1917. The minimum of one year of high school demanded by the Missouri State Board was simply too high for the German women, who frequently lacked any high school education and whose religious community's "poverty made it impossible to pay salaries for instructors and by the same token prevented the sisters from taking adequate time for study."[35] Until 1917 the sisters were forced to obtain licensure circuitously—sisters registered in Wisconsin, a less arduous proposition, then gained Missouri licensure through reciprocal recognition agreements.

German-American Rift[36]

Mother Odilia died in 1880, soon after ecclesiastical approval for the community had been received and she was finally able to make her vows.[37] The priest Mother Odilia trusted so much, Father Faerber, had enormous input in the formation of this community, its title, and the development of its rule, and considered himself their founder, giving himself this title on all their correspondence. It was through him that the Immaculate Virgin asked the community to adopt the title "Sisters of St. Mary," and through him that Mother Odilia, on her deathbed, appointed a successor, and no vote was taken to elect a superior to replace her (as the rule dictated).[38] Her choice was unpopular; twenty-nine-year-old Mother Seraphia Schloctemeyer was considered tyrannical and unpredictable, dismissing sisters "right and left."[39] In her leadership of the community she relied heavily on the advice of the Father Faerber, who continually modified the rule to prepare it for papal approbation, apparently little concerned with maintaining its Franciscan nature.[40] In fact, after Mother Odilia's death Father Faerber began to call himself "Superior and rector of the Order."[41] In 1897 Mother Seraphia went to Germany to recruit women. She returned with thirty women and immediately reordered the community in a way that privileged German over American-born women. This was the cause of great unhappiness to the individuals who were now deposed as novice mistress and from other responsible posts in the community. A group of American-German and American-Irish women left the Sisters of St. Mary and, with approval from their bishop, non-German Bishop Burke, established themselves as the Sisters of St. Francis.[42]

Sisters of St. Francis: In Search of the "Free Spirit of Franciscanism"

Sister Augustine Giesen assumed the direction of this new community, which dedicated itself to the Franciscan direction of their foundress, Mother Odilia. The rebel sisters felt that this Franciscan spiritual orientation had suffered in the Sisters of St. Mary under the new superior, and under the "undue influence and control by spiritual director Father Faerber," had lost "the free spirit of Franciscanism."[43] They accepted an invitation to teach in Maryville, Missouri. This proved a challenge for a group of nurses, and they were assisted by a better educated and experienced Benedictine sister until they could organize teacher training for a new recruit.[44] However, nursing remained their central mission and skill. Sister Augustine had spent nine years as the surgery nurse at Sisters of St. Mary hospitals, including two years as superior of the Missouri Pacific Hospital in Sedalia, and Sister Salesia had been superior at St. Mary's Hospital, Chillicothe.[45] Bringing their previous experience to bear, they were successful in securing more railroad hospital contracts.[46]

The Sisters of St. Francis embraced English from the outset.[47] In contrast to the reticence of the Sisters of St. Mary in training and nursing professionalization, the Sisters of St. Francis began a nursing school at St. Anthony's, Oklahoma City. Opened for both sisters and lay women in 1908, in 1912 it became the first school of nursing to be accredited by the State of Oklahoma.[48]

For the German community in North America, the nursing work of such sisterhoods was valued across sectarian lines, with the surprising phenomenon of Catholic sisters nursing in non-Catholic German hospitals, as at the Kansas City German Hospital.

The Germans were the most numerous non-English-speaking immigrant group, and whereas Polish and Italian immigrants were virtually all Catholic, and the Scandinavians all Lutheran (or at least Protestant), the German community was distinctive in that it included both Catholics and Protestants. Most notably, the German community was also distinctive in that it had developed a Protestant equivalent to the Catholic sisterhoods. These women, the deaconesses, were to have a major impact upon the development of nursing and hospitals in the United States, and on the secularization and professionalization of nursing as a whole.

Kaiserswerth: The Impetus Behind the Deaconess Movement

The circumstances in Germany that stimulated the development and revitalization of Catholic communities of women to work among the needy also stirred the Protestant German community. The conventional story is that the Kaiserswerth deaconesses, formed in 1836, sprang from the observations of war of Pastor Fliedner during his travels. Some thirty years before the Crimean War, Fliedner was struck by the lack of a Protestant equivalent to the Sisters of Charity, and he was moved by the spontaneous work of village women to help the injured following battle.[49] It is interesting this frequently quoted background to the establishment of Kaiserswerth conspicuously avoids the key impetus.[50] This area of Germany was, as we have seen, to be the site of the Catholic rebirth in the 1850s. Under the French, the Daughters of Charity model was introduced to Germany, and sisters established a motherhouse and a hospital in Strasbourg in Alsace.[51] According to Prelinger, the "spirit that sustained the Protestant female diaconate was . . . designed to contain the

Catholic renascence in the Rhine Province."[52] In fact, the Sisters of Charity revival so concerned Fliedner that he complained to the English philanthropist, Elizabeth Fry, that the Sisters of Charity "flood everywhere . . . in Protestant countries and hospitals . . . where they endeavor artfully to place their church in the best possible light to make proselytes of the sick and poor."[53]

It was at this time that the notion of a social apostolate became an influential reform movement within Lutheranism. The "Inner Mission" movement, under the leadership of Johann Henrich Winchern (1808–81), addressed the moral and social responsibilities of Protestants to prevent the "dechristianization" of Germany. The Denkschrift statement of 1849, in response to the Communist Manifesto, was a call for evangelism and social action in the cities and towns of Germany.[54] The deaconess movement was one response to this call. It formed part of a concerted program of social reform among Lutherans that countered socialist and liberal criticisms of Christian apathy. It matched the energies of evangelical Christians in Britain and Ireland, North America, and Australia who in the nineteenth century worked tirelessly in philanthropy and social reform.

Theodur Fliedner was an impassioned visionary. He rejected what he considered to be the intellectualism and secularity of established Lutheranism. As an evangelical he sought to affirm the spirit and sense of God's immediacy in Christian life. He sought a simplicity and a powerful sense of service and compassion. His little parish at Kaiserswerth was a Protestant outpost in a Catholic part of Germany. When he took up this impoverished parish as a young man, he had only thirty families to care for. But he became committed to the parish, subsequently declining more prosperous appointments. Early in his ministry it appeared that the parish would fail through lack of funds. Fliedner traveled Protestant Germany, Switzerland, the Netherlands, and Britain, successfully raising ample resources for its rescue. On these travels he observed many social reform movements (including Anabaptist deaconesses in the Netherlands); he was determined to implement these programs in Kaiserswerth and to trust in Providence that they would succeed.

Fliedner's prison work, influenced by Quaker Elizabeth Fry's work in England, was the first prison visiting mission in Germany. Fliedner persuaded the local priest also to visit the prison and conduct services for Catholic prisoners, while Fliedner conducted the services for Lutherans.[55] In fact, in many areas his social mission drove him to ecumenical acts. For instance, the first doctor whose charitable services he obtained for the Kaiserswerth hospital was a Catholic. Coupled with his radical scheme to form religious communities of deaconesses, it is perhaps unsurprising that Fliedner's opponents accused him of championing Catholicism instead of Lutheranism.[56]

There were certainly elements of the deaconess model that were recognizable as Catholic in origin. The term "sister" was used for the deaconesses, and it remained the generic German title for nurse into the twentieth century. The deaconess institute revolved around its motherhouse (*Mutterhaus*), where all recruitment and training of women took place. The motherhouse model continued to be a highly efficient means to regulate recruits, respond to demands, and coordinate operations. Moreover, Fliedner understood that if women were to forgo marriage and family they needed a supportive community. Even more pragmatically, the women needed to be looked after once they became too old to work. The motherhouse achieved these goals for Catholic sisters: training, organizational efficiency, security, and companionship; they were no less essential for deaconesses. The motherhouse was under the direction of the pastor, Fliedner, and the sister superior (*Frau Oberin*). The novice mistress or training sister was the *Probemeisterin*. Under her guidance new deaconesses received twelve months training in Scripture, theology, and nursing. After this year of study the title of sister was conferred and the distinctive deaconess dress assumed. After several years of probation a consecration service to the calling of deaconess took place.[57] Not surprisingly, Pastor Fliedner was conscious to distance his deaconesses from nuns. The links with the Vincentian model were carefully downplayed and the sisters adopted the dress and demeanor of Protestant widows of the Rhineland. Fliedner banned the use of black, preferring a nonecclesiastical blue dress for deaconesses.[58]

It is important to acknowledge that Fliedner was not the only one to call for Protestant Sisters of Charity. In fact, there had been several influential moves in this direction, again largely stimulated by the success of the French Daughters of Charity and their many Catholic imitators.[59] Amalie Sieveking, founder of the Female Association for the Care of the Poor and the Sick, produced another way to harness German female energies in a social apostolate. In fact, Sieveking rejected Fliedner's invitation to lead the first community of women at Kaiserswerth. She disliked both the Catholic framework of the deaconesses and Fliedner's superintendence.[60] But it was Fliedner who, like Vincent de Paul, possessed the abundant energy and simple faith that were able to overcome resistance to the idea, and who finally succeeded in having the female diaconate formally recognized by the Lutheran Synod and adopted by the different branches of Lutheranism.[61] He was also successful in gaining the royal family as enthusiastic sponsors of the deaconesses, and Kaiser Friedrich Wilhelm IV opened the Bethany Institute in Berlin.[62] This official patronage was critical in the rapid development of the movement in Germany.

The rest of Protestant Europe watched closely. In Scandinavia Lutheranism was the official religion, and the deaconess model was able to function on a path parallel to that of the Catholic sisterhoods in Catholic countries. For instance, the official endorsement of the deaconess sisterhood allowed for the successful reform of public institutions that were dominated by Lutheran board members. The figures are quite staggering. By 1884 there were deaconess houses in Germany, France, Switzerland, and Scandinavia. Fifty years after the foundation of Kaiserswerth, by 1884, there were 60 houses with a total of nearly 6000 deaconesses.[63] Throughout Lutheran Europe, hospitals run by deaconesses became organized and respectable institutions. They were places where medicine was safely practiced and all care given by trained women.

The Kaiserswerth experiment encompassed the Protestant social apostolate among the sick, elderly, those in prison, and so forth, with proven successful methods for training and organizing women.[64] Within the space of a few decades, the deaconess model had spread throughout Germany and Protestant Europe, matching the rapidity and energy that characterized the emergence of secular nursing in Britain, North America, and Australia. Moreover, the impact of the model was not confined to Europe. For the German and Scandinavian immigrants to the United States, this experience of deaconesses was of prime importance when these communities came to establish hospitals in the New World.

Deaconesses in America

> *Question 3: What are some of the necessary conditions for entering Deaconess Work?*
> *Answer: A clear experience of salvation, good physical health, normal and healthy intelligence, the acquiescence of one's parents and the firm determination to give oneself unreservedly to this noble calling.*[65]

The first deaconesses in the United States were imported by Pastor William Passavant to Pittsburgh. Following a tour of Germany, Pastor Passavant was inspired by the visionary work of Pastor Fliedner. Passavant could immediately see the great need for deaconess hospitals in the industrial cities of America. He appealed directly to Fliedner, who finally responded in 1849 by personally accompanying four deaconesses to the United States. The deaconess tradition in the United States thus directly connects with the German tradition and Fliedner himself. But, this first attempt to establish the tradition in North America was not a great success. For, although the hospital was provided for the deaconesses in its entirety, by 1854 three-quarters of the German recruits had left to settle in America or returned home to Germany. Even more critically, their numbers were not sustained by American recruits. In the thirty-five years between 1849 and 1884 there were only sixteen candidates.[66]

Some decades later, in the 1870s, the board of the German Hospital, Philadelphia, which was comprised of German citizens, including three Lutheran pastors, supported its president John Lankenau in his attempt again to establish deaconesses in the United States. Lankenau appealed directly to a group of deaconesses unconnected with Fliedner and Kaiserswerth, and in 1884 secured seven deaconesses under the direction of Oberin Sister Marie Kruger, from Westphalia.[67] Established in one of the key centers of American Lutheranism and stoutly supported by the wealthiest German in Philadelphia, the Philadelphia motherhouse was able to consolidate its position and finally establish an American deaconess movement.[68]

The deaconess model had enthusiastic proponents in nearly all branches of Protestantism. In Protestant Europe, England, Australia, and North America, Anglican, Methodist, and various evangelical groupings set up deaconess movements. Within the deaconess model there were and are many variations, and nursing was not the main activity of all deaconess groups. Lutheran deaconesses in the nineteenth century were called "sister" and were consecrated to work until marriage. This freedom to marry was the key distinction between deaconesses and Catholic and Anglican (Episcopalian) sisters.[69] English-speaking Methodist deaconesses did not use the term "sister" (while German Methodists did), and by the twentieth century were able to marry and continue their role as deaconesses.[70] In the United States it appears that nursing was the core activity of most nineteenth-century deaconesses, and most deaconess training involved some degree of practical nursing training.[71]

Philadelphia: The Center of the American Deaconess Movement

The Lutheran deaconesses in Philadelphia had been imported to the United States to assume control of the German Hospital. This entailed a difficult transition for the existing staff — particularly the medical staff. It is clear from the statements made by Lankenau to the hospital board that the deaconesses experienced marked difficulties in the handover of the hospital to their care, difficulties that stemmed from a lack of cooperation from medical staff. Lankenau moved to consolidate the position of the deaconesses, arguing strongly to the board that it was the deaconesses who were the experts. Both Lankenau and German consul and fellow board member Charles H. Meyer placed papers before the board to resolve the matter formally.[72] According to Meyer,

They [the deaconesses] did not come to learn from us the best modes of governing a hospital, ..but they came to us as TEACHERS, to give us the benefit of their experience. To LEARN, of course, our language and customs, in order to adapt their knowledge to American circumstances. (emphasis in original)[73]

Lankenau, for his part, moved to have the authority of the Oberin (superior of the motherhouse) confirmed within the administrative structures of the hospital, and he formalized her role as hospital head. The system of resident medical officers was abolished, and two resident physicians subordinate to the Oberin were appointed. This radical change, Meyer argued, effectively "put us in condition to dispense entirely with the Medical Board of Visiting Physicians, if these gentlemen could not be brought to give their consent to the changes proposed."[74] The Oberin was to "be looked upon as executive head of the hospital and household. All admissions and discharges of patients, or permits for temporary absence must pass through her hands."

Yet despite this strong support from the board the deaconesses did not have board representation, nor did they have any public face for those outside the hospital. In fact, the 1895 Annual Report of the German Hospital does not mention the deaconesses until page twenty-nine, and then only for one paragraph.[75] The public face of the hospital deemphasized the role and importance of the deaconesses, and focused instead on the largesse of Lankenau and the board prestige.[76]

The subordinate position of the deaconesses within their own organizational structure was underlined by the fact that the formal agreement between the German Hospital of Philadelphia and the Mary Drexel Home and Philadelphia Motherhouse of Deaconesses, in March 1899, was signed by John Lankenau as president of the German Hospital and Lankenau again as president of the Mary Drexel Home and motherhouse.[77] Frederick Wischan and Hugo Grahn were cosignatories as secretaries of the respective institutions; no deaconess signatures were required.[78]

With the establishment of the motherhouse in the United States, new recruits were eventually forthcoming from the local population. Moreover, the motherhouse served as a critical center for the training of non-German Lutheran women to establish deaconess movements within the Swedish, Norwegian, and Danish communities. However, numbers were still sustained by German imports, and the attrition rate to marriage remained high. Pastor Wilhelm Lowe, who had supplied German deaconesses to Milwaukee in the 1890s, eventually refused any further requests, claiming that he was "tired of providing wives for American pastors!"[79] The German character of the Philadelphia motherhouse was maintained in all training, correspondence, and administration. It was not until the first decade of the twentieth century that debate ensued over whether the German identity of the motherhouse interfered with the success

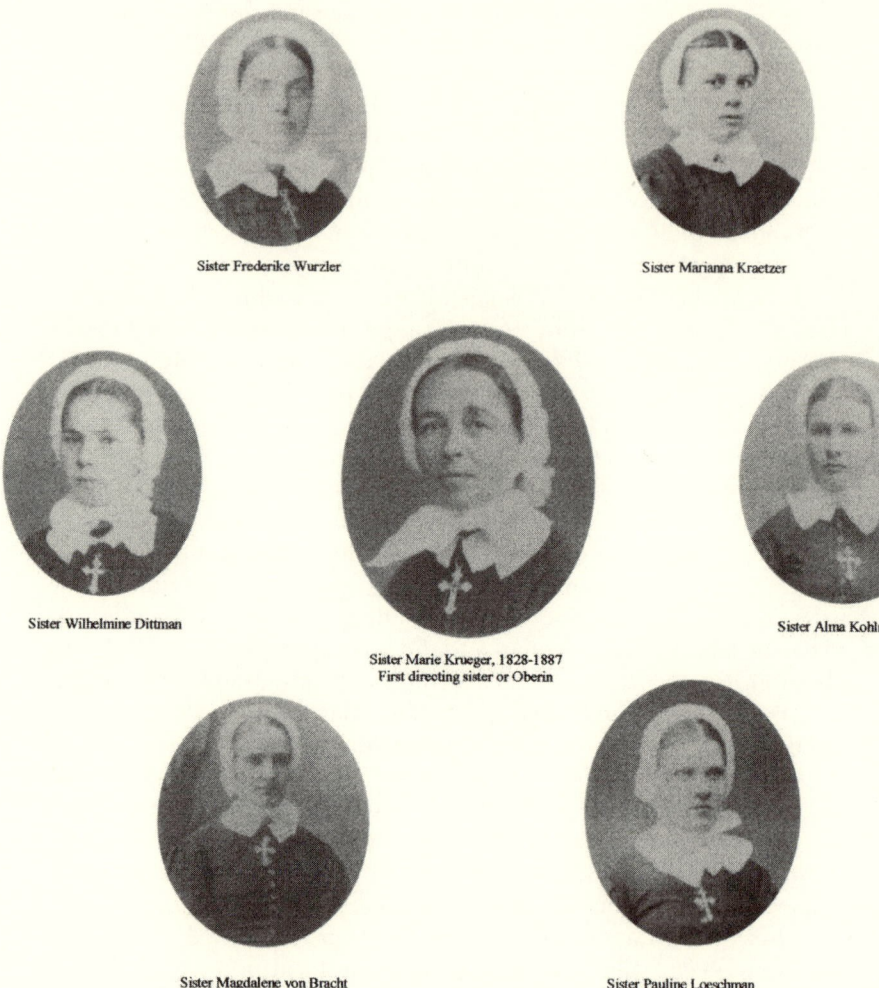

Sister Frederike Wurzler

Sister Marianna Kraetzer

Sister Wilhelmine Dittman

Sister Marie Krueger, 1828-1887
First directing sister or Oberin

Sister Alma Kohlmann

Sister Magdalene von Bracht

Sister Pauline Loeschman

Figure 8. The original seven Lutheran deaconesses to Philadelphia: Sister Marie Krueger (1828–87), first directing sister (*Oberin*); Sister Frederike Wurzler (1846–87); Sister Marianna Kraetzer (1850–1924); Sister Alma Kohlmann (1859–92); Sister Pauline Loeschman (1861–?); Sister Magdalene von Bracht (1850–1941); Sister Wilhelmine Dittman (1849–1922). Reprinted with permission of the Deaconess Community, Evangelical Lutheran Church of America, Gladwyne, Pennsylvania.

of the American mission. The hospital changed its name from the German Hospital to the Lankenau Hospital in 1917, but it was not until 1919 that motherhouse meeting minutes began to appear in English.[80]

German Methodist Deaconesses

The Methodist revivals of the late nineteenth century "saved" many throughout the country. In the Midwest, so many Germans were saved that they established their own tradition within Methodism, creating parishes and institutions for German immigrants and their children, mounting overseas missions, and even evangelizing back to Germany.[81] The complex history of American Methodism led to divisions between the English-speaking (white) church, the African-American church, and the German-speaking church.[82] In 1873 Methodists proposed the opening of deaconess institutes at their Conference in Scaffenhausen, Switzerland.[83] In 1887 Isabella Thoburn, sister of Bishop Thoburn of Chicago, began Methodist deaconess work in the United States.

One influential deaconess movement in the Methodist tradition was centered in Cincinnati.[84] In 1888 the Elizabeth Gamble Deaconess Home Association and Christ Hospital were established in Cincinnati by English- and German-speaking Methodist deaconesses. In 1896 brother and sister Christian and Louise Golder founded the motherhouse of the Central German Conference, and Christian's wife, Ida Golder, commenced the Bethesda Society which began the Bethesda Hospital.

The Cincinnati Methodist deaconesses were immigrant women or daughters of immigrants. The applications for admission were for the most part in German, and the few English-speaking inquiries requested information on the level of German literacy necessary for deaconess training.[85] These were common, working women, converted during revival meetings and filled with evangelical conviction. The application process required the women to express their call from God and their experience of salvation. As working women, domestic servants, seamstresses, and so forth, becoming "set apart" as a deaconess allowed them the financial freedom and security to perform good work.[86] For instance, in her application Miss Bay laments,

Dear Sister Golder
I feel Jesus has called me to do this work for I love to care for the sick. I was converted last October, I sew from 7 to six every day (no time for parish work). I am a German but all the knowledge of the language I have learned at Sunday School and Church. I long to be able to do God's work.[87]

It was only in the German Methodist community that the motherhouse structure was established. Christian Golder concurred with Fliedner, arguing that the aim of the motherhouse was to provide education, training, protection, a home, and care in sickness and old age. Fliedner saw that neither Church Board nor high salaries would satisfy a woman's longing and need for a protecting home and its fellowship. The motherhouse, in large measure, replaced the parental home in the life of a deaconess.[88]

Clearly for German Protestants the risk of the "cloister" was less than that of female autonomy. Despite the very high profile of Miss Golder, the deaconesses at the Bethesda Hospital in Cincinnati held what appears to have been a relatively minor role in hospital management with very little power of admission and review. Pastors were directors of key committees, including the deaconess ruling committee.[89] The Charter des Mutterhauses (13 April 1896) and Articles of Incorporation were signed by eleven members of the founding board, all men.[90] Moreover, hospital management roles were carved out clearly between the board and medical staff.[91] In this model, the deaconesses supplied an effective, respectable, and trained workforce of humble women for the German community.

The Limits of the Movement

The limits of a German movement on American soil were evident in the numbers of recruits. By 1962 the Lutheran Church had produced 515 deaconesses, of whom 108 had left the sisterhood and 223 had died in service.[92] American women obviously had a great many more options than their European counterparts, not the least of these the greater number of German male than female settlers in the New World. Given the commitment to the sanctity of marriage that is central to Lutheranism, it is not surprising that the critical mass of women was simply not available in the German-American community. Addressing the low numbers of deaconess recruits, the Lutheran conference decided that America was not fertile soil for this calling. With clearheaded regret, the conference reported that, aside from an American desire for independence, the lure of marriage (particularly to a pastor), and the rising status of nursing generally, American Lutheran women (and their parents) were simply not drawn to the unpaid working life of a *hausfrau* that was the core of deaconess work.[93]

Northern European Deaconesses

As immigration patterns shifted by the late century, different newcomers began to outnumber the Irish Catholic immigrants of the previous decades. Norwegian, Swedish, and Danish Lutheran communities all established deaconess houses and hospitals, serving their communities in their own language. There was an interplay of training and expertise as deaconesses were sent to the Philadelphia motherhouse for training, then perhaps back to Denmark or Sweden for further training. This was the case with the Omaha deaconesses founded by yet another charismatic and determined pastor. Pastor Erik Fogelstrom, evangelical Swedish pastor, devoted himself in 1879 to the hard and unreceptive territory of Nebraska, just as Fliedner had to the backwater of Kaiserswerth.[94] Inspired by the Swedish deaconess Elsa Borg's mission at Hvita Bergen, Fogelstrom founded the Immanuel Deaconess Institute, in the belief that the female diaconate represented God's answer to American corruption, selfishness, and profanity.[95] The Immanuel Deaconess Institute at Omaha began by sending one woman to the Philadelphia motherhouse for training, followed by two years of training in Sweden at Sigtuna, the home of the Swedish diaconate.[96] In 1889 four more women were sent to Pennsylvania for training; they returned in 1890 to open the new Immanuel Hospital.[97] The board of trustees was made up of American and Swedish men, but there was conflict. Finally, in 1894, in an effort to bolster the support of the Swedish community for the hospital, a new board was established comprised fully of Swedes, including two women — Sister Bothilda and Mrs. Helin.[98]

Fogelstrom was concerned that the Catholics monopolized charitable institutions — where he complained that he was unable to visit his parishioners or even, on occasion, to get them admitted. But of more serious concern to Fogelström was the way Catholics had effectively grasped the evangelical opportunities afforded by acts of mercy and left Protestants so far behind. Note Fogelstrom's admiration for the economy of the sisters in the following passage:

The Catholics are systematically doing great work among the masses. In their institutions money goes far and does so much good by reason of their personal sacrifice of labor in connection with their expenditure of money. The Catholic sisters train the children and the young; they nurse and care for the sick and unfortunate. We do not blame them for doing all they can, but we fear, if they only are to do this work, there is nothing that can prevent this great republic from eventually coming more and more under the influence of Rome.

But what are the Protestants doing? They are doing a great missionary work both home and abroad. They spend large sums of money in building all kinds of state institutions of so-called mercy and charity. Great efforts are made to relieve the sick, the poor and the suffering, but very little thoroughly organized and self-sacrificing work like that of the Catholics is done by the Protestants in America — perhaps with the exception of the Salvation Army.[99]

To Fogelstrom it was the conflation of evangelical self-sacrifice and the economy and efficiency of administration of the sisterhoods that was such an effective agent of Catholicism. Boards of good men and wealthy philanthropists simply could not deliver the same returns as a group of determined, efficient, and altruistic women. It was this possibility that he opened up to Swedish Lutheran women, and he was convinced it would bring salvation to America and save the Christian cause. Fogelstrom is distinctive in that his ideas on the value of deaconesses hinge on their evangelistic power. Although Fliedner observed that this was a feature of the Sisters of Charity, and hence that Protestants needed to match the efforts as they were making "proselytes of the sick," his deaconesses' role was less evangelistic.[100] He argued that it was important for a Christian society to do this work, and who better to do it than women. The women worked among the sick, took care of orphans, assisted the pastor with parish work and prison work. But it was always an adjunct role — bearing witness and serving God.[101] Fogelstrom, on the other hand, expressed views far more in line with Vincent de Paul's original mission for the Daughters of Charity. For both Vincent de Paul and Fogelstrom, the women were a remedy for a social and spiritual malaise. By answering God's call their work was in itself something that brought God to the hearts of those they cared for.[102]

Germanic Identity and Female Piety

The conservatism of both Catholic and Lutheran Germans in response to growing liberalism, socialism, and secularism in Germany was the backdrop for the emergence of sisterhoods — Protestant and Catholic. In America, the ties of language and community and the drive for preservation and continuity were equally strong on both sides of the confessional divide. A shared commitment to German religious traditions and social organizations made the confessional issues to some extent subordinate to cultural issues.

The forces that resulted in 3.4 million Germans settling in the United States in the nineteenth century are complex and varied. For instance, the Missouri Synod, the center of Lutheran orthodoxy in the United States, was established when a group of High Lutheran clergy, appalled at what they deemed to be increasing heresy and liberalism in Germany, set forth in 1839 to establish a home for the true faith.[103] Founded in 1847, it was the spiritual and cultural home of millions of German Lutheran settlers in the mid- and far west. For these devout immigrants their cultural and linguistic identity was inextricably linked with their religious expression. Luther's divinely inspired writings were in German; these, it was felt, could not be translated. Theirs was a German religion, their prayers, liturgy, and, of course, sermons were all in German. It was a close knit though geographically dispersed community. Interaction with outsiders, even other German Lutherans, was actively discouraged. Not until well into the twentieth century did this group begin the slow process of translating their religion into English.[104]

The Missouri Synod did not promote the role of deaconesses or support large public institutions such as hospitals to any great extent in the nineteenth century. Theirs was a religion of the patriarchal home, and Christian marriage the goal for women.[105] Moreover, the Missouri Synod predated wide acceptance in Germany of the female diaconate and Pastor Fliedner's innovations in Kaiserswerth.[106] So for this group of Lutherans the woman's role in the care of the sick was an extension of her domestic and community role, and something to be undertaken informally. Moreover, for rural Lutherans, the epidemics and public health disasters that stimulated the rise of religious and public philanthropy were less significant. Nonetheless, the Missouri Synod did eventually embrace the deaconess movement, and women were given an active and outward role in their community in 1919.[107]

The Missouri Synod Lutherans exemplify the distinctiveness of the German immigration experience. In one sense they represented a quintessential American impulse — the pursuit of religious freedom and community autonomy — yet at the same time their linguistic distinctiveness and their hard won sense of separateness placed them as outsiders to American society. This sense of community, interestingly, brought them into coalition with Catholic Germans to fight state proposals to ban foreign language schools.[108]

A sense of cultural homogeneity among German immigrants can also be illustrated by the story of the North and South Dakota Germans, Catholic and Protestant, who came from the Odessa region of Russia. This community has an extraordinary history of dislocation. Displaced by Napoleon's armies at the beginning of the nineteenth century, entire villages moved intact as colonists to the Russian territories around the Black Sea. Language and religion remained stable and central to their lives as they prospered in their transplanted German communities. In the 1870s, when the Russian Army began to conscript their men, whole communities began the process of transplanting their villages to the wild plains of Dakota, Kansas, Nebraska, and Canada.[109] For over a century these Germans had been anchored by the solidity of culture and language. As rural communities they had neither the financial resources nor the surplus labor that allowed for institution building (such as hospital formation) during the nineteenth century. But again by the early twentieth century it was German models of health care that they turned to when the need became apparent and hospital building began.[110]

But, of course, for the many millions of Germans who flooded into the United States it was a case not of transplantation but of displacement. The instability of Germany and the European wars and blockades meant disaster for the German economy, especially manufacturing. In addition to the migrations of rural Germans to the American heartlands, Germany's skilled workers and urban poor also moved to the industrial north of the United States, working in mills and factories, making German towns in American cities.

In the 1870s, when Bismarck's Kulturkampf was declared, Catholic clergy were expelled, church property seized, and Catholic religious communities persecuted. America offered the hope of religious freedom. But for German Catholics this religious freedom was inextricably linked to the freedom to celebrate the German character of their liturgy.[111] In St. Louis, Missouri, side by side with the Lutheran Missouri Synod, a movement began among German Catholics that fought for religious equality within the American Church. The local German priests were angered by the fact that German Catholic parishes "did not enjoy the same rights and privileges as English-language parishes, which were virtually all Irish." This anger was fueled by the paper *Pastoral-Blatt*, edited by the pastor of the Sisters of St. Mary, Father Faerber.[112] German resentment led to a petition to Rome in 1884 by eighty-two priests, who requested equal rights with the English-language American Catholics. This movement, coined by Archbishop John Ireland as "Cahenslyism," after the German layman who appealed to the Vatican in 1891 to support German Catholicism, created a furor that lasted well into the twentieth century. Jay P. Dolan explains:

On the one side . . . were a host of bishops who wanted Catholic immigrants to become American; they favored the Americanization of the foreign-born and abhorred any . . . "spirit of nationalism" among diverse groups of immigrants in the church. On the other side were the German clergy and people, who wanted recognition of their needs and equal rights in the church, their common enemy was the Irish, whom they feared "would Americanize everything."[113]

Nor was it only the clergy who adhered to German traditions, valuing their distinctive religious tradition. Catholic women brought to America their love of the Franciscan tradition.[114] In addition to the notable asceticism of St. Francis, his love of the poor and his preference for the "simple" provided a powerful motive for women to enter a life of self-denial and good works.[115] The Sisters of St. Mary continued this ascetic tradition. Mother Odilia slept on straw and practiced long vigils to the Blessed Sacrament, and during the long train journey from St. Louis to Kansas City the sisters exhausted themselves trying to sit straight without leaning back to rest.[116] Religious traditions most closely identified with nursing, such as the Augustinian or Vincentian traditions, expressly forbade extra ascetic practices, demanding that the sisters eat well, rest well, and conserve their strength and energy for their work.[117] Nonetheless, the German communities of women in these early years were distinguished by their nursing work, which offered more spiritual and ascetic opportunities than teaching. Second, German women were often relatively uneducated, so despite the demand for German teachers, their ability to function as teachers in a society with quite high levels of literacy, such as the United States, was limited.[118]

Thus, from patriarchal communities of the Lutheran Missouri Synod, to the Catholic and Protestant German hamlets of the Dakota plains, to the Catholic parishes of the German-American church in St. Louis, imported religious traditions flourished in conservative communities of German settlers, with German identity and German religious expression inextricably linked. The deaconess tradition took some decades to reach the rural settlements of the Missouri Synod and the Dakotas, but there, too, women were called for service to the sick of their communities, and the deaconess model successfully provided that avenue for women without threatening the authority of the family patriarch or devaluing the importance of Christian marriage.

Catholic women's service was not confined to the German community. The financial self-reliance prerequisite for all Catholic communities of women meant that, even in St. Louis, the sisterhoods were independent financial and legal entities. To be financially viable and to evangelize among non-Catholics (or lapsed Catholics), the sisters had to overcome both their language difficulties and German cultural expectations of women, to interact directly with the wider community of patients, doctors, railroad companies, state licensure boards, and so forth. Even in the most restrictive of environments, where few women spoke English, the doctors were mainly German, and the pastor was extremely interventionist, it was still a bigger role in the world than their non-Catholic counterparts were offered.

Role of the Pastor

> *Needless to say, this sketch has not been written in vain laudation of the Sisters' work, or in eulogy of their achievements. There are many Religious Orders and Congregations of men and women, whose origins was more humble, and start more difficult; whose hardships were greater, and obstacles more trying; whose progress was more rapid, and results more significant; with activities more widespread, and success more glorious.*
>
> *— W. Keuenhof, Chaplain, St. Mary's Hospital, Kansas City, Missouri, 5 March 1921[119]*

At the anniversary of the Sisters of St. Mary, the faint praise of Father Keuenhof (who saves his glowing testimonial for Pastor Faerber, self-proclaimed founder of the community), reveals a significant element in the experience of German religious nurses. The communities that have been examined here — the Sisters of St. Mary, the deaconesses of Kaiserswerth, the Philadelphia Evangelical Lutheran Deaconesses, the German Methodist deaconesses of Cincinnati, the deaconesses of Pittsburgh, and the Omaha deaconesses — all possessed forthright and commanding male leadership. They were established in the context of their ethnic / religious / cultural community largely due to the determined efforts of a pastor who believed firmly in their contribution to the social apostolate. Rarely is it possible to hear the voices of these women. Within the hospital they may have ruled, but the public face of the institution, its board and committees, and its annual reports mention them almost in passing.[120]

Louise Golder, sister of the prominent German Methodist pastor Christian Golder and an author in her own right, is something of an exception to this ghostly presence.[121] But the fact is the organization of deaconesses in Cincinnati offered even less scope and authority for deaconesses than the Philadelphia model — no Cincinnati deaconesses were ever proclaimed as "teachers" to medical men on matters of efficient hospital administration. For their part, the Sisters of St. Francis had to move beyond the German clergy to achieve the religious life that they sought and which they believed their Franciscan rule demanded of them.

German Nurses in America

The efforts of the Catholic sisterhoods and deaconesses in the nineteenth-century United States were remarkable when one considers that Germany had produced no counterpart for the "widespread collaboration of women in Christian charity in the eighteenth and nineteenth centuries."[122] Catherine Prelinger argues that the breakthrough for German women into the public sphere of Christian philanthropy was the direct result of the erosion of the nineteenth-century family structure, producing large numbers of displaced rural women of peasant and artisan background, along with idle women from the ruling classes.[123] This was the context for the German recruits for the Catholic sisterhoods. But most significantly, this combination of displaced women and Catholic resurgence also empowered Fliedner to reverse a 300-year Lutheran tradition and provide a means to incorporate women into a public philanthropic role. Interestingly, while the centrality of marriage in the Lutheran consciousness prevented women from moving beyond the patriarchal home, Fliedner's innovation was to transpose that marital and parental hierarchy at the core of Lutheranism into the structure for the deaconess institutes.[124] Unlike the Catholic convent where virgins are consecrated as "brides of Christ" to live in a female domain under an earthly mother superior, the deaconesses were virgin daughters who lived in a patriarchal family home with a mother (the pastor's wife) and father (pastor). Of course Catholic convent discourse is also rife with mothers and fathers — heavenly and temporal. The domestic discourse of the deaconess motherhouse, however, laboriously reasserted the centrality of the Protestant family.

The overwhelming male representation in documents of incorporation, deeds of trustees, and so forth in deaconess institutes, too, reasserts the prominence of the father, or pastor, central to Protestantism — particularly German Protestantism. Nineteenth-century German women did not have civil rights under Prussian law. This meant that women were not permitted to sign legal documents or enter into contracts without their father or husband's consent, regardless of their age.[125] In the United States deaconesses operated hospitals owned by the German community, or their church.[126] This was not how Catholic women (American, German, Irish, French, or Québecoises) did business in the New World. Even under the firm patriarchal hand of orthodox German Catholicism in St. Louis, the women were signatories on their own contracts, trustees of their own hospitals. This independence protected the diocese and the wider church from legal and financial responsibility — it was in the end a limited paternalism. Catholic sisterhoods took their own risks.

The slow, reactive progress of the Sisters of St. Mary into the professional realm of nursing training and licensure should not be seen as a reflection on all German sisterhoods. After all, one of the most famous centers of clinical excellence in the United States, St. Mary's, Rochester, Minnesota, was the result of a progressive partnership between a community of German women (a different group of Sisters of St. Francis) and Dr. William Worrall Mayo — a partnership initiated by Mother Mary Alfred Moes.[127] However, Rochester, Minnesota was not the heart of conservative German Catholicism, as was St. Louis, nor were the sisters under the pastoral direction of the men who led the German-speaking Catholic Church's attempt to achieve separation and independence of administration in the United States. For the St. Louis German Catholic hierarchy, German identity was a product of their liturgical and spiritual heritage. In Philadelphia, too, the monopoly of German-born (or descent) deaconesses over the German Hospital was a cause of celebration rather than concern. Even in the twentieth century, at least some deaconesses refused, or were unable, to recognize that linguistic and cultural distinctiveness inhibited recruitment.[128]

Yet despite the long arm of clergy protection, in the United States German women successfully entered the public domain as champions of philanthropy and social service. Notwithstanding the relatively constrained role of the nineteenth-century deaconesses and German Catholic sister-hoods in comparison with organizations such as the Daughters of Charity or the Sisters of Providence, the call to nurse in God's service broke through the patriarchal family's control of its daughters. For Catholic women, the free enterprise nature of American society meant that the sisters had to function as businesswomen and corporate directors, what-ever the limitations of language and experience. For Lutheran and Meth-odist women, the role of deaconess may have begun as a circumscribed and tentative role within the church; however, as the twentieth century wore on, recognition of the female apostolate in Protestantism gained acceptance and power. Deaconesses overwhelmingly abandoned nursing in the twentieth century, choosing instead to create for themselves a role in ministry and not allow "the devotion of Mary to be put aside for the service of Martha."[129]

Nursing, therefore, was a stepping stone to a share in Christian minis-try for Protestant women. It also trained and provided experience to generations of German women, Catholic and Protestant, in the newly emerging profession of nursing. Their work gave the role respectability and credence in the German community, but, most important, it edu-cated that same community on the talents and competence of women working in the world.

Chapter 8

The Twentieth Century
"Every Day Life Got Smaller"

When Elizabeth Ann Seton, foundress of the American Sisters of Charity, struggled with her call from God during the first decade of the nineteenth century, she could scarcely have dreamed that by the century's end Catholic women would have built the largest health care network in the country. By 1917 their hospitals accounted for half the American health care system.[1] But a century after Seton, Catholic sisters were not the only women to perform nursing work with dignity and diligence. The stage was by then crowded with Protestant religious nurses — the Anglican nuns and the Lutheran and Methodist deaconesses, and great numbers of secular nurses, led by educated, articulate, and political women. Of this final group a great deal is known, and their story has successfully obscured that of the religious nurses. All earlier versions of nursing were to fall under the shadow of Florence Nightingale and be dismissed — the religious nurses as unprofessional and the nonreligious nurses (the poor Sarah Gamps) as beneath contempt.[2]

But how important were the religious nurses — Catholic sister-nurses, Anglican sisterhoods, and Methodist and Lutheran deaconesses — to the shaping of modern nursing? To answer that question it becomes necessary to move beyond the nursing legends and enter the gendered religious domain of Christian charity and the nineteenth-century European diaspora. The first nurses outside Catholic Europe were the women of eighteenth-century New France — Jeanne Mance and Marguerite D'Youville were the pioneers of nursing in the New World.[3] In the Anglophone world it was the Irish nuns — Sisters of Mercy and Sisters of Charity. There were also non-Irish nuns such as Elizabeth Seton, the American convert who founded the American Sisters of Charity — but many of her nuns were Irish too.

The efforts of these women are conspicuously absent from accounts of nursing history and the history of women and work. By ignoring these women we are ignoring the way modern care of the sick came into being. We are displacing it from its place within a broad pastoral mission among the poor of the nineteenth century. Care of the sick was both a skilled practice and an evangelizing opportunity. The nursing nuns were a hybrid form — pragmatic and worldly, vocation-driven and deeply religious at the same time. It was this hybrid form of life, pious nursing, that crossed such a significant boundary, the boundary between the secular and the religious domains, and colonized new territory — gendered professional territory.

This book has taken up the hybrid positioning of nineteenth-century nursing to examine the relationship between vocational ethos and the emergence of a role for women as part of a professional work force. This aspect of nursing history has received very little attention from either women's studies scholars or feminist historians. But how did women begin to develop professional lives in the nineteenth century — what shift in "mentalité" occurred? How important was care of the sick in bridging this distance between the home as the women's sphere and the hospital or home of the sick? How important were the nursing nuns in opening up this space for women? What is at issue here is the emergence of a mass profession for women and the social/ethical challenges that this role transformation occasioned.

The persona of the professional woman was a *new* creation, and for women to be abroad in the world as autonomous agents they required protection — if not of the veil, at least of its equivalent in decorum and vocational bearing. It is in this area of professional/vocational shaping that the influence of the nursing nuns is so critical, and the continuities in training and ethical shaping from the cloister to the nurses' home become intelligible. The persona of the new nurse emerged from this hybrid pious and pragmatic space complete with the evangelical and corporeal duties of the nursing nun. Nursing's caring ethic was embedded in gendered religious practices. That said, these gendered religious practices also built the health systems within which nurses still work. Even today, for nurses the demands and ambiguities of being, as Susan Reverby put it, "ordered to care in a society that does not value caring," remain overwhelming.[4]

This book has been an attempt to move beyond the separation of religious and secular history and to integrate the work of religious women, principally Catholic vowed women, into the history of the rise of professional nursing. The nineteenth century began with a couple of solitary beacons, Elizabeth Seton in the United States and Mary Aikenhead in Ireland. Both women were moved by the plight of the poor, filled with a sense of social apostolate, and driven by the conviction that God required them to act in His name. To follow this call Seton and Aikenhead converted from Protestantism to Catholicism. Both women were encouraged and fostered by influential men. Elizabeth Seton was supported by Bishop Carroll of Maryland, the man largely responsible for the establish-

ment of the American Catholic Church. Mary Aikenhead's mentor was
Bishop Murray of Dublin — another builder. Murray led the church during its reestablishment in Ireland following the repeal of the penal codes.
Both established communities of women, the American Sisters of Charity
and the Irish Sisters of Charity which owed strong (but informal) allegiance to the (French) Daughters of Charity of St. Vincent de Paul, and
both communities trained women as hospital builders and nurses par
excellence.

For both communities of women, too, their hospital work provided a
means for the church to integrate itself into a society that had formerly excluded Catholics. In the United States, epidemics, medical support, and
state and county funds enabled the sisters (in the name of the Church) to
provide an essential service to all Americans — regardless of religion. In
Ireland the sisters' nursing ability gave the Church the means to seize
back control of services from the Protestant ascendancy. Epidemics provided a "foot in the door" to the workhouse infirmaries for the sisterhoods, and when workhouse infirmaries finally evolved into public hospitals, the sisters stayed in charge.[5]

As the utility of these communities of religious women became evident, the chord was struck among Protestants who struggled to find a
similar path for their own motivated and energized women. The most
successful and extensive program of religious life for Protestant women
was that established by Theodur Fliedner in the German Rhineland in
1836. The revival of the female diaconate provided the established Lutheran Church with a formal mechanism to develop its social program in
the Lutheran confessional states of Northern Europe. Sanctioned by the
official church, with the blessing of the crown and the aristocracy, the
deaconesses became the means for the reform of hospitals and nursing in
these countries.

The story of Lutheranism in North America was somewhat different.
While it was not the established church, it did have generous private
benefactors such as John Lankenau of Philadelphia. Nonetheless, the
deaconess movement remained marginal to the Lutheran mission in the
United States. After all, American women had plenty of other options,
and the deaconess movement was caught between maintaining the Lutheran Church's commitment to Christian marriage and valuing a sancti-
fied life of celibacy for women. The deaconesses were important in the
United States, though, because they provided a means for the development of health care services that were distinctively German, Norwegian, Swedish, and Danish. However, these services failed to be sustained
by American deaconesses, relying instead upon the import of foreign
women. They therefore functioned as a transitional service for these
immigrant communities.

For non-Lutheran deaconesses the issues were different again. The Methodist revival of the late nineteenth century converted many a girl — including German women. These women were moved to God's work but also commonly bound to earn their keep. Louise Golder's files in Cincinnati reveal a class of woman who worked as servants or seamstresses, women who were keen to trade that life for one in God's glory, God's security, and God's respectability. To be a deaconess at that time meant to be a nurse, but the role began to extend beyond hospital work and into the community, as had in fact been Fliedner's intention. This parish work was not for simple serving girls but for competent women who could support the work of the minister. As resistance to such work by women began to lessen, the nursing aspect of their role lessened too, and the deaconesses moved gradually into an apostolic role within their churches.

The numbers of Anglican or Episcopalian sisters also peaked early in the twentieth century. This group of women had many more difficulties than the deaconesses because they were under suspicion of being crypto-Catholic. Nonetheless, in mid-nineteenth-century Britain the Anglican sisterhoods were of great importance in developing the ground for trained secular nurses. As Anne Summers's work has made clear, these women were significant in establishing the need for trained nurses, upgrading the level of nursing skills expected in hospitals and at the private bedside, and demonstrating the combination of clinical excellence and ethical deportment that was so vital to the gentrification of nursing.[6] This gentrification allowed for educated, ambitious women to choose leadership in nursing as their career path, to become the reformers of nursing and the founders of its professional associations and training and accreditation processes.

But for both the Protestant sisterhoods and the deaconesses, the efforts of the women were limited by the lack of consensus surrounding their chosen life and its place within their respective churches. It was in this regard that Catholic religious (nuns, priests, and brothers) were so advantaged. Catholic families faithfully produced children who became dedicated members of the church. The Catholic community consensus revered the religious and considered their work to be God's own. Furthermore, the Church's institutions were structured to produce successive generations of strong Catholics. The tight school system and intense parish structure were highly successful in keeping the numbers of women prepared to vow themselves to God's service very high until the mid-twentieth century.

In addition to the local community structures that privileged a "call" to God by any individual, the Catholic Church relentlessly exploited its Old World connections and provided opportunities for immigrant girls to come to the New World as nuns or novices. Extensive recruitment drives in Ireland supported the English-speaking Catholic Church well into the twentieth century.[7] Irish seeking employment commonly expected to go to England or further. Opportunities at home were scarce — until 1950 the major occupation for Irish women was still domestic service.[8] Such a big step to the New World was perhaps not such a leap for Irish women, who, unlike other women, had been making the journey alone in great numbers throughout the nineteenth century. In fact, Ireland still boasted the highest level of female migration in Europe for the period 1945–60.[9] Finally, to become a member of a religious community in Ireland required a dowry. This could be a goodly sum — in the nineteenth century dowries were between 300 and 500 pounds. However, volunteering to join an overseas mission, such as in the United States or Australia, generally meant that the dowry requirement was waived.

German women, too, provided fresh recruits for the German sisterhoods, and recruitment drives back to Catholic Germany were an important means of sustaining the German identity of some of the communities under study in previous chapters. French women did not migrate to the English-speaking world in very great numbers, but where they did their education and experience often inclined them to the teaching of elite girls, rather than hospital work. The latter remained very much the domain of Irish and German immigrant women or children of immigrants. The Sisters of the Incarnate Word and the Sisters of the Holy Cross are good examples of the phenomenon of a French community gradually becoming an Irish one.[10] French Canadians were something of an exception to this rule. They felt called to proselytize both the Native American peoples and the godless Americans who went west with the opening of the continent to miners, traders, and settlers. The Canadian women were clearly missionaries. Bound to home and sustained by fresh recruits, they remained missionaries until well into the twentieth century. They had a very different consciousness from that of the French or German women who were driven from their homelands by political conflict and persecution, or the pragmatic Irish women who filled the ranks of American communities — building an Irish empire in the New World.

Female Religious Life

In the first half of the nineteenth century it had been simply impossible for women without veil and vow to move abroad among the poor and wretched and provide for their care. As we have seen, even for those set apart as religious women, the Protestant worlds of North America, Australia, Britain, and Germany were extremely hostile to the sisters' work.

Even in Catholic communities the lives of vowed women were frequently trials of persecution and harassment by clergy. The nineteenth-century bishop, literal prince of the church, considered it mere female impudence on the part of sisters to struggle to maintain their independence in order to follow the example of their holy foundress and the rule they had vowed to serve.

The status of women in the church was complicated. During the first half of the nineteenth century, the extent to which the often high-born sisters felt obliged to obey the (male) clergy was mediated by social class. In Sydney well-born Sisters of Charity were most reluctant to be bullied by ignorant Irishmen who were far from their social equals. For the French Canadian Daughters of Providence and the French Sisters of the Incarnate Word, the issue of obedience was personally resolved in the light of the sister's individual interpretation of God's will. Thus in Seattle the Sisters of Providence acted without approval on the rationale that if God had wanted them to take the pastor's advice, he would not have sent them this opportunity when the pastor was so far away. Similarly, in San Antonio, Mother Saint Pierre looked into her heart, to her rule, and to the spirit of her vows to give her the strength to rebuke a bullying Polish priest.

Thus through personal and spiritual negotiation the sisters overcame the obstacles and restrictions placed in the way of their vocation and the destiny they felt God had called their holy community to fulfill. The modus operandi of religious profession that made all things possible was "first things first and trust the rest to Divine Providence."[11] What worked in the sisters' favor was the lack of clarity from Rome and the wide discrepancy in viewpoint on the role of religious communities, their relationship with their pastor and with the diocese. For bishops in need of a workforce the solution to difficult communities of independent women was to set up their own, with rules that served the needs of the diocese. The plethora of new nineteenth-century communities was the result of pious women answering these local needs. Under pressure from bishops to make communities of religious women diocesan, large and centrally organized communities of women (such as the Daughters of Charity, or the Irish Sisters of Charity) became increasingly difficult to establish — almost impossible by the twentieth century. However, the field was already well supplied with such communities, which, as a result of the Herculean efforts of the early women, had acquired a substantial asset base and extensive experience in the field of health care. It was certainly no disadvantage to the position of the Catholic Church in North America and Australia that it could boast such major public institutions, all firmly within the bosom of the Catholic community.

Fossilization

However, caught up in the impetus to bring the Catholic flock under the umbrella of Catholic institutions, sisters, too, found themselves by the turn of the century increasingly governed. At the beginning of the twentieth century the Vatican decreed that active communities of religious women needed to embrace the cloister as a defining characteristic of religious life. Following the gradual increase of restrictions on women religious that began with the papal decrees of 1900 and 1901, the green fields of the nineteenth-century landscape of the New World began to disappear. Active communities became known as apostolic communities, to emphasize their missionary importance. They were also formally redefined as "religious" and subject to many of the same prohibitions and limitations as cloistered nuns. As one sister put it, "every day life got smaller. Religious life had become the celebration of the trivial."[12] Incrementally but inexorably the cloister "doors" closed, until Vatican II blew them off their hinges in 1962 and religious women once more came face to face with the world.[13]

Canon Law — A Decision from Rome

The uncertainties that had surrounded the precise position of active communities of women for more than two hundred years were starkly defined when canon law was finally codified and promulgated in 1917.[14] The church determined that the lives of sisters needed to be sharply defined by externalized structures: set times for prayers and daily Eucharist began to be imposed. The imposition of these traditional markings of religious life in the cloister reaffirmed the view from Rome that religious life takes place in the convent, as opposed to the streets, hospital wards, and homes of the poor.[15] Travel restrictions came into place and the sisters were forbidden to stay in hotels — a major issue that restricted travel. They were also forbidden to go out alone.

In making these decrees the Vatican was responding to a century of urging by bishops that sisterhoods should be under diocesan control. The slow but relentless grinding of the Vatican bureaucracy meant that the nineteenth-century dynamic outpouring of female pious energy was steered toward rationalization and administrative control. With this shift opportunities for extraordinary work, for full participation in policy and planning roles became severely curtailed as more and more of the sisters' authority devolved to priests acting in their stead. As prohibitions on movement increased, the pioneering achievements of the nineteenth century became less and less possible to repeat.[16]

The American Catholic Church lost its missionary status in 1908. Now the largest religious body in the United States, and formally under direct Vatican administration, the Church's pioneering days faded into a period of consolidation. Meanwhile the "Catholic world" created by the plethora of Catholic institutions continued to grow. Canon law expressly forbade Catholics from attending non-Catholic schools. With this ruling, providing the parochial school system with teachers became the primary task of religious women. By 1966 63 percent of all Catholic sisters were involved in teaching or teaching administration.[17] Large numbers of women continued to join the ranks of the sisterhoods to support this effort, and social and material opportunities enhanced the spiritual rewards on offer for members of religious communities. As Helen Ebaugh argued, "For Catholic girls, nuns provided the role model, and Catholic orders the vehicle, for upward mobility both out of the working class and from the restrictions and low status of the traditional wife-mother role!"[18]

As the twentieth century progressed and power within the church centralized, the Vatican began to take a closer interest in the daily activities of the sisters. Every five years communities were required to report on their conformity to the new codes. With this process the emphasis of religious life turned from responsiveness and initiative to obedience to the "letter of the law."[19] According to Patricia Byrne, the archives "abound" with evidence of surveillance following the invocation of canon law. For instance, one letter from the diocese to the Sisters of Charity of Nazareth in 1922 complained of "violation of Canon 607 of the new code, which requires a companion for sisters outside their houses." Apparently, "priests and others" had seen "sisters of the different communities alone in the most crowded streets of the city . . . in office buildings and department stores, going from room to room and counter to counter unescorted."[20]

For working sisters this new set of expectations constituted an onerous burden. In addition to their demanding work schedules, the newly imposed regimen of prayer, chant, and meditation constituted hours of extra work in an already overextended day. Travel restrictions impeded the performance of the sisters' duties and their ability to undergo further training and qualifications. These restrictions came into force at the same time that the wider community was increasing its expectations of professional workers. The sisters were under pressure to give primary focus to their religious life, and their professional obligations now needed to fit into their religious schedule. The call for regular prayers led the sisters away from the wards, while the need for daily Eucharist kept them close to the chapel. The net result of these changes was that, for the first time, the sisters' professional life became something of a compromise with their religious life.[21]

A further outcome of these changes was the absorption of the Catholic hospital firmly into the Catholic world, transforming the sisters' hospitals into Catholic monoliths.[22] The ecumenical position nineteenth-century sisters had frequently found for themselves, with Protestant doctors, Protestant supporters and fundraisers, and Protestant women in charge of training schools, was difficult to maintain in the twentieth-century climate of Catholic totality. By mid-century the Catholic identity of the hospitals and their nursing schools was reaffirmed at every opportunity. For instance, nurses' graduation ceremonies increasingly took on the appearance of a first holy communion ceremony, complete with graduation mass.

The Catholicity of their hospitals was constantly affirmed by the incorporation of Catholic rituals in the training of nurses, and the scrutiny of the nurses' behavior was carried out as a Catholic pastoral responsibility. Moreover the nursing practice of the sisters within the hospital now required clear justification. In common with all trained nurses of the time, the supervisory role of the nursing sister (or registered nurse) freed religious nurses from the necessity for direct patient care. This was convenient where, in the Vatican's view, such care compromised their modesty. Rules of nursing communities took an explicit character; for instance, the 1928 Customary of the Daughters of Providence required that as "a general rule the sister will make use of students to catheterize women."[23] This recommendation was followed by the recurrent caveat that "discretion inspired by charity will always trace out the line to be followed by the supervisor in such delicate circumstances."[24] Whether the sisters took to heart the stringency of canon law and its enforcers, or merely satisfied their scrutinizers that their nursing practice was appropriate and defensible, the net result of these pressures was the accommodation of papal concerns into rules and customaries and the downplaying of the sisters' contribution to clinical practice. Effectively, by the mid-twentieth century, the autonomous and separate realm that typified the hospital world run by Catholic religious women of the nineteenth century had ceased to exist.[25]

Hospital Organization

The nineteenth century witnessed the rise of scientific medicine and the modern hospital. It was a period of rapid advancement in technology and skill. The religious communities that had been managing hospitals (or networks of hospitals) for almost the length of the century had presided over medicine's entry to the hospital. The advent of germ theory and improvements in anesthesia resulted in the transformation of the hospital into a surgical institution — complete with all the changes in operating theater technology and practice and post-surgical nursing care this entailed. They presided over hospitals where patient observations were transformed from complex and individualized measures of the physician to standardized technologically based regimens. Patient charts and medical records ordered both patient and practitioner (physician and nurse), while X-ray and pathology technology revolutionized diagnosis and treatment. The simple wards of the 1830s were light years away from the postoperative wards of the 1890s. The care of patients had become complex, and to remain financially viable the sisters had to demonstrate that their institutions welcomed the best doctors in the field and boasted the best care.

As the nursing profession emerged and training became routine, the sisters presided over a further revolution — the revolution in nursing. When the sisters first began establishing hospitals they did all the work themselves. The hierarchical structure of their communities provided for the demarcation of responsibility and delegation of manual labor. Although there are plentiful anecdotes that refer to the mother superior working in the laundry or scrubbing the entry halls of the hospital, in general these tasks were left to novices and postulants.[26] Nonetheless, communities were always short of workers, and the virtue in hard work that was at the core of religious training for sisters certainly had ample opportunity for demonstration in hospital work.

All these changes required substantial organizational reform and increased capital. For a hospital to remain financially viable, then as now, it needed to keep abreast of changes and adapt to new demands — demands of patients, funders, and the professions. To meet this challenge, Charles Moulinier, a Jesuit, established the Catholic Hospitals Association (CHA) in 1915. Moulinier was determined that North America's large network of Catholic hospitals, which accounted for 50 percent of all hospitals in the United States and Canada at that time, should be positioned to take advantage of the accreditation movement to build public confidence in Catholic hospitals, silence their critics, and dominate health care service provision.

In the first decades of the twentieth century there was great variation in the standards of nursing care and hospital organization. This was the case for Catholic and non-Catholic hospitals alike. The American College of Surgeons (ACS) initiated the standardization movement with the development of minimum standards for hospital practice. The four key elements to these standards were

1. operating privileges restricted to surgical staff who were trained and approved;
2. regular staff meetings;

3. efficient record system;
4. laboratory and X-ray facilities and staff.[27]

A good many Catholic hospitals already met these standards — the Buffalo Hospital of the Daughters of Charity had been the site of a major showdown between the sisters and medical practitioners over these very issues during the last decade of the nineteenth century.[28] However, for other communities, conformity with secular standards for hospital management, such as the requirement that nursing sisters wear a washable white habit, precipitated a crisis.[29]

Moulinier anticipated the emergent standards movement and cooperated with the ACS to promote the standards and build support for them in the Catholic hospital system. Moulinier wanted the CHA to be a sisters' organization with a sister president. But conservative views within the church prevailed. Under the impetus of the standardization movement in the 1920s the CHA worked with medical leaders and clergy to form policy and set guidelines for Catholic hospitals, and much of the leadership role in this movement evolved away from women. In response to these initiatives the relative indifference of the diocese toward the management of hospitals conducted by women religious within the diocese was replaced by keen interest.[30] In fact, Kauffman reports how the CHA in its early years became yet another means to control the sisters — concerned with limiting sisters' contact with non-Catholics and male patients, controlling their movement, and reinforcing canon law.

The church also became embroiled in controversy over the type of services provided by Catholic hospitals. From the Church's point of view, the care of women in labor had long been problematic for nursing nuns — their practice was formally prohibited in this field (although loosely policed in the nineteenth century).[31] In 1901 a new set of norms was drawn up by the Sacred Congregation of Bishops and regulars (in Rome) which prohibited approval for institutes of sisters engaged in the care of "infants in the cradle" or women in childbirth. These norms were reaffirmed in 1921, as such care was considered "unbecoming for virgins consecrated to God and wearing a religious habit."[32] This trend was finally reversed in 1936, when midwifery training for those in missionary countries was formally sanctioned by Rome.[33] Furthermore, as Kate Joyce has pointed out, the ethical issues surrounding gynecological surgery that resulted in female sterilization were immensely controversial in the early twentieth century, foreshadowing later pro-choice / pro-life debates. One powerful camp within the CHA was comprised of clerics who objected, in principle, to standards for Catholic hospitals set by medical men.[34] Nonetheless, by 1929 over half of all Catholic hospitals had met minimum standards as compared to only a quarter of non-Catholic hospitals.[35]

The Nursing Profession

SISTER-NURSES

Meanwhile, professional expectations of the sisters as major health care providers were rising just as the Vatican was hardening its attitude toward women religious in "active" roles. One motivation of Moulinier in founding the CHA was to provide the sisters with a safe forum to improve their nursing and management skills in a climate of increased restriction.[36] And despite the difficulties, a good many communities had no intention of losing professional or corporate ground. In 1890, when there were only thirty-five training schools in the United States, the Sisters Hospital, Buffalo, the Mercy in Chicago, and Saint Mary's, Brooklyn had opened training schools for nurses.[37] Doyle's 1929 survey of state nursing associations, reported in her series of articles on religious nurses in the *American Journal of Nursing*, found that all twenty-one state associations that responded to her survey reported involvement by religious nurses in state professional associations.[38] Large nursing communities such as the Sisters of Providence and the Daughters of Charity had even created a designated role for a sister-nurse supervisor whose responsibility it was to conduct additional educational programs for graduate sister-nurses.[39] Doyle reported the involvement of nursing sisterhoods in pushing through nursing registration legislation in states such as Alabama and Utah.[40] Sisters were also active as members of state boards of examiners and as training school inspectors.[41] The "dual engagement in professional life" of the sisters meant by mid-century that, despite the onerous regimen of canon law, the demands of their institutional roles, their low public and professional profile, the sisters were among the best-educated cohorts of women in the country and highly active in their professions.[42]

NON-VOWED NURSES

Meanwhile, as the sisters moved out of the professional limelight, forced out by canon law, the non-vowed women who followed them continued to operate in their place. Negotiating the same space of work, male bodies, and respectability, ordinary women mobilized the same arsenal of gender and vocation. The fact that this territory had been colonized decades before by religious women laboring within particular constraints and possibilities in turn defined and bounded the mode of professional evolution for other women who came, toward the end of the nineteenth century, to join and transform nursing.

From the inception of nursing reform, the moral attributes of the nurse were considered to far outweigh any clinical competence or experience she might possess. As Rafferty points out, "Character rather than theory or intellectual talents became the touchstone of nursing skill and qualifications."[43] In the early nineteenth century nursing was only respectable when conducted by nuns. Women who were like nuns (such as Anglican women and deaconesses) found a way to do this work too without loss of status. Nightingale's achievement was to find a means to generalize this form — nursing as moral work — to a wider, nonsectarian group of women. This movement intersected with the rapid rise of hospitals and modern medicine and, by the end of the century, nursing skills found a ready market as hospitals moved from the care of the poor to the middle class. However, the vocational underpinning of nursing — an indisputable legacy of the religious nurses — continued to complicate the professional agenda of twentieth-century nurses. As Barbara Melosh has argued, in the first decades of the twentieth century, the "ministry" of nursing hindered the recognition and respect for nursing skill demanded by the more progressive sections of the nursing leadership.[44]

This much is understood and acknowledged by historians. But such an account lacks depth and specificity as to the importance of the sisterhoods. It implies a "natural" progression from the religious to the secular world that undercuts the achievements of religious women and their role, not as precursors, but as collaborators in the regulation and professionalization of nursing. It also erases from view the fact that religious women were cofounders of the American health care system. A final important feature of nursing in North America and Australia was the tension that existed between religious hospitals and their nursing sisters and competing hospitals and nonreligious nurses. This tension was a positive and productive force that made both groups of nurses acutely aware of the criticisms of their opponents and determined to demonstrate their competitive edge and clinical competence.

The story of nursing is not one of parallel paths requiring two histories. It was the relationship between these two important groups of women, the determined and competent vowed women (Catholic and Protestant) on one side, and the equally determined and ambitious non-vowed women on the other, that created modern nursing in North America and Australia. For just as it is impossible to understand nursing, its history or its present, without a working understanding of gender, the premise of this book has been that it is equally implausible to omit religion from the frame.

Nearly two hundred years after Elizabeth Seton and Mary Aikenhead, nursing remains a moral practice — people trust nurses. It is equally true that as a female profession it is underpaid and undervalued. Without the religious vocational framing of the nineteenth century or the patriotic and civic imperatives of the first half of the twentieth century, it is difficult today to express why nursing is important. Yet the demands of the health reform agenda make it more important than ever before to argue the case for nursing, and to persuade men and women that it is a good thing to be a nurse. To do this successfully we need to understand how nursing is gendered — why does it appeal to so few men? But equally important we need to understand the vocational imperatives that still attract so many women to nurse, that make them endure poor conditions and hard work, and that leave them full of guilt and inadequacy when they have not managed the unmanageable, or achieved the unachievable at the end of a shift.

For better or worse, these are the legacies of the religious nurses. It was they who turned care of the sick into an uplifting task for good women. They were the convincing proof that good nurses were worthwhile and women had a great deal to offer. But most important of all, they pioneered the path for women through the moral contagion of sickness. They showed how to work among male bodies and the sick poor without loss of status — in fact with increased status. They left the cloister and led women into the world. Once in the world they showed that women could do business, and women could take charge. Catholic sisters did not suffer the same trials as other nurses; the contests with medicine featured in European hospitals were not such an issue in the New World. In the New World the Catholic sisters owned their hospitals and medical men had to learn their place — a few were slow. But the occasional skirmish with medical men pales into insignificance when compared to the real danger — male clergy. But in their struggles to achieve sovereignty over their communities, to live according to their rule and act out their mission, the sisters learned a great deal. They acquired political skill, business acumen, and a corporate understanding without equal among their sex. Catholic women needed these skills when the Vatican crackdown of the twentieth century commenced.

Nursing needs to look beyond the veil and see that its progenitors were not the meek and obedient slaves to medicine that Florence Nightingale and Dorothy Dix would have us believe. The religious nurses were leaders, they were professional pioneers, and they created entire health care networks owned and conducted by women. Nursing would not be what it is today without them.

Abbreviations

ADCELCA	Archives of the Deaconess Community of the Evangelical Lutheran Church in America, Gladwyne, Pennsylvania
AMIW	Archives, Sisters of the Incarnate Word, Motherhouse, San Antonio, Texas
BL	British Library
CHSNCGM	Cincinnati Historical Society, Nippert Collection of German Methodism, Cincinnati, Ohio
CSNH	Center for the Study of Nursing History, University of Pennsylvania, Philadelphia.
DOCA	Daughters of Charity Archives, Albany, New York.
LMSP	Letters of Mother Saint Pierre Cinquin, trans. Sister Kathleen Garvey (1977), AMIW
MJSH	Mother Joseph of the Sacred Heart Personal Papers Collection, SPA
SPA	Sisters of Providence Archives, Sacred Heart Province, Seattle, Washington

Notes

Chapter 1. "Say Little, Do Much"

1. The sacred vows of poverty, chastity, and obedience have defined religious life since the days of the early Christian church. But there are degrees of vow — solemn and simple, private and public, and varieties of religious rules under which men and women could live fully enclosed within a convent (never to leave), or live temporarily therein, or live under a modified form of the rule, or live piously in the world. My use of the term "vowed women" in the nineteenth-century context reflects and acknowledges these ancient variations.

2. "Government" in the sense developed by Michel Foucault, which referred to mechanisms of state for the management and discipline of the populace. Foucault, "Governmentality," in *The Foucault Effect: Studies in Governmentality*, ed. Graham Burchell, Colin Gordon, and Peter Miller (Chicago: University of Chicago Press, 1991), 87–104. See the application of these ideas in Nikolas Rose, *Governing the Soul: The Shaping of Private Life* (London: Routledge, 1990) and Mitchell Dean, *The Constitution of Poverty: Towards a Genealogy of Liberal Governance* (London: Routledge, 1994).

3. "Say little, do much" has been associated with Vincent de Paul as a line from the popular 1948 Academy Award film *Monsieur Vincent*, directed by Maurice Cloche. It evokes the spirit of de Paul, though it is unlikely that he ever used these words.

4. Secular is used in the sense "of the world" as opposed to "of religion." This is the sense used in the nineteenth-century secularism movement — which worked to separate church and state in every aspect of society. I use the term "secular nurses" to refer to nurses who were not members of a religious community or formally affiliated with any religious group. As with the word vow, secular has historically layered meanings. Technically in Catholicism, secular means religious men and women living outside the cloister. Secular priests (and bishops) are those who live "in the world," as opposed to living in monasteries. They live relatively independently in parishes and own property.

5. Marvin O'Connell, "The Roman Catholic Tradition Since 1545," in *Caring and Curing: Health and Medicine in the Western Religious Traditions*, ed. Ronald L. Numbers and Darrel W. Amundsen (New York: Macmillan, 1986), 108–45, 137.

Chapter 2. Martha's Turn

1. S. B. Mansell, *English Sisterhoods: An Address Delivered at the Re-opening and Benediction of St. Peter's Home, Brompton Square, 5 May 1863* (London: Joseph Masters, Aldergate Street, 1863).

2. Nancy F. Cott, *The Bonds of Womanhood: "Woman's Sphere" in New England, 1780–1835* (New Haven, Conn.: Yale University Press, 1977), 140.

3. Ibid., 202.

4. Marilyn J. Westerkamp's bibliographical essay charts this territory of "Reformation Faiths and the Gender Dynamic," in *Women and Religion in Early America, 1600–1850: The Puritan and Evangelical Traditions* (London: Routledge, 1999), 202–14. Linda Gerber, "Separate Spheres, Female Worlds, Women's Place: The Rhetoric of Women's History," *Journal of American History* 75, 1 (1988): 9–39 examines the impact of the notion of separate spheres on women's history.

5. See Lori D. Ginzberg, *Women and the Work of Benevolence: Morality, Politics, and Class in the Nineteenth-Century United States* (New Haven, Conn.: Yale University Press, 1990), 11–35, on feminine moral authority. In the Women's Christian Temperance Union, Frances Willard (leader, 1879–98) pursued a "Do Everything Policy" that made issues as diverse as the living wage and the India policy part of the WCTU platform. See Joseph R. Gusfield, *Symbolic Crusade: Status Politics and the American Temperance Movement* (Urbana: University of Illinois Press, 1986), 75–77.

6. Westerkamp observes that " 'disturbers of the peace' are the most popular subjects," *Women and Religion in Early America*, 204.

7. I use the term "vowed women" to emphasize the fact that these women were simply women living under a voluntary vow to a particular rule. In this way Anglican sisterhoods can be included in this categorization.

8. Margaret Susan Thompson, "Women, Feminism, and the New Religious History: Catholic Sisters as a Case Study," in *Belief and Behavior: Essays in the New Religious History*, ed. Philip R. VanderMeer and Robert P. Swierenga (New Brunswick, N.J.: Rutgers University Press, 1991), 137. Thompson discusses difficulty with data on nuns. They were not counted in the same way as priests, and the historian must rely on community figures which are not in consistent format if they exist at all. Aggregate figures, therefore, are notoriously difficult to determine.

9. Maria Luddy, *Women and Philanthropy in Nineteenth-Century Ireland* (Cambridge: Cambridge University Press, 1995), 23. Luddy's writing reveals discomfort with the religious language of humility and vocation, see 26–27. Thompson, "Women, Feminism, and the New Religious History," 141, argues that it is possible to read through the code and the rhetoric of religious writings to gain a useful source on the women's lives. Luddy's view sharply contrasts with the more recent work of Mary Peckham Magray, *The Transforming Power of the Nuns: Women, Religion, and Cultural Change in Ireland, 1750–1900* (New York: Oxford University Press, 1998), whose detailed analysis of the work and community of Catholic women in nineteenth-century Ireland shows the massive social impact of Irish women on the social, economic, and religious landscape of Irish society.

10. There have been some rather heroic efforts to argue that the Catholic and Anglican sisterhoods were to some extent pursuing a feminist agenda. See Helen Rose Fuchs Ebaugh, "Patriarchal Bargains and Latent Avenues of Social Mobility: Nuns in the Roman Catholic Church," *Gender and Society* 7, 3 (September 1993): 400–414 and Magray, *The Transforming Power of the Nuns* on the Catholic sisterhoods; Susan Mumm, *Stolen Daughters, Virgin Mothers: Anglican Sisterhoods in Vic-*

torian Britain (London: Leicester University Press, 1999); and Judith Moore, *A Zeal for Responsibility: The Struggle for Professional Nursing in Victorian England, 1868–1883* (Athens: University of Georgia Press, 1988) on the Anglican sisterhoods.

11. There is of course plentiful evidence that the sisters did not break ties with family, retained their own identities, and pursued their interests with nothing resembling indifference — but the ideal of religious life should not be confused with its reality.

12. This desexualization had its limits. With the Catholic resurgence in the first half of the nineteenth century in Britain and the United States, the Gothic imagination of the time intensely sexualized convent life and the nun. Maria Monk and her ilk sponsored a puritan pornography around the topic. However, the titillation rested in the nun's obedience to the clergyman, her own fall the result of his wickedness. Much has been written on this salacious topic. Jenny Franchot, *Roads to Rome: The Antebellum Protestant Encounter with Catholicism* (Berkeley: University of California Press, 1994) is one of the best on the genre.

13. See Mary Denis Maher, *To Bind Up the Wounds: Catholic Sister Nurses in the U.S. Civil War* (New York: Greenwood Press, 1989).

14. Among the 2,115,815 employed RNs in the United States in 1996, an estimated 113,683 were men, 5.4 percent of the total, a substantial increase over 1992 (79,557 of 1,853,024, 4.3 percent). Notes from the National Sample Survey of Registered Nurses, March 1996, Health Resources and Service Administration, Bureau of Health Professionals, Department of Health and Human Services, Washington, D.C. ⟨www.hrsa.dhhs.gov/bhpr/dn/dn.htm⟩.

15. It is difficult to generalize, but in many instances the sisters were keen to promote the professionalization of nursing: they were forward thinking on the registration question, members of state licensing boards, and so forth. See Suzy A. Farren, *A Call to Care: The Women Who Built Catholic Healthcare in America* (St. Louis: Catholic Hospitals Association, 1996).

16. Thompson, "Women, Feminism, and the New Religious History," 137.

17. Mary Ewens, *The Role of the Nun in Nineteenth-Century America* (New York: Arno Press, 1978), one of the first scholarly attempts at the subject of sisterhoods in America, examines their representation in literature.

18. Marvin O'Connell, "The Roman Catholic Tradition Since 1545," in *Caring and Curing: Health and Medicine in the Western Religious Tradition*s, ed. Ronald L. Numbers and Darrel W. Amundsen (New York: Macmillan, 1986), 136.

19. His treatment of the split of the American Daughters and the New York sisters certainly reads as a fight between men. George C. Stewart, Jr., *Marvels of Charity: History of American Sisters and Nuns* (Huntington, Ind.: Our Sunday Visitor, 1994), 97–99.

20. Jo Ann Kay McNamara, *Sisters in Arms: Catholic Nuns Through Two Millennia* (Cambridge, Mass: Harvard University Press, 1996).

21. Magray, *The Transforming Power of the Nuns.*

22. Susan O'Brien, "French Nuns in Nineteenth Century England," *Past and Present* 154 (1997): 142–80.

23. Carol K. Coburn and Martha Smith, *Spirited Lives: How Nuns Shaped Catholic Culture and American Life, 1836–1920* (Chapel Hill: University of North Carolina Press, 1999). Also Coburn and Smith, " 'Pray for Your Wanderers': Women Religious on the Colorado Mining Frontier, 1877–1917," *Frontiers* 15, 3 (1995): 27–52.

24. Suellen Hoy, "The Journey Out: The Recruitment and Emigration of Irish

Religious Women to the United States, 1812–1914," *Journal of Women's History* 6, 4 (1995): 64–98.

25. Elizabeth Smyth, "Professionalization Among the Professed: The Case of Roman Catholic Women Religious," in *Challenging Professions: Historical and Contemporary Perspectives on Women's Professional Work*, ed. Elizabeth Smyth, Sandra Acker, Sandra Bourne, and Alison Prentice (Toronto: University of Toronto Press, 1999), 234–54.

26. Coburn and Smith, *Spirited Lives*. Their book's examination of nursing takes only fourteen pages.

27. Smyth, "Professionalization Among the Professed."

28. Joan Lynaugh, *The Community Hospitals of Kansas City, Missouri, 1870–1915* (New York: Garland Press, 1989); Jean Richardson, "Catholic Religious Women as Institutional Innovators: The Sisters of Charity and the Rise of the Modern Urban Hospital in Buffalo, N.Y., 1848–1900," dissertation, State University of New York at Buffalo, 1996; Bernadette McCauley, " 'Sublime Anomalies': Women Religious and Roman Catholic Hospitals in New York City, 1850–1920," *Journal of the History of Medicine and Allied Sciences* 52 (July, 1997): 289–309.

29. Kathleen M. Joyce, "Science and the Saints: American Catholics and Health Care, 1880–1930," dissertation, Princeton University, 1995; Barbra Mann Wall, "Unlikely Entrepreneurs: Nuns, Nursing, and Hospital Development in the West and Midwest, 1865–1915," dissertation, University of Notre Dame, 2000.

30. Martha Vicinus, *Independent Women: Work and Community for Single Women, 1850–1920* (Chicago: University of Chicago Press, 1985); Susan P. Casteras, "Virgin Vows," in *Religion in the Lives of English Women, 1760–1930*, ed. Gail Malmgreen (London: Croom Helm, 1986); and Mumm, *Stolen Daughters, Virgin Mothers*.

31. Moore, *Zeal for Responsibility* is an exception to this as she focuses on nursing sisterhoods.

32. Catherine M. Prelinger is a notable exception here; see "The Nineteenth-Century Deaconessate in Germany: The Efficacy of a Family Model," in *German Women in the Eighteenth and Nineteenth Centuries: A Social and Literary History*, ed. Ruth-Ellen B. Joeres and Mary Jo Maynes (Bloomington: Indiana University Press, 1986), 215–30; Rima Lunin Schultz, "Woman's Work and Woman's Calling in the Episcopal Church: Chicago, 1880–1989," in *Episcopal Women: Gender, Spirituality, and Commitment in an American Mainline Denomination*, ed. Catherine M. Prelinger (New York: Oxford University Press, 1992), 19–71.

33. Mary Ewens, "The Leadership of Nuns in Immigrant Catholicism," in *Women and Religion in America*, vol. 1, *The Nineteenth Century*, ed. Rosemary Radford Ruether and Rosemary Skinner Keller (San Francisco: Harper and Row, 1981), 103.

34. The Irish Sisters of Charity assumed an Australian identity early and did not recruit from Ireland. However, the Australian community founded by Mary McKillop was most notably not Irish, yet it attracted Irish women in great numbers. See Janice Tranter, "The Irish Dimension of an Australian Religious Sisterhood: The Sisters of St. Joseph," in *The Irish World Wide*, vol. 5, *Religion and Identity*, ed. Patrick O'Sullivan (London: Leicester University Press, 1996), 234–55. In the United States, the Sisters of the Incarnate Word are one of the best examples of the Irish and German influence on a French community. See Sister Margaret Patrice Slattery, *Promises to Keep: A History of the Sisters of Charity of the Incarnate Word*, 2nd ed., 2 vols. (San Antonio: Sisters of the Incarnate Word, 1998).

35. "Secular" societies were comprised of ordinary citizens as opposed to priests or nuns. The *dévots* were not members of any religious community but "lay

persons," that is, ordinary communicants in the Catholic Church. It was both a male and female movement characterized by the pious devotions of wealthy families. See Elizabeth Rapley, *The Dévotes: Women and Church in Seventeenth-Century France* (Montreal: McGill University Press, 1995).

36. Colin Jones, *The Charitable Imperative: Hospitals and Nursing in Ancien Régime and Revolutionary France* (London: Routledge, 1989).

37. Ibid., 93.

38. Female groups such as the Beguines became widespread prior to the Reformation. These groups of women commonly took care of the sick but did not work in hospitals. In medieval times and during the Renaissance tertiaries were employed nursing in hospitals. These nurses were commonly widows and lived devout modest lives attached to particular institutions under the Augustinian rule.

39. Owen Hufton and Frank Tallet, "Communities of Women, the Religious Life, and Public Service in Seventeenth Century France," in *Connecting Spheres: Women in the Western World, 1500 to the Present,* ed. Marilyn H. Boxer and Jean H. Quatraert (New York: Oxford University Press, 1987), 75–85.

40. Vincent de Paul, in Rapley, *The Dévotes,* 86

41. Jones, *Charitable Imperative,* 116.

42. Ibid., 101.

43. Ibid., 147.

44. Dora B. Weiner, *The Citizen-Patient in Revolutionary and Imperial Paris* (Baltimore: Johns Hopkins University Press, 1993), 110.

45. Dora B. Weiner, "The French Revolution, Napoleon, and the Nursing Profession," *Bulletin of the History of Medicine* 46, 3 (1972): 274–305.

46. Claude Langlois, *Le Catholicisme au féminin: Les congrégations françaises à supérieure générale au XIXe siècle* (Paris: Éditions du Cerf, 1984), 307–13.

47. Even at the height of anticlericalism with the Third Republic, the state "was not yet prepared to provide the paramedical services, particularly nursing . . . closed down schools . . . would still call on religious orders to provide nursing staff for hospitals." Ralph Gibson, *A Social History of French Catholicism, 1789–1914* (London: Routledge, 1989), 109. In 1911 "the lay personnel necessary to replace in quantity and quality the *religieuses* currently employed does not exist."

48. Sheridan Gilley calls it "The Irish empire beyond the seas"; see "The Roman Catholic Church and the Nineteenth Century Irish Diaspora," *Journal of Ecclesiastical History* 35, 2 (1984): 188.

49. Caitrona Clear, *Nuns in Nineteenth Century Ireland* (Dublin: Gill and Macmillan, 1897), 37.

50. Hoy, "The Journey Out," 77, 79. So many probably came to Australia because Mother Michael, the founder, a Sister of Mercy, was cousin to Patrick Moran, archbishop of Sydney. One sodality in Dublin, George's Hill, sent out nearly 60 women to the U.S. Texas community Sisters of the Incarnate Word and produced seven superiors of the order from one parish!

51. Catherine M. Prelinger, *Charity, Challenge, and Change: Religious Dimensions of the Mid-Nineteenth-Century Women's Movement in Germany* (New York: Greenwood Press, 1987).

52. Florence Nightingale to H. E. Manning, 1852, BL Add Mss 9095/10.

53. There had been successive attempts throughout the centuries by women to establish a religious path that involved good works in the world. Each movement failed as the church continually imposed the cloister rule on female communities and refused to allow them a role in the world. See Jones, *The Charitable Imperative,* 97–99.

54. For detail on the innovations of the Vincentian model, see Sioban Nelson, "Entering the Professional Domain in Seventeenth Century France," *Nursing History Review* 7 (1999): 171–88.

55. Magray, *The Transforming Power of the Nuns*, 36–37.

56. Ewens, "The Leadership of Nuns," 103.

57. M. R. McGinley, *A Dynamic of Hope: Institutes of Women Religious in Australia* (Sydney: Crossing Press, 1996), 70

58. These texts were also read by Nightingale and were the subject of correspondence between herself and Mother Mary Moore of the Bermondsey Sisters of Mercy, who accompanied Nightingale to the Crimea and who remained something of a spiritual confessor to Nightingale in the years following. See Mary C. Sullivan, *The Friendship of Florence Nightingale and Mary Clare Moore* (Philadelphia: University of Pennsylvania Press, 1999).

59. Jones, *The Charitable Imperative*, 106–8 for a discussion of the conference system.

60. The conferences entered the religious literature with texts such as the *Imitatio Christi* as standard fare in religious training. They were particularly useful for nursing communities.

61. Magray, *The Transforming Power of the Nuns*, 119, offers examples of the lengths sisters went to have their own choice of priest appointed.

62. Cited in ibid., 118.

63. This was a long legal process that involved scrupulous documentation in Latin. It was always a great moment for a community when this was granted.

64. The Community of the Sisters of St. Joseph were another community with a motherhouse structure; Mother Seton's Sisters of Charity, too, had a motherhouse structure from the beginning. When they merged with the French Daughters of Charity in 1850 they of course assumed the original model of St. Vincent. The Irish Sisters of Charity have a motherhouse model, as do the French Canadian Daughters of Providence.

65. See Magray, *The Transforming Power of the Nuns*, 107–30; Coburn and Smith, " 'Pray for Your Wanderers'"; Ewens, The Leadership of Nuns," 128–37; and Thompson, "Women, Feminism, and the New Religious History," 142, 147 for a sample of the stories of hardship, exploitation, and downright cruelty that so many sisters endured.

66. Thompson, "Women, Feminism, and the New Religious History," 148.

67. For instance, Coburn and Smith relate the extraordinarily complex business dealings and negotiations that preceded the move of the Sisters of St. Joseph Carondelet into Colorado. They ensured that, unlike other sisterhoods, their property would be secure from the notorious bishop, who always did negotiations with lawyers in tow. See Coburn and Smith, " 'Pray for Your Wanderers.'"

68. See Stewart, *Marvels of Charity*, 97–99.

69. Catherine Prelinger's work is one of the few scholarly sources available in English on this period on women and religion in Germany. See *Charity, Challenge, and Change*, 10.

70. Fliedner was originally influenced by Elizabeth Fry's prison work; the nursing side of the operation, however, dominated from the early days. Abdel Ross Wentz, *Fliedner the Faithful* (Philadelphia: Board of Publications of the United Lutheran Church in America, 1936), 34.

71. Casteras, "Virgin Vows," 129–60.

72. Elizabeth Fry's group, called the Sisters of Mercy, were simply women who

undertook nursing duties after some training; they had references from their minister.

73. Monica E. Baly, *Florence Nightingale and the Nursing Legacy* (London: Croom Helm, 1986).

74. Ibid., 1–4.

75. Ibid., 34.

76. Monica E. Baly, "The Nightingale Nurses: The Myth and the Reality," in *Nursing History: The State of the Art*, ed. Christopher Maggs (London: Croom Helm, 1987), 33–59.

77. For an analysis of this revisionism see Sioban Nelson, "Reading Nursing History," *Nursing Inquiry* 4, 4 (1997): 229–36.

78. Anne Summers, "Ministering Angels," *History Today* 39 (February 1989): 31–37.

79. Anne Summers, Judith Moore, and Carol Helmstadter have contributed to our improved awareness of the importance of the St. John's House nurses in gaining credence for the notion of trained nursing. See Anne Summers, "The Cost and Benefits of Caring: Nursing Charities, c 1830–1860," in *Medicine and Charity Before the Welfare State*, ed. Jonathan Barry and Colin Jones (London: Routledge, 1991), 133–48 and Anne Summers, "Frameworks or Straitjackets? Secular and Religious Models in the Historiography of Nursing," in *Past Is Present: The CAHN/ACHN Keynote Presentations, 1988–1996*, ed. Sheila J. Rankin Zerr (Vancouver: Canadian Association for the History of Nursing, 1997), 31–37; Moore, *Zeal for Responsibility*. See also Carol Helmstadter, "Robert Bentley Todd, Saint John's House, and the Origins of the Modern Trained Nurse," *Bulletin of the History of Medicine* 67, 3 (1993): 282–319.

80. F. B. Smith, *Florence Nightingale: Reputation and Power* (London: Croom Helm, 1982), 27.

81. Summers, "Frameworks or Straitjackets?" 219.

82. See Summers, "The Cost and Benefits of Caring" and Helmstadter, "Robert Bentley Todd."

83. Colleen Adele Hobbs, *Florence Nightingale* (New York: Twayne, 1997), 12–13, 26.

84. Smith, *Reputation and Power*, 25–68.

85. Magray, *The Transforming Power of the Nuns*, 77–78.

86. Maher, *To Bind Up the Wounds*.

87. Katrin Schultheiss, " 'La Véritable médicine des femmes': Anna Hamilton and the Politics of Nursing Reform in Bordeaux, 1900–1914," *French Historical Studies* 19, 1 (Spring 1995).

88. The Sisters of Providence and Sisters of the Incarnate Word both delivered babies when need arose. In Buffalo the Daughters of Charity ran the maternity hospital.

89. Clear, *Nuns in Nineteenth Century Ireland*, 91, 127.

90. In my own nursing experience, when I worked at a major (non-Catholic) teaching hospital in Australia in the 1980s all male preoperative shaves and even catheterizations were performed by male "dressers."

Chapter 3. Free Enterprise and Resourcefulness

1. The Board that "sanctioned" building or considerable repair was made up of the sister servant as President and two other Daughters of Charity as secre-

tary and treasurer. Daughters of Charity Archives, Albany (hereafter DOCA), 11-33-01; A-1.

2. This figure does not include hospitals managed by the sisters but owned by the county or diocese. See George C. Stewart, Jr., *Marvels of Charity: History of American Sisters and Nuns* (Huntington, Ind.: Our Sunday Visitor, 1994), Appendix C, 515 for a complete list of these hospitals.

3. There have been French, French Canadian, and German communities of women inspired by the Daughters of Charity. Mother Seton was the first in what was to become an Irish, English, American, and Australian flood of English-speaking communities to follow this path, from Mary Aikenhead a decade later in Ireland to Mother Teresa in twentieth-century Calcutta.

4. By 1890 American Catholics constituted the largest denomination in the country, with over seven million members, or 12 percent of the population. See Charles Morris, *Saints and Sinners* (New York: Times Books, 1997), 84–85.

5. See Winthrop S. Hudson, *Religion in America: An Historical Account of the Development of American Religious Life* (New York: Scribner's, 1981) for a discussion of the Great Awakening in eighteenth-century New England, especially exemplified by the revivals led by George Whitefield (1714–70), and the decades of the Second Great Awakening in the early nineteenth century. These meetings certainly stirred commitment to the forces of Reformation and enmity toward Catholicism. Preacher Lyman Beecher delivered anti-Catholic sermons to the Boston crowds, days before a mob burned a convent to the ground. See Stewart, *Marvels of Charity*, 84.

6. Ibid., 94–95.

7. Maria Monk, *The Awful Disclosures of Maria Monk, or the Secrets of a Nun's Life in a Convent Exposed* (1836; New York: D.M. Bennett, 1878).

8. See Jenny Franchot, *Roads to Rome: The Antebellum Protestant Encounter with Catholicism* (Berkeley: University of California Press, 1993) for a discussion of this nineteenth-century "pulp fiction."

9. Christopher J. Kauffman, *Ministry and Meaning: A History of Catholic Health Care in the United States* (New York: Crossroad, 1995), 80.

10. See Joseph G. Mannard, "Converts in Convents: Protestant Women and the Social Appeal of Catholic Religious Life in Antebellum America," *Records of the American Catholic Historical Society of Philadelphia* 104, 1–4 (1993): 79–90. It would appear that in antebellum America the teaching sisters were very successful in "turning" some of their wards toward the Church and attracting recruits for their own communities.

11. See Franchot, *Roads to Rome* for an examination of Protestant representations of Catholicism in nineteenth-century America.

12. Mannard, "Converts in Convents," 79.

13. See Sioban Nelson, "Entering the Professional Domain in 17th Century France," *Nursing History Review* 7 (1999): 171–88.

14. This personal recollection from the author of a history of the Troy Hospital. Handwritten, c. 1891. DOCA, 11-23-01; 12-2/10 #2a.

15. Stewart, *Marvels of Charity*, 99.

16. The Sulpicians were a French community of priests who established the first seminary in the United States and acted as spiritual directors of the Emmitsburg motherhouse for a period.

17. Ibid.

18. Bernadette McCauley, " 'Sublime Anomalies': Women Religious and Ro-

man Catholic Hospitals in New York City 1850–1920," *Journal of the History of Medicine and Allied Sciences* 52 (July 1997): 60.

19. The five communities, in addition to the Daughters unified with France, were the Sisters of Charity of St. Vincent de Paul, New York; Sisters of Charity of St. Vincent de Paul, Halifax; Sisters of Charity, Cincinnati; Sisters of Charity of St. Elizabeth, Convent Station; Sisters of Charity of Seton Hill, Greenburg. See Stewart, *Marvels of Charity*, 103.

20. Margaret Susan Thompson, *To Serve the People of God: Nineteenth Century Sisters and the Creation of a Religious Life*, Cushwa Center Working Papers ser. 18, 2 (South Bend, Ind.: Cushwa Center for the Study of American Catholicism, University of Notre Dame,1987).

21. In the case of the Sisters of St. Joseph, their reorganization from diocesan communities to a centralized structure in 1860 placed the bishop of St. Louis, Bishop Kenrick, in the position of authority over all their American houses. Bishops from several dioceses, such as Buffalo, refused permission for their Sisters of St. Joseph even to attend the meeting to discuss the proposed changes in their constitution. The resulting split was devastating to the community. See Carol K. Coburn and Martha Smith, *Spirited Lives: How Nuns Shaped Catholic Culture and American Life, 1836–1920* (Chapel Hill: University of North Carolina Press, 1999), 56–60.

22. Stewart argues that the tension was also the result of French men, Sulpician and Vincentian priests, and Irish men, bishops and secular clergy. See Stewart, *Marvels of Charity*, 128.

23. Stewart, though a champion of the sisters, appears to fall into this trap. He writes as if the division of the American Sisters of Charity was a clash between men and the sisters were slightly dazed victims.

24. In Ireland there was utter disbelief (and fury) among the episcopate when the Christian Brothers won from Rome independence from clerical interference. The bishops declared that the Brothers would be banned from dioceses forthwith — it did not happen. See Emmet Larkin, *The Roman Catholic Church and the Creation of the Irish State* (Philadelphia: American Philosophical Society, 1975), 10–11.

25. Sister Bernadette Armiger, "The History of the Hospital Work of the Daughters of Charity of St. Vincent de Paul in the Eastern Province of the United States, 1823–1860" (Master of Science in Nursing Education thesis, Catholic University of America, 1947), 106.

26. Charles E. Rosenberg, *The Cholera Years: The United States in 1832, 1849, and 1866* (Chicago: University of Chicago Press, 1962).

27. See Sister Mary Gabriel Henninger, *Sisters of St. Mary and Their Healing Mission* (St. Louis: Sisters of St. Mary of the Third Order of St. Francis, 1979), 1, for a discussion of this process with the German Sisters of St. Mary, and Gerald A. Kelly, *The Life of Mother Hieronymo* (Rochester, N.Y.: Christopher Press, 1900) (DOCA, 11-33; 19-5/14 #1 5a, 2) for this process with the Daughters of Charity in the Northeast.

28. Kelly, *The Life of Mother Hieronymo*, 3.

29. See Peter Brown, *The Body and Society: Men, Women, and Sexual Renunciation in Early Christianity* (London: Faber and Faber, 1990).

30. Rosenberg, *The Cholera Years*, 139, cites correspondence for Richard Henry Dana to Mrs. Dana, 11 August 1848, Dana Papers, Massachusetts Historical Society: "In spite of all you say, I believe that if anybody goes to heaven from Boston it will be the Sisters of Charity and the Roman Catholic clergy."

31. It was a strategy that failed in Australia. First, the long sea voyage to Sydney functioned as a natural quarantine and epidemics were never as severe in Australia as elsewhere. Second, the state authorities quite rudely declined any offers from the sisters when the occasion did arise. They were most concerned that they would not be able to remove them afterward. But in the United States the epidemics were of such a severe nature that any assistance at all was impossible to refuse.

32. David Ward, *Cities and Immigrants: A Geography of Change in Nineteenth-Century America* (New York: Oxford University Press, 1978), 55.

33. Eulogies for the epidemic nurses abound. See Kauffman, *Ministry and Meaning*, 50–63 for the story of cholera nursing.

34. Timon to Rev. Louis Deluol, 10 April 1849, cited in Jean Richardson, "Catholic Religious Women as Institutional Innovators: The Sisters of Charity and the Rise of the Modern Urban Hospital in Buffalo, NY, 1848–1900" (PhD dissertation, State University of New York at Buffalo, 1996), 117–18.

35. *Buffalo Medical Journal*, quoted by Richardson.

36. Ibid.

37. Robert M. T. Hunter, Editorial, *Washington Sentinel*, 9 August 1855, cited by Armiger, "The History of the Hospital Work," 83.

38. Armiger, "The History of the Hospital Work," 86.

39. Ibid.

40. The Timon correspondence includes a letter from Thaddeus Amat to Timon, 26 February 1844, which discusses the proposal to put forward a petition to the legislature at New Orleans to ask for a portion of the land that is to be given to the Sisters of Charity, to include seven acres for a seminary because the sisters will need confessors. He says, "The legislature appears that all are generally well disposed to help us, particularly for the novitiate for the sisters." Vincentians Collection, IV3-N1, Archives of the University of Notre Dame.

41. Altogether thirty-five million European immigrants entered the United States in 1830–1930. In the peak year of 1854, 427,833 immigrants entered, of whom 215,000 were German and 102,000 Irish; see Philip Taylor, *The Distant Magnet: European Emigration to the U.S.A.* (London: Eyre & Spottiswoode, 1971), 62–63. The Irish sent by far the largest proportion of their emigrants to America (about five million). With the Great Famine, poor Catholic peasants vastly outnumbered the skilled Protestants who had previously represented the majority of Irish immigrants. See Patrick Blessing, "Irish Emigration to the United States, 1800–1920: An Overview," in *The Irish in America: Emigration, Assimilation, and Impact*, ed. P. J. Drudy (New York: Cambridge University Press, 1985).

42. David Gerber, *The Making of an American Pluralism, Buffalo, New York, 1825–60* (Urbana: University of Illinois Press, 1989), 311–13.

43. Ibid., 182–84.

44. Jean Richardson, "A Tale of Two Nineteenth Century Hospitals: Buffalo Hospital of the Sisters of Charity and Buffalo General Hospital," in *Medical History in Buffalo, Collected Essays*, ed. Lilli Stentz (Buffalo: School of Nursing and Biomedical Sciences, State University of New York at Buffalo, 1996), 47–60.

45. Ibid. The Annual Report for 1856 shows the importance of immigrant funding: of 487 patients, 216 are from Ireland, 144 from Germany, and only 63 from the United States. House Surgeon and Physician's Semi-Annual Report to the Board of Physicians and Surgeons, and staff of the Buffalo Hospital of the Sisters of Charity, October 1, 1855–April 1, 1856. *Buffalo Medical Journal* 12 (June 1856): 62.

46. Richardson, "Catholic Religious Women," 101.

47. The disbursement of public funds into hospitals owned by the sisters was not a move welcomed by all. Sisters in Buffalo received their funds unchallenged in 1849. Their 1850 application stirred anti-Catholic controversy, but they were funded in 1851. See Richardson, "Catholic Religious Women," 109–10. In fact, this payment was the subject of restrictive legislation in various states. Nonetheless, even where legislation did exist prohibiting taxpayers' funds from going to a Catholic foundation, it did in fact occur. The practice was even to survive a 1920 court challenge under the First Amendment. See Rosemary Stevens, *In Sickness and in Wealth: American Hospitals in the Twentieth Century* (New York: Basic Books, 1989), 315–16; and Kathleen M. Joyce, "Science and the Saints: American Catholics and Health Care, 1880–1930" (PhD dissertation, Princeton University, 1995), 76–116.

48. Richardson, "Catholic Religious Women," 112.

49. Ibid., 113.

50. DOCA, 11-23-01; 12-2/10 #2a.

51. Armiger, "The History of the Hospital Work," 78.

52. Kelly, *The Life of Mother Hieronymo*, 3; see also Armiger, "The History of the Hospital Work," 88.

53. Gail Farr Casterline, " 'Twice as Irish': History of St. Joseph's Hospital, Philadelphia, PA, 1849–1900" (paper, American Medical History, University of Pennsylvania, 1982), 22. DOCA 11-34; 1-2/2 #1. See also Gail Farr Casterline, "St. Joseph's and St. Mary's: The Origins of Catholic Hospitals in Philadelphia," *Pennsylvania Magazine of History and Biography* 108, 3 (1984): 291–314.

54. Ibid., 94.

55. Sister Celeste Cummings, "History of the Hospital Work and the Development of the Schools of Nursing of the Sisters of Charity in the Eastern Province (1860–1900)" (Master of Science in Nursing Education thesis, Catholic University of America, 1948), 17.

56. Ibid.

57. Ibid., 20.

58. Ibid.,12.

59. Stewart, *Marvels of Charity*, 76.

60. The role of the resident medical officer was problematic, as the sisters felt it was impossible for them to stay at the hospital with a young man.

61. For a discussion of marine hospitals, see John Jensen, "Before the Surgeon General: Marine Hospitals in Mid-19th Century America," *Public Health Reports* (November–December 1997): 112, 525–27.

62. The medical students were also a source of income for the sisters. See 125th Anniversary of Sisters Hospital, DOCA, 11-27-04; 7-2/5A #14, 6. See also significant dates for the Buffalo Hospital of the Sisters of Charity, DOCA, 11-27-00; 1-11 #1 a.

63. Richardson, "Catholic Religious Women," 222, 225–29.

64. Ibid., 233–34.

65. Ibid., 236–38.

66. Ibid., 238–39.

67. Charities Buffalo Annual Report, 1903, DOCA, 11-27-00, 1-11 #5, income from county patients $12,000, from private patients $39,000.

68. Casterline, "St. Joseph's and St. Mary's," 303.

69. Ibid., 297–98.

70. Ibid., 303.

71. St. Joseph's Hospital, 49th Annual Report, 1897, 36, DOCA 11-34-00; 1-1/2 #4.

72. Report of the Training School, St. Joseph's Philadelphia, 1897, 37, DOCA 11-34-00; 1-1/2 #5.

73. Mary Ewens, *The Role of the Nun in Nineteenth-Century America* (New York: Arno Press, 1978), 250–51.

74. R. Martin, "They Served the Sick, in North and South," *Military Medicine* (July 1961): 575, for a table of all military hospitals served by the Daughters during the war.

75. Kauffman, *Ministry and Meaning*, 83; Mary Denis Maher, *To Bind Up the Wounds: Catholic Sister Nurses in the U.S. Civil War* (New York: Greenwood Press, 1989).

76. However, for others hospital nursing opened up new possibilities, and orders for whom nursing had not been a primary focus, such as the Sisters of the Holy Cross, became enthusiastic hospital nurses. See Barbra Mann Wall, "Religion, Ethnicity, and Nursing: The Americanization of Irish Catholic Sister Nurses," in *Proceedings of the Conference on the History of Women Religious*, Loyola University, Chicago, June 1998 (Chicago, 1998).

77. Dorothy Dix was not a supporter of the nuns. They were not under her authority and had an untroubled relationship with the military that must have infuriated her. See Ewens, *The Nun in Nineteenth-Century America*, 221–40; Jane E. Schultz, "The Inhospitable Hospital: Gender and Professionalism in Civil War Medicine," *Signs* (Winter 1992): 367. The charges of proselytism appear to have foundation, but it is difficult to know which sisters responded in this way. It is possible that women more used to nursing a mix of Catholics and Protestants would be more sensitive to the sectarian issues and just do their job. The accounts of war nursing do not assist in clarifying this question.

78. Ewens, *The Nun in Nineteenth-Century America*, 221.

79. Grant had expressed a preference for a nursing sister to perform the honor as he felt their work had not been properly recognized, and his personal train was dispatched for Mother Josephine, veteran of the Battle of Perryville, Kentucky. See Stewart, *Marvels of Charity*, 185.

80. For instance, see the eulogies for Sister Hieronymo O'Brien of St. Mary's, Rochester. Hieronymo was something of a champion and hero for the thousands of soldiers she nursed. She saw them through a smallpox epidemic, had an officer dismissed for torturing the men, and refused to allow guards to be placed on soldiers in her hospital. See Kelly, *The Life of Mother Hieronymo*.

81. Ursula Stepsis and Dolores Liptak, eds., *Pioneer Healers: The History of Women Religious in American Health Care* (New York: Crossroad, 1989), 287.

82. *Daily National Intelligencer*, 5 June 1861, cited in Cummings, "History of the Hospital Work," 1.

83. *Washington Evening Star*, 29 June 1861, quoted in ibid., 3.

84. Ibid., 5. Moreover, when Congress decided to build a contagious hospital, the sisters offered the land and in return were given the contract to manage the institution. See *Washington Post*, 26 September 1899, quoted in ibid., 7. In 1901 they received a further $50,000 from Congress for an extension.

85. Kelly, *The Life of Mother Hieronymo*, 5.

86. The rate for these patients was $1.50 per week. Sister Hieronymo kept scrupulous records to back her applications for funding.

87. Sister Mary Edmund, "Brief History of St. Mary's Hospital Rochester," 1979. Archives of St. Mary's, Rochester, 3. DOCA, 11-33-00, 2-2/1 #2g.

88. Kelly, *The Life of Mother Hieronymo*, 10.

89. City Hospital opened in 1864 but was too small to take many soldiers. See Sister Delphine Steele, Historical sketch, St. Mary's, Rochester, DOCA, 11-33 2-21 #3, 12.

90. Ibid. See also the register of Civil War soldiers at St. Mary's, Rochester, 1864, DOCA, 11-33-00; 2-2/2 #2a; Edmund, "Brief History of St. Mary's Hospital Rochester," 4, DOCA, 11-33-00; 2-21/#2g.

91. Ibid., 15.

92. Elizabeth Blackwell and Emily Blackwell, *Medicine as a Profession for Women* (New York: W.H. Tinson, 1860), 11–12, quoted in Mannard, "Converts in Convents," 81.

93. Undated communication from Emmitsburg to St. Mary's Rochester. DOCA 11-33-00; 2-2, #2b.

94. Correspondence, St. Mary's Rochester Emmitsburg, 12 January 1875, DOCA, 11-27-02; 6-1/1 #3.

95. See minutes of St. Mary's Rochester directors' meetings, 1857–1949: gas stock purchase, 25 May 1889; authorize president (sister servant) to pay off floating debt, 1 May 1890. DOCA 11-33-01; Box A 1 #17.

96. Sisters Hospital at Buffalo was also very professionally conducted. See, for instance, the material on Sisters Hospital at Buffalo, Bond of Corporation, signed by Sister Ann Louise, DOCA, 11-27-02; 2-8 #1a; architect contract signed by Sister Alberta, 5 June 1861, 11-27-02; 2-9 #1a; mortgage documents, 11-27-01; 4-9 #2.

97. Sister Arcania, "This is the ground where the sisters have been burying medals for years — so they seem to be growing." St. Vincent's Asylum, 28 May 1884. DOCA, 11-43-00; 1-3/1 #1.

98. See Sister Mary Gabriel Henninger, *Sisters of Saint Mary and Their Healing Mission* (St. Louis: Sisters of St. Mary of the Third Order of Saint Francis, 1979), 362–64, for a collection of letters to St. Joseph and to the Blessed Virgin from Mother Odilia of the Sisters of St. Francis.

99. Armiger, "The History of the Hospital Work," 82.

100. 125th Anniversary of Sister Hospital, DOCA, 11-27-04; 7-2 5A #14, 10–11.

101. Armiger, "The History of the Hospital Work," 75.

102. Providence Hospital, Detroit, Archives, cited in Cummings, "History of the Hospital Work," 34. See also Armiger, "The History of the Hospital Work," 72–74.

103. Florence Nightingale to Manning, 1852, cited in Seymer, *A General History of Nursing* (London: Faber and Faber, 1932), 80.

104. For instance, Sister Hieronymo O'Brien saved the leg of a man she nursed in Buffalo. His gratitude was lifelong. He loaned her $1200 for the new hospital building, sent her a horse and a cow, and came down from Buffalo weekly to cut wood and tidy the hospital grounds. See Kelly, *The Life of Mother Hieronymo*, 7.

Chapter 4. Behind Enemy Lines

1. Colleen Adele Hobbs, *Florence Nightingale* (New York: Twayne, 1997), xiii.

2. A fact acknowledged by historians such as Monica Baly and Anne Summers, whose work emphasizes the contemporaneous movements that gradually increased in momentum and resulted in the formal reform of nursing and the establishment of nursing training in the final quarter of the nineteenth century. See Monica E. Baly, *Florence Nightingale and the Nursing Legacy* (London: Croom

Helm, 1986); Anne Summers, "The Mysterious Demise of Sarah Gamp: The Domiciliary Nurse and Her Detractors," *Victorian Studies* 32 (1989): 365–86; Anne Summers, "Ministering Angels," *History Today* 39 (February 1989): 31–37.

3. The next nursing foundation was that of Elizabeth Fry, established in 1840; see Anne Summers, "The Cost and Benefits of Caring: Nursing Charities, c 1830–1860," in *Medicine and Charity Before the Welfare State*, ed. Jonathan Barry and Colin Jones (London: Routledge, 1991), 133–48.

4. The Sisters of Mercy were established in Dublin on 12 December 1831, *Harvest of Mercy*, Convent of Mercy, Bermondsey (London: Winchester Press, n.d.).

5. In 1850, amid great controversy, the church hierarchy was formally reestablished, under Cardinal H. E. Wiseman. See Sheridan Gilley, "Protestant London, No-Popery and the Irish Poor, 1830–1860," *Recusant History* 10, 4 (1969): 210–30.

6. For a discussion of Ireland under the Penal Code, see Edward Brynan, *The Church of Ireland in the Age of Catholic Emancipation* (New York: Garland, 1982).

7. See John Bossy, *The English Catholic Community, 1570–1850* (London: Darton, Longman, and Todd, 1976), 295–390; or Sheridan Gilley's abundant work on English Catholicism, such as "The Roman Catholic Mission to the Irish in London," *Recusant History* 10, 3 (1969): 123–45 or "Protestant London."

8. Ultramontanism reasserted the "Rome" in Roman Catholicism. This emphasis was of particular importance in Britain with its increasingly prominent Anglo-Catholic tradition.

9. Infallibility, of course, also implied a political and social view of the world. The declaration of papal infallibility heightened tensions between Catholic conservative and liberal, socialist and nationalist movements in Europe. These apparently tangential events were keenly observed and given heightened meaning in the sectarian context of England. Unlikely as it may seem, tensions erupted in the so-called Garibaldi Riots between Irish pro-Vatican mobs and liberal mobs of nationalist Garibaldi supporters. See Sheridan Gilley, "The Garibaldi Riots of 1862," *Historical Journal* 16, 4 (1973): 697–732.

10. See Susan P. Casteras, "Virgin Vows," in *Religion in the Lives of English Women, 1760–1930*, ed. Gail Malmgreen (London: Croom Helm, 1986), 129–60, for a discussion of the power of the convent on the English social imagination.

11. Florence Nightingale to H. E. Manning, 15? July 1852, BL Add Mss 9095/10, photocopy Wellcome Institute, London.

12. John Henry Newman was a major figure in the Oxford movement, and his spiritual journey from Oxford don to Catholic cardinal was emblematic of Catholic pride and the conviction that its time had come in Britain. See Hugh McLeod, *Religion and Society in England, 1850–1914* (New York: St. Martin's Press, 1996), 39.

13. Conditions in Ireland under the Penal Codes in the eighteenth century were extremely severe; see Brynan, *The Church of Ireland*.

14. See Graham Davis on the "high spirited revelry" associated with Irish religious customs, in Davis, *The Irish in Britain, 1815–1914* (Dublin: Gill and Macmillan, 1991), 127.

15. Jean Delumeau, *Catholicism Between Luther and Voltaire: A New View of the Counter-Reformation*, trans. John Bossy (London: Burns and Oates, 1977), 4–16.

16. In France the number of vocations following the restoration of the monarchy was phenomenal. In 1878 there were 135,000 religious in France, seven for every thousand French women. See Ralph Gibson, *A Social History of French Catholicism, 1789–1914* (London: Routledge, 1989),109.

17. There is debate over the nature of Irish Catholicism and its measure. Those

who would call themselves Catholic as opposed to those who practice is just one important distinction. See Gerard Connolly, "Irish Catholic Myth or Reality? Another Sort of Irish and the Renewal of Catholic Professional Among Catholics in England, 1791–1918," in *The Irish in the Victorian City*, ed. Roger Swift and Sheridan Gilley (London: Croom Helm, 1985), 225–54 for a discussion of the measure of Catholicism.

18. Those who moved to Britain before 1861 tended to be more customary in their practice according to Davis, *The Irish in Britain*, 132.

19. Friedrich Engels, *The Condition of the Working Class in England* (1844; Oxford: Blackwell, 1971), 104.

20. The Irish population in England and Wales was 291,000 in 1841, 520,000 in 1851, and 602,000 in 1861 (3 percent of the total population, 5 percent of London, 25 percent of Liverpool). In Scotland the figures were 128,000 in 1841 and 207,000 in 1851 (7 percent of the total population,18 percent of Dundee). See Sheridan Gilley, "Irish Catholicism in Britain," in *Religion, State, and Ethnic Groups*, ed. Donal A. Kerr (Aldershot: Dartmouth Publishing, 1992), 229. It is important to note that Irish immigration was not numerically, religiously, economically, or socially homogeneous. See David Fitzpatrick, "A Curious Middle Place: The Irish in Britain, 1871–1920," in *The Irish in Britain, 1815–1939*, ed. Roger Swift and Sheridan Galley (Savage, Md.: Barnes and Noble, 1989), 14.

21. The *Times* asked, "is every English workingman always to carry an Irish family on his shoulders?" Davis, *The Irish in Britain*, 154.

22. See Sheridan Gilley, "Protestant London," for a discussion of the sanitation issues and reference to official reports on sanitation, cholera, and the Irish, 223; also Davis, *The Irish in Britain*, 154.

23. See Davis, *The Irish in Britain*, 109 for a discussion of the 1838 J. P. Kay report to the Board of Health.

24. See Steven Fielding, *Class and Ethnicity: Irish Catholics in England, 1880–1939* (Buckingham: Open University Press, 1993), 5–18 for a discussion of anti-Irish attitudes.

25. See M. A. G. O'Tuathraigh, "The Irish in Nineteenth-Century Britain, Problems of Integration," in *The Irish in Britain*, ed. Swift and Gilley, 13–36.

26. *Punch* was full of just such cartoons. L. P. Curtis, Jr., *Anglo-Saxons and Celts: A Study of Anti-Irish Prejudice in Victorian England* (Bridgeport, Conn: University of Bridgeport Conference on British Studies, 1968) and *Apes and Angels: The Irishman in Victorian Caricature* (Washington, D.C.: Smithsonian Institution Press, 1971) studies this issue; Noel Ignatiev, *How the Irish Became White* (New York: Routledge, 1995) deals with these issues in the much more racialized American context.

27. There were only five Irish speakers among the twenty-one Irish-born priests in London in 1842. See Gilley, "Roman Catholic Mission," 141. Irish-speaking congregations such as Bermondsey were the subject of enthusiastic proselytism from Irish-speaking Protestants; see Alan Bartlett, "From Strength to Strength: Roman Catholicism in Bermondsey up to 1939," in *The Church and the People: Catholics and Their Church in Britain, c.1880–1939* (Warwick: Centre for the Study of Social History, University of Warwick, 1988), 30.

28. In 1851 40 percent of the seats in London Catholic churches were paid for by pew rents and not free to members of the congregation. Davis, *The Irish in Britain*, 148.

29. For instance, Belgian Joseph Buggenoms "dedicated himself to the Irish in London," Bartlett,, 138. Often, however, the Irish insisted on Irish priests,

frequently coming into conflict with others. The Belgian-led Redemptorists organized spectacularly successful retreats conducted in the East End by Redemptorists brought from Limerick for the occasion; see Gilley, "Roman Catholic Mission," 141.

30. The appointment of prelates was tricky. Rome appeared to favor some kind of rationalization of the complex Irish and British hierarchy; however, their suggestion that they appoint a nuncio for England who would be in charge of Ireland was shouted down in rare unison by the Irish bishops. Rome of course was anti-revolutionary and very suspicious of Irish nationalism. See Emmet Larkin, *The Roman Catholic Church and the Creation of the Modern Irish State, 1878–1886* (Philadelphia: American Philosophical Society, 1975). See also Gilley, "Irish Catholicism in Britain," 240.

31. There had long been an Irish community at Bermondsey. According to Bartlett, "From Strength to Strength," 30, one subdistrict reached 15 percent Irish-born in 1851.

32. A vicar apostolic was a bishop appointed by the Congregatio Propaganda Fide (Congregation for the Propagation of the Faith) in Rome to an area not yet created as a territorial diocese. I am grateful to Rosa MacGinley for explaining this to me.

33. Cork was thought to be a more discreet site for such celebrated postulants. Miss Agnew was the niece of Sir Andrew Agnew and the author of a popular three-part religious novel called *Geraldine, a Tale of Conscience* (Philadelphia: E. Cummiskey, 1819); see Denis G. Murphy, *Terra Incognita or the Convents of the United Kingdom* (London: Longmans, 1873), 165. These aristocratic converts were a major coup for the newly established church: they provided a high profile with excessive media coverage, they offered a counter to the ignorant Irish Paddy image of Catholicism, and they gave a great deal of money to the Church. See Mary Austin Carroll, RSM, *Leaves from the Annals of the Sisters of Mercy*, 3 vols., vol. 2, *Concerning Sketches of the Order in England, Crimea, Scotland, Australia, and New Zealand* (New York: Catholic Publication Society, 1883), 27.

34. It was an apprehensive time for the sisters. As Mother McAuley wrote, "nine masses to be offered for us tomorrow, thank God! Father O'Hanlon is alarmed at the angry things said in the English papers." They traveled as unobtrusively as possible; Reverend Mother was addressed as "friend Catherine" for the journey. Carroll, *Leaves from the Annals*, 2: 53.

35. Pugin's work personified the Gothic and romantic obsessions of the period. Mother McAuley was unmoved, declaring it not to her taste. " I do not like Mr Pugin's taste, though so celebrated. . . . He was determined we should not look out of the windows — they are in the ceiling." Mother McAuley, letter from Bermondsey to Charleville, 26 December 1839. Archives of the Sisters of Mercy, Bermondsey.

36. Moore is a good example of the impressive experience a young and able woman could build up over a short period of time. She joined the Sisters of Mercy as Georgiana Moore at the age of seventeen and was fully professed at just under nineteen; she was often consulted by Mother McAuley when compiling the Holy Rule; at about twenty-one she was sent as local superior to the first branch house at Kingston near Dublin; at twenty-four she set up the new establishment in Cork. At twenty-six she accompanied two English sisters she had trained back to England for twelve months to oversee the establishment of a convent in England and governed that house for thirty-three years. See Life of Mother Mary Clare Moore,

Annals of the Convent of Our Lady of Mercy, Bermondsey, 216–20, Archives of the Sisters of Mercy, Bermondsey.

37. Carroll, *Leaves from the Annals*, 62–63.

38. One of the women entering the community was Lady Barbara Eyre, daughter of the earl of Newburgh. "The Convent of Mercy, Bermondsey," *Southwark Record*, January 1932, 15–19. Archives of the Sisters of Mercy, Bermondsey. According to the *Annals*, "several bishops and about forty priests were . . . in all the richest robes. The church was gay with the court-dress of the ladies . . . [and] foreign ambassadors." At the breakfast following the long ceremony the fire had to be rekindled and Lord Augustus Fitzclarence, son of William IV, insisted on making the fire for the sisters. Carroll, *Leaves from the Annals*, 62, 66.

39. Carroll, *Leaves from the Annals*, 65.

40. Ibid., 57. "That convent [Bermondsey] has never been without persons under instruction for reception into the Church. In the early days they came by hundreds."

41. In 1840 the sisters' first "martyr" fell victim to a "malignant fever."

42. See Carroll, *Leaves from the Annals*, 5. But the Mercies were not the only community to establish convents in England. In fact convents proliferated to such an extent that by 1900 there were 600 convents in England and Wales with 8,000–10,000 nuns. McLeod, *Religion and Society in England*, 166.

43. In London the various establishments of the Sisters of Mercy worked hard among the poor, visiting workhouses and hospitals and caring for the indigent. By their own account they were warmly received in these institutions. Carroll, *Leaves from the Annals*, 288. They opened a night refuge in 1860 (296); the House of Mercy in Blandford Square for homeless girls with a creche for the infants of the working poor was opened in 1873 (285–87).

44. According to Carroll, the nuns on occasion were summoned to the deathbed of a benefactor, perhaps at the request of a bishop (83).

45. The story of Nightingale in the Crimea has been told and retold from many perspectives. Important to this narrative are the accounts by the Sisters of Mercy of their work in Crimea, which are critical of Nightingale; see Evelyn Bolster, *The Sisters of Mercy in the Crimean War* (Cork: Mercier Press, 1964) and more recently the excellent work of Mary Ellen Doona, "Sister Mary Joseph Croke: Another Voice from the Crimean War, 1854–1856," *Nursing History Review* 3 (1995): 3–41, which brings to light the clinical competence of the nuns as a consequence of their experience and discipline.

46. Carroll, *Leaves from the Annals*, 89.

47. In 1840 three sisters died of typhus after caring for an afflicted family. The letter of condolence from Bishop Griffiths demonstrates the heroic approach to such deaths: "Dear Reverend Mother: I seize the first opportunity to congratulate with you and all the dear sisters on this first martyr of charity offered to Almighty God." Ibid., 73.

48. Ibid., 84.

49. Carroll writes delicately of the strange behavior at Bermondsey when the convent was under the leadership of Sister Clare Agnew, author of *Geraldine*. Their superior required them to be of the same height, distressed at their uneven appearance in church. To solve this dilemma she ordered padding to be worn under the habits of certain sisters to make them taller. She also implemented a seating arrangement over meals that avoided eye contact between women — she had them seated back-to-back. Ibid., 87–88.

50. Lady Barbara Eyre joined with a full wardrobe of garments. As her humility developed she gradually gave away all her possessions. Ibid., 78–79.

51. In 1840, in addition to the aristocratic connection, new recruits included Miss Louisa Birch, the granddaughter of Zephaniah Holwell, governor of Calcutta of Black Hole of Calcutta fame; Miss Celeste Beste was the daughter of a Protestant minister. Ibid., 67.

52. See Bolster, *The Sisters of Mercy in the Crimean War*, 14.

53. Rome took the Irish part in this drama, chastising the English Catholic hierarchy for allowing Mother Moore to be under Miss Nightingale's authority; see Bolster, *The Sisters of Mercy in the Crimean War*, 21.

54. The goal of the Irish contingent was not to make a public relations coup for Catholic tolerance in Britain, but to support the one-third of the British Army who were Irish. Wiseman claimed in 1863 that a quarter of the army in the Crimea had been Catholic and without chaplains. See Nicholas Patrick Stephen Cardinal Wiseman, address to the Catholic Congress of Malines, Belgium, 21 August 1864, in *The Religious and Social Position of Catholics in England* (Dublin: James Duffy, 1864), 183.

55. See Walter L. Arnstein, *Protestant Versus Catholic in Mid-Victorian England: Mr. Newdegate and the Nuns* (Columbia: University of Missouri Press, 1982).

56. Carroll, *Leaves from the Annals*, 135.

57. As Cardinal Wiseman declared in his speech to the Catholic Congress of Malines, 1864, "since then we have had no more attempts to interfere with ladies who have proved themselves as patriotic as they are virtuous,"183.

58. See Louis Marteau, *The Hospital of St. John and St. Elizabeth* (London: Hospital of St. John and St. Elizabeth, 1992), 5.

59. In fact, after Wiseman died Manning assumed control of the hospital and tried to replace the Sisters of Mercy with French Sisters of Charity. Nightingale was incensed and applied all the direct and indirect pressure she could to have them keep the hospital. In the end they kept the hospital but their sister in charge left the institution. See Mary C. Sullivan, *The Friendship of Florence Nightingale and Mary Clare Moore* (Philadelphia: University of Pennsylvania Press, 1999), 149–51.

60. Their work among homeless women and children was something they undertook with special enthusiasm. See Carroll, *Leaves from the Annals*, 285–301.

61. Susan Mumm claims they did not wear their habit in public, but this is misleading. Mumm, *Stolen Daughters, Virgin Mothers: Anglican Sisterhoods in Victorian Britain* (London: Leicester University Press, 1999), 78. The early travels of the Sisters of Mercy were not in habit but incognito (1840s). By the time of the Crimea (1854) they were wearing habits abroad. See Fanny M. Taylor et al., *Eastern Hospitals and English Nurses: The Narrative of Twelve Months' Experience in the Hospitals of Koulali and Scutari*, 2 vols. (London: Hurst and Blackett, 1856), 316.

62. T. Bowman Stephenson, *Concerning Sisterhoods* (London: C.H. Kelly, 1890), 78.

63. There was constant confusion among Protestants over the names of Catholic religious communities. Even Nightingale, normally well informed about such matters, thought the Sisters of Mercy ran St. Vincent's Hospital in Dublin, whereas it was the Sisters of Charity. The French Soeurs de Charité commonly referred to, actually the Filles de Charité (Daughters), had no connection with the Irish community.

64. This popularity of Vincent de Paul is discussed in Gilley, "Heretic London, Holy Poverty, and the Irish Poor," *Downside Review* 89 (1971): 72.

65. For a discussion of the Victorian intersection of the moral and physical

worlds, see Richard Helmstadter and Paul T. Phillips, eds., *Religion in Victorian Society: A Sourcebook of Documents* (Lanham, Md.: University Press of America, 1985), in particular, Phillips, "Converting the Working Classes," 211–63; and F. K. Prochaska, "Body and Soul: Bible Nurses and the Poor in Victorian London," *Historical Research* 60, 143 (1987): 336–34.

66. Pusey and his young daughter—who unfortunately died at fifteen before fulfilling their joint wish that she establish a sisterhood—visited Ireland in 1841–42. See Thomas Jay Williamson, *Priscilla Sellon, the Restorer After Three Centuries of the Religious life in the Anglican Church* (London: SPCK, 1950), 11, 12.

67. Hobbs, *Florence Nightingale*, 12.

68. Anna Jameson's public lecture is much cited secular comment on this internal debate. See Anna Jameson, *Sisters of Charity, Catholic and Protestant, Abroad and at Home* (London: Longmans, 1855). See also J. Master, "A Few Words to Some of the Women of the Church of God" (London, 1850, reprinted in Dale A. Johnson, *Women in English Religion, 1700–1925* (New York: Edwin Mellen, 1983), 17–23.

69. William Augustus Muhlenberg, ed., *Thoughts on Evangelical Sisterhoods* (London: S.W. Partridge and Co, 1872), 3.

70. John Henry Newman, *Apologia Pro Vita Sua* (1864; New York: Penguin, 1994), 50.

71. Peter Frederick Anson, *The Call of the Cloister: Religious Communities and Kindred Bodies in the Anglican Communion* (London: SPCK, 1955) remains one of the best general texts on this subject. See also A. M. Allchin. *The Silent Rebellion: Anglican Religious Communities, 1845–1900* (London: SCM, 1958).

72. Christopher Wordsworth, Bishop of Lincoln, *On Sisterhoods and Vows: A letter to the Ven. Sir George Provost* (London: Rivingtons, 1879), 20.

73. The life of the deaconess was never as popular as that of the sister, although this astounded many (male) church leaders. Mumm estimates that there were 3000 to 4000 members of sixty Anglican sisterhoods in 1900. Deaconess figures are harder to determine and of course extend beyond Anglicanism; however, contemporary sources agree with Mumm that there were far fewer deaconesses than sisters. See Rev. Leighton Coleman, "English Sisterhoods and Deaconesses," *Church Magazine* (1886): 425; and Mumm, *Stolen Daughters, Virgin Mothers*, 152.

74. See Coleman, "English Sisterhoods and Deaconesses," 429–30 and Sean Gill, *Women and the Church of England: From the Eighteenth Century to the Present* (London: SPCK, 1994), 165.

75. Gill, *Women and the Church of England*, 166.

76. This community, however, slipped steadily toward Anglo-Catholicism, and in 1887 the Head Sister became Mother Superior. Ibid., 165.

77. North London Deaconess Institute, *The Second Annual Report and Balance Sheet of the North London Deaconess Institute* (London: Printed by Varty,1863), 6.

78. Ibid., 8.

79. It adds that those who "possess exceptional spiritual and mental force" will not be excluded. Prospectus of the Institute, published in Stephenson, *Concerning Sisterhoods*, 95.

80. Stephenson, *Concerning Sisterhoods*, 426.

81. Edward Bouverie Pusey in Bishop Lidden's *Life of Pusey*, cited in Lucy Ridgely Seymer, *A General History of Nursing* (New York: Macmillan,1932), 73.

82. Stephenson, *Concerning Sisterhoods*, 48 claims that Sellon had carpet laid for her as she walked up her spiral staircase and then pulled up—several times a day.

83. Ibid.

84. Mumm does not give details as to who wrote the rule or who acted as confessor.

85. The Order of the Holy Cross was founded by Pusey in 1845. St. John's House was another male initiative in 1848. Once these early foundations created the precedent, the women were quite capable of doing it on their own.

86. Mumm, *Stolen Daughters, Virgin Mothers*, 137–65. The fluidity of the Anglican sisterhoods in the nineteenth century mirrors that of the Catholic sisterhoods in the first few decades of the century. As a new and growing phenomenon the sisterhoods were able to take advantage of the lack of clarity from Rome if they were Catholic, from the diocese if they were Anglicans.

87. Neale apparently thought of the community as "his." He claims in a letter of 1 February 1855 that "my little cub was beginning to take good properties; the next thing was to feed him. Just then came the scutter business, on this I took courage and wrote to everyone in our part of the diocese. . . . I had not a single demurer to the scheme," *Letters of John Mason Neale*, ed. daughter Mary Sackville Lawson (London: Longmans, 1920), 235.

88. See Mumm, *Stolen Daughters, Virgin Mothers*, 186.

89. Gill, *Women and the Church of England*, 81.

90. Ellen Schell, "Nurses Under Attack: The Lewes Riot and the Society of St. Margaret," *Nursing Research* 41, 1 (1992): 33–38 and Mumm, *Stolen Daughters, Virgin Mothers*, 186 give full details of the scandal and the funeral riot.

91. Mumm, *Stolen Daughters, Virgin Mothers*, 82–83.

92. Ibid., 21.

93. Mumm found instructions so detailed that she argued that the well-born novices must have been exceedingly ignorant of practical matters such as "shut window when it rains." Ibid., 24.

94. Ibid., 20.

95. Mumm's data claim that 34 percent of women who left communities did so to become Catholics. Ibid., 223.

96. The Gorham judgment on infant baptism caused great controversy — the decision was that nonbaptized infants were condemned to hell. Ibid., 143. Nightingale was appalled; see Hobbs, *Florence Nightingale*, 43–46.

97. The actual length of training was variable, from a few weeks to some months. Ladies were considered to require less training.

98. Mumm, *Stolen Daughters, Virgin Mothers*, 114; Carol Helmstadter, "Old Nurses and New: Nursing in the London Teaching Hospitals Before and After the Mid-Nineteenth-Century Reforms," *Nursing History Review* 1 (1993): 43–70, 58; Helmstadter, "Robert Bentley Todd, St. John's House, and the Origins of the Modern Trained Nurses," *Bulletin of the History of Medicine* 67 (1993): 282–319, 319; and Summers, "The Cost and Benefits of Caring" agree on this point.

99. Summers, "The Cost and Benefits of Caring."

100. Helmstadter discusses his reforms of medical teaching at King's; see "Robert Bentley Todd," 286–90.

101. Judith Moore, *A Zeal for Responsibility: The Struggle for Professional Nursing in Victorian England, 1868–1883* (Athens: University of Georgia Press, 1988), 7.

102. By 1873 they had rejected five other hospitals. Ibid.

103. Sister Mary Jones, Minute Book of the Council of St. John's House, July 1864–January 1876, 99. Cited in Moore, *A Zeal for Responsibility*, 9.

104. Moore, 136.

105. Ibid., 130.

106. Ibid., 152.

107. Ibid., 165. Many requests came from New Zealand, the Sandwich Islands, and so forth. They did pursue their nursing and remained influential, particularly for missions.

108. See Summers, "The Cost and Benefits of Caring" and Anne Summers, "Frameworks or Straitjackets? Secular and Religious Models in the Historiography of Nursing,"*Past Is Present: The CAHN/ACHN Keynote Presentations, 1988–1996*, ed. Sheila J. Rankin Zerr (Vancouver: Canadian Association for the History of Nursing, 1997), 215–39.

109. Mumm, *Stolen Daughters, Virgin Mothers*, 115.

110. This is not to say that there were no new hospitals in England in the nineteenth century. However, England had experienced successive waves of hospital foundation from Norman to Georgian times. On the other hand in the United States there were only three hospitals by 1821. According to J. Vogel, "When Boston's first general hospital opened in 1821, there were only two other such institutions in the United States." Vogel, *The Invention of the Modern Hospital* (Chicago: University of Chicago Press, 1980), 1. In Colonial New South Wales there was one hospital in 1820.

111. Dora B. Weiner shows how Napoleon made an exception for the nursing sisterhoods; see *The Citizen-Patient in Revolutionary and Imperial Paris* (Baltimore: Johns Hopkins University Press, 1993), 4. Kulturkampf decrees, too, exempted nursing sisterhoods; see Jonathon Sperber, *Popular Catholicism in Nineteenth-Century Germany* (Princeton, N.J.: University Press, 1984), 223.

112. For a discussion of the dilemma of Victorian women, and Florence Nightingale in particular, see Martha Vicinus, *Independent Women: Work and Community for Single Women, 1850–1920* (Chicago: University of Chicago Press, 1985); Mary Poovey, *Uneven Developments: The Ideological Work of Gender in Mid-Victorian England* (Chicago: University of Chicago Press, 1988); Florence Nightingale, *Ever Yours, Florence Nightingale: Selected Letters*, ed. Martha Vicinus and Bea Nergaard (London: Virago Press, 1989); Elaine Showalter, "Florence Nightingale's Feminist Complaint: Women, Religion, and *Suggestions for Thought*," *Signs: Journal of Women in Culture and Society* 6, 3 (1981): 395–412 .

113. Nightingale to Manning, 15? July 1852, BL Add Mss 9095/10, Photocopy Wellcome Institute, London. Manning did not consider her good material for conversion, as she valued her own interpretation of Christianity too highly, and he apparently thought the obedience required of the religious life would not be possible for her to attain. She seemed to agree with his assessment and recovered from her flirtation with conversion.

114. Nightingale's correspondence can be quoted as anti-nun or as very supportive and admiring. Nursing nuns were not all the same, and Nightingale understood this. It was the context, their professionalism, and their work ethic that mattered to her. As a young woman in Alexandria she found "nineteen Sisters of Charity doing the work of ninety." "On Different Systems of Hospital Nursing," appendix to *Notes on Hospitals* (1859), reprinted in *Florence Nightingale on Hospital Reform*, ed. Charles E Rosenberg (New York: Garland, 1989), 181–87.

115. With Manning's assistance she was able to gain permission to enter the Maison de la Providence in Paris as a "postulant" to receive nursing training. She was to wear a habit and work under the direction of the sisters. She was to take meals and sleep separately from the nuns. She caught measles within two weeks and was forced to abandon the exercise. Denis G. Murphy, *They Did Not Pass By: The Story of the Early Pioneers of Nursing* (London: Longmans, 1956).

116. The religious tension in the Crimea came as much from Nightingale as

anyone else. Mother Bridgeman's diary records harmonious relationships with the doctors, most of whom she describes as "Protestant dissenters." The sisters even starched the ministerial collars for the chaplains when they laundered their own veils. See Bolster, *The Sisters of Mercy in the Crimean War*, 140–41.

117. See, for instance, Taylor et al., *Eastern Hospitals and English Nurses* and Elizabeth Davis, *The Autobiography of Elizabeth Davis, a Balaclava Nurse, Daughter of Dafydd Cadwaladyr*, ed. Jane Williams, 2 vols. (London: Hurst and Blackett, 1857).

118. See Anne Summers, *Angels and Citizens: British Women as Military Nurses, 1854–1915* (London: Routledge, 1988).

119. Ibid.,71.

120. Bolster, *The Sisters of Mercy in the Crimean War*, 15.

121. Florence Nightingale to Benjamin Jowett, 1889, BL Add. Mss 45,785, cited in JoAnn G. Widerquist, "Dearest Rev'd Mother," in *Florence Nightingale and Her Era: A Collection of New Scholarship*, ed. Vern Bullough, Bonnie Bullough, and Marietta P. Stanton (New York: Garland, 1990), 302.

122. Edward Cook claims that Nightingale thought nursing "the least important of all the functions into which she had been forced." Cook, *The Life of Florence Nightingale*, 2 vols. (London: Macmillan, 1913),1: 234.

123. Helmstadter, "Robert Bentley Todd," 310; see also Seymer, *A General History of Nursing*, 20–23.

124. I am grateful to Carol Helmstadter for pointing out the fact that improvements in accommodation for nurses had been underway since the 1830s, predating the "moral reform" issues that later dominated nurses' residences.

125. Florence Nightingale, cited in Desiree Edward-Rees, *The Story of Nursing* (London: Constable Young Books, 1965), 60.

126. Monica Baly, "The Nightingale Nurses: The Myth and the Reality," in *Nursing History: The State of the Art*, ed. Christopher Maggs (London: Croom Helm, 1987).

127. As the font of all knowledge she was consulted on the establishment of hospital services for the U.S. government during the Civil War, and as a result of her efforts in the Franco-Prussian War she was, incredibly, decorated by both sides. She was awarded the Bronze Cross by the Société de Secours au Blessés by the French and the Prussian Cross of Merit by the Kaiser in 1871; see Florence Nightingale, *As Miss Nightingale Said: Florence Nightingale Through Her Sayings: A Victorian Perspective*, ed. Monica Baly (London: Scutari Press, 1991), 36.

Chapter 5. At the Margins of the Empire

1. It was an expensive trip from England. It took four months; passengers had to provide for their own sustenance and required enough changes of clothing to allow for a clean outfit each week (no water wasted on laundry). See A. W. Martin, *Henry Parkes: A Biography* (Carlton, Vic.: Melbourne University Press, 1980), 10–25.

2. The rectresses of St. Vincent's hospital were women of education and substance, according to Catherine O'Carrigan, "Australian Catholic Hospitals in the Nineteenth Century," *Journal of the Australian Catholic Historical Society* 7, 4 (1964): 20–36. "The four rectresses of the nineteenth century St. Vincent's were its foundress, Mother Baptist de Lacy, trained in Dublin St. Vincent's; Mother Joseph O'Brien; her sister Mother Veronica O'Brien, both educated in France and first cousins of Sir Dominic Corrigan, the eminent Dublin physician. The first

Australian-born nurse and long-serving rectress, Mother Xavier Cunningham, in contrast, was the granddaughter of convicts" (22).

3. Anti-Catholicism and sectarian rivalry was no small issue in colonial Sydney, but it was still mild compared to North America. There were no "Know-nothings" or Nativist movement equivalents in Australian history. Nonetheless there were notable anti-Catholic figures, and Henry Parkes gave a famed "Immigration Speech" that tried to tap into the voting powers of those frightened that the colony was becoming Irish. Despite the rhetoric and inflammatory speeches, the nursing Sisters of Charity were often exempt from much of this hatred.

4. The Royal Prince Alfred Hospital was opened late in 1882 and took some years to become established. There was a lunatic asylum, and regional hospitals appeared with settlement. However St. Vincent's and the Sydney Infirmary remained the only major hospitals until the 1890s.

5. As the British government intended, New South Wales, so remote an outpost, was a place of exile from which few could expect to return.

6. B. R. Mitchell, *International Historical Statistics: Africa, Asia and Oceania, 1750–1988*, 2nd rev. ed. (New York: Stockton, 1995), 63; and Mitchell, *International Historical Statistics: The Americas and Australasia* (Detroit: Gale Research, 1983), 77, 95.

7. Van Diemen's Land is the island known as Tasmania after 1855.

8. The settlement of New South Wales involved the dispossession of its Aboriginal population. See Henry Reynolds, *Dispossession: Black Australians and White Invaders* (Sydney: Allen and Unwin, 1989).

9. This was to change by the 1870s, when women (in particular Irish women) in Sydney for a while outnumbered men. The story up country was quite different, and men continued to outnumber women significantly in overall terms. See Shirley Fitzgerald, *Rising Damp: Sydney 1870–90* (Melbourne: Oxford University Press, 1987), 179.

10. If the women's babies survived to the age of two they were transferred to the Orphan School. Ruth Teale, ed., *Colonial Eve: Sources on Women in Australia, 1788–1914* (Melbourne: Oxford University Press, 1978), 18.

11. Rosa MacGinley, *A Dynamic of Hope: Women Religious Institutes in Australia* (Sydney: Crossing Press, 1996), 702.

12. They also brought music. Such was the joy in singing that, according to legend, one woman escaped the Refectory one evening to serenade the sisters in appreciation before returning to her dormitory. Private communication with Sister Catherine O'Carrigan, historian of the Sisters of Charity, Potts Point, Sydney.

13. Miriam Dixson, *The Real Matilda: Women and Identity in Australia, 1788–1975* (Sydney: Penguin Books, 1976), 119–20. No convict women were sent to Van Diemen's Land from Ireland.

14. Patrick O'Farrell, *The Irish in Australia*, rev. ed. (Kensington: New South Wales University Press, 1993), 23.

15. Polding to Propaganda Fide, October 1839. *The Letters of John Bede Polding*, ed. M. Xavier Compton et al. (Sydney: Good Samaritan Sisters, 1994), vol. 1, 146

16. This move was in conformity with their rule. The sisters considered that their vow of poverty prevented them from receiving payment.

17. Sister O'Brien was particularly incensed at this. Her poverty in Sydney was beyond her worst expectations. Her dowry had been £1,300 — a substantial sum — and to be begging from the bishop and surviving on donations of food was very hard. Maureen M. K. O'Sullivan, *A Cause of Trouble? Irish Nuns and English Clerics* (Sydney: Crossing Press, 1995), 62.

18. MacGinley, *Dynamic of Hope*, 67.

19. Rule formulated with Jesuit assistance. The other Jesuit influence comes from the York House of Mary Ward, where Mary Aikenhead undertook her novitiate in preparation for establishing the Sisters of Charity. See MacGinley, *Dynamic of Hope*, 70.

20. However, the permission of the bishop was always required for works within his diocese.

21. *A Century of Service: The Record of One Hundred Years*, published for the Centenary of St. Vincent's Hospital, 23 January 1934 (Dublin: Browne and Nolan, 1934), 20–21.

22. The Mother Rectress controlled the hospital — nurses and medical men. "It is to her that the Medical staff are responsible for all that concerns the scientific welfare of the hospital. She also ratifies the nomination of all medical officers, though bestowal of staff appointments is reserved for the Head Superior (of the community). Disbursement is entirely in her hands," Ibid., 30.

23. Ibid., 64–66.

24. Sister de Sales (Catherine O'Brien) had trained at the Hôpital de la Piétie, run by the Hospitalières of Thomas de Villeneuve. Her 1833 notebook (in French) contained medical and nursing information. She also spent a month at Le Havre Children's Hospital and had a knowledge of dispensing. O'Brien went to Hobart in 1847 to escape Polding's persecution. Sister Baptist (Alicia de Lacy) trained at St. Vincent's in Dublin. See "200 Years of Nursing, a Photographic History," Bicentennial lift out, *The Lamp*, April 1988.

25. See Anne-Maree Whitaker, "The Convict Priests: Irish Catholicism in Early Colonial New South Wales," in *The Irish World Wide: History, Heritage, Identity*, vol. 5, *Religion and Identity*, ed. Patrick O'Sullivan (London: Leicester University Press, 1996), 25–40. Particularly during the French Wars these Catholic convicts and their priests were regarded with considerable suspicion. For a discussion of Christian churches in eighteenth- and nineteenth-century Sydney see Geoffrey Partington, *The Australian Nation: Its British and Irish Roots* (Melbourne: Australian Scholarly Publishing, 1994), 1–28.

26. O'Carrigan, "Sisters of Charity," 2.

27. There were three deaths in 1835. See O'Sullivan, *A Cause of Trouble?*, 235.

28. Ibid., 123 for a discussion of the attempted dispossession of the sisters of Charity of their Parramatta convent.

29. In 1854 Miss Mary Ann Cunningham, who was to become the first Australian trained nurse, and its longest serving, dying as rectress of St. Vincent's Hospital in 1903, arrived to join the community and be trained as a nurse. She was sent away until the community had a home of their own. Catherine O'Carrigan, "St. Vincent's Hospital, Sydney, Pioneer in Nineteenth Century Health Care" (MA thesis, University of Sydney, 1986).

30. Polding was overseas and Gregory as second in command was in charge. The Sisters considered Gregory "common." They were not inclined to be ordered about by a man they considered their social inferior. See O'Sullivan, *A Cause of Trouble?*, 228.

31. Father Gregory to Sister Williams, 16 April 1847, Correspondence, Gregory to Williams, 16 April 1847, quoted in O'Sullivan, 111.

32. (John Hubert Plunkett), *A Brief Sketch of the Pious Congregation of Sisters of Charity, Carefully Selected from Authentic Sources* (Sydney: Kemp and Fairfax, 1855), quoted in O'Carrigan, "St. Vincent's Hospital, Sydney."

33. *Sydney Morning Herald*, 8 February 1855.

34. Geoffrey Serle, *The Golden Age: A History of the Colony of Victoria, 1851–1861* (Melbourne: Melbourne University Press, 1971), 10–12.

35. Opposition to the transportation of convicts had become increasingly vocal in Victoria and New South Wales, but the end of transportation was finally sealed with the gold rush. As the British Secretary of State dryly remarked, "It would appear a solecism to convey offenders, at the public expense, with the intention of at no distant time setting them free, to the immediate vicinity of those very goldfields which thousands of honest labourers are in vain trying to reach." Manning Clark, *A Short History of Australia* (Melbourne: Penguin, 1995), 131. Transportation to Western Australia did, however, continue until 1867.

36. The papacy was very nervous about nationalist movements. This caused problems for the hierarchy in Ireland, who endeavored to explain that Irish independence was not a left-wing revolutionary movement. But by the 1920s, while only five of a hundred Catholics were Irish, three of four priests were Irishmen. See O'Farrell, *The Irish in Australia*, 293. In Australia the long twentieth-century reign of Archbishop Mannix in Melbourne dramatically shaped Australian political history through both world wars and the Cold War. See Michael Hogan, "Whatever Happened to Australian Sectarianism," *Journal of Religious History* 13, 1 (1984–85): 83–91.

37. Whether the sisterhood was Irish or not in character and foundation, communities of religious women in the nineteenth century in Australia, and to a great extent in North America, almost inevitably became Irish in number—Irish women ran almost all the sisterhoods. Even the (non-Irish) Australian foundation of the Sisters of St. Joseph, under the rebellious Mother McKillop, was taken over by Irish women. See Janice Tranter, "The Irish Dimension of an Australian Religious Sisterhood: The Sisters of St. Joseph," in *The Irish World Wide*, vol. 5, ed. O'Sullivan, 234–55.

38. The best illustration of this Australian nature of the Sydney community is that St. Vincent's proudly provided Australia's first nursing volunteer to World War I. The Irish in Australia were overwhelmingly against involvement in the war, a significant factor in the defeat of the two national referenda on conscription. For the political Irish, the issue of military service for Britain was linked to dramatic events back home, such as the defeated 1916 Easter Rising in Dublin, and the 1917 execution of Irish patriots.

39. Polding to Propaganda Fide, 20 June 1859, *Polding Letters*, 287.

40. Sir Charles Nicholson, described by Dublin's Archbishop Cullen as a "benefactor of the nuns and an admirer of their work," was typical of the kind of non-Catholic philanthropist who valued the work of the sisters. He was a man of enormous wealth and a substantial historical figure in the economic development of Australia. In 1857 he returned to England where he became a key adviser to the British government on all matters Australian.

41. Ibid. He was to continue to support the hospital with gifts from Europe of stained glass and religious art.

42. Ibid. To be paid in £500 installments at 7 percent interest.

43. (Plunkett), *A Brief Sketch of the Pious Congregation Called Sisters of Charity.*

44. Polding to Propaganda Fide, 20 June 1859, *Polding Letters*, 287.

45. Ibid.: "contrary to my judgement, but in deference to Mrs de Lacy, a Dr Robertson had been appointed medical attendant."

46. St. Vincent's Hospital, *First Annual Report*, 1857–61 (Sydney).

47. Polding to Propaganda Fides, 13 May 1859. "The finance of the Archdiocese has been greatly strained by a debt of £1000." *Polding Letters*, 284.

48. It was the cause of great resentment and dismay to the sisters. However, although Sister Scholastica Gibbons is revered as the founder of the Australian community of the Sisters of the Good Shepherd, she refused ever to renounce her status as a Sister of Charity and remained a Sister of Charity until she died. See MacGinley, *A Dynamic of Hope*, 92.

49. Sisters of Charity, *A History of the Sisters of Charity in Australia*, 118.

50. *Sydney Morning Herald*, 2 June 1859.

51. *Sydney Morning Herald*, 6 June 1859.

52. She was certainly not punished, despite the fact that Polding had arranged for the Sisters of Charity to be formally severed from their Dublin house. See O'Sullivan, *A Cause of Trouble?*, 91–105 for a discussion of the change of the Sisters of Charity rule that Polding secretly obtained from Rome, which separated them from Dublin and put them under his authority. It was clear that de Lacy had not wished to return to Ireland and loved Sydney and the hospital greatly. A letter she wrote to the sisters in Sydney many years later reflects how much she had missed her "dear friends in the sunny south." Annals of the Sisters of Charity, Sisters of Charity Archives, Dublin.

53. O'Sullivan, *A Cause of Trouble?*, 239.

54. Polding to Cardinal Barnabo at Propaganda Fide, 16 April 1860. *Polding Letters*, 317.

55. And perhaps he was. Certainly an Irish bishop, Dr. Quinn, shamelessly persecuted a group of Sisters of Mercy in Brisbane at this time without censure. See Edmund Campion, *Rockchoppers: Growing Up Catholic in Australia* (Melbourne: Penguin, 1982), 73.

56. None of the five original Sisters of Charity remained in Sydney when de Lacy returned to Ireland in 1859. See MacGinley, *A Dynamic of Hope*.

57. Until the twentieth century, when the hospital became increasingly successful at gaining public funds. See Brian Dickey, "St. Vincent's Hospital, Sydney: A Note," *Journal of the Royal Australian Historical Society* (8 September 1978): 131–33.

58. Such was the number of foreigners who came to St. Vincent's that there was a call for embassies to assist the sisters to defray the cost of burial of foreigners without family. St. Vincent's Hospital, *Annual Report*, 1872 (Sydney).

59. Henry Parkes, *Fifty Years of Australian History* (London: Longmans, 1892), vol. 2, 28.

60. O'Carrigan, "Australian Catholic Hospitals in the Nineteenth Century," 20–36.

61. *Medical Gazette* 1 (1871): 110.

62. Ibid.

63. Parkes was not about to miss the opportunity to bask in the reflected glory of one of the real stars of the Victorian era. He continued a cordial correspondence with Nightingale and he was even so honored as to be granted an audience by the lady on her invalid couch in 1888. Parkes, *Fifty Years of Australian History*, 209–10.

64. Florence Nightingale to Henry Parkes, 24 October 1866. *Copy of correspondence between the Colonial government and Miss Florence Nightingale and others with reference to the Introduction of Trained Nurses for the Sydney Infirmary and Dispensary* (Sydney: Joseph Cook, 1867), 8. Mitchell.

65. J. Frederick Watson, *The History of the Sydney Hospital from 1811 to 1911* (Sydney: W. A. Gullick, 1911), 50.

66. James Mileham was court-martialed for neglecting this woman. Thereafter, attending surgeons were allowed limited private practice at the Sydney Infirmary.

See C. J. Cummins, "The Colonial Medical Service," *Modern Medicine of Australia* (7 January 1974): 16.

67. Bartz Schultz, *A Tapestry of Service: The Evolution of Nursing in Australia* (Melbourne: Churchill Livingstone, 1991), 77; and Douglas Miller, *Earlier Days: A Story of St. Vincent's* (Sydney: Angus and Robertson, 1969).

68. It was a dreadful scandal for Australia. Prince Alfred was the first member of the royal family to visit the continent and his visit had caused a frenzy of patriotism at each stop. Freda McDonnell, *Miss Nightingale's Young Ladies* (Sydney: Angus and Robertson, 1970), 31.

69. The Fenians were a secret nationalist group formally called the Irish Republican Brotherhood. They were named after a mythic Celtic hero and branches were formed simultaneously in New York and Dublin in 1858. They were famous for, among other things, an ill-conceived assault on Canada in 1866. Henry Parkes was most hysterical about the threat of the Irish and withheld the information that O'Farrell was an unfortunate disturbed individual who was most likely acting alone. Indeed, he had attempted to assassinate the Catholic bishop of Melbourne a short time before the attempt on Prince Alfred. The truth did not come to light until after the execution. A. W. Martin, *Henry Parkes: A Biography* (Melbourne: Melbourne University Press, 1980), 240–41.

70. See Judith Godden and Sue Forsyth, "Defining Relationships and Limiting Power: Two Leaders of Australian Nursing, 1868–1904," *Nursing Inquiry* 7 (2000) for a discussion of the power struggles between trained nurses and medical men in New South Wales.

71. In fact, when the model new hospital was opened, the Prince Alfred, Roberts pointedly avoided appointing a trained nurse as matron. This was a snub to Osburn, who returned to England in 1884. The untrained matron was also unsatisfactory, "exceeding her authority" by appointing nurses as head nurses. Roberts appointed another trained nurse, Susan McGahey, to the position in 1891, but again refused to give her the authority to function properly. Ibid.

72. Mary Barker to Florence Nightingale, 30 May 1868, BL Add. Mss. 47,757, ff 235–36. Mitchell. Library.

73. Lucy Osburn to Florence Nightingale, 20 May 1869, BL Add. Mss. 47,757, ff 73–75, Mitchell Library.

74. Ibid. Osburn is quoting Miller's grumbling to Nightingale here.

75. Osburn to Nightingale, 26 February 1869, BL Add. Mss. 47,575, ff 101–4, Mitchell Library.

76. Osburn to Nightingale, 4 December 1868, BL Add. Mss. 47, 757, ff 95–100, Mitchell Library.

77. Henry Mayhew observed that Irishwomen "having been accustomed to their hoods — they seldom wear bonnets." Mayhew, *London Labour and the London Poor* (1861–12; reprint Harmondsworth: Penguin, 1985), 57.

78. Ibid.

79. In addition to the "makeover" of the nurses' hair, Osburn immediately introduced prayers in the wards. Barker to Nightingale, 30 May 1868, BL Add. Mss. 47, 757, ff 235–36, Mitchell Library.

80. Public Charities Commission, *Commission Appointed to Inquire into and Report Upon the Working and Management of the Public Charities, First Report*, 18 September 1873 (Sydney: Thomas Richards, 1973), 76.

81. Ibid., 73.

82. Beverley Kingston, *My Wife, My Daughter, and Poor Mary Ann: Women and Work in Australia* (Sydney: Nelson, 1975), 29–55.

83. Register of Nursing, Sydney Hospital 1868–84, Sydney Hospital Archive.

84. Osburn to Nightingale, 24 March 1870, BL Add. Mss. 47,757, ff 127–32, Mitchell Library.

85. D. G. Boud, *Lucy Osburn, 1836–1891* (Windsor: Hawksbury Press, 1968), 19.

86. Ibid.

87. Lucy Osburn to Florence Nightingale, 24 March 1870, Add. Mss. 47,757, ff 127–32, Mitchell Library.

88. At the end of their three-year contract four of the five were not continued. See Boud, *Lucy Osburn*, 20.

89. Osburn to Nightingale, 24 March 1870, BL Add. Mss. 47, 757, ff 127–32, Mitchell Library.

90. Osburn to Nightingale, 16 June 1869, BL Add. Mss. 47,757, ff 113–18, Mitchell Library.

91. Ibid., 119–22.

92. Osburn to Nightingale, 26 February 1869, BL Add. Mss. 47 575, ff 101–4, Mitchell Library.

93. Public Charities Commission, *First Report*, 72.

94. Because of this difficulty, there was no sister in training at the time of the 1873 inquiry. Ibid., 34.

95. Osburn to Nightingale, 16 June 1869, BL Add. Mss. 47,757, ff 113–18, Mitchell Library.

96. Osburn to Nightingale, 12 May 1873, BL Add. Mss. 47,757, ff 140–45, Mitchell Library.

97. See Partington, *The Australian Nation*, 28–45.

98. Lillian James, "Horse-Breaking Preferred! Lucy Osburn of Sydney Hospital," in *Lives Obscurely Great: Historical Essays on Women in New South Wales*, ed. Patricia Thompson and Susan Yorke (Sydney: Society of Women Writers (Australia) New South Wales Branch, 1980), 92.

99. McDonnell, *Miss Nightingale's Young Ladies*, 103.

100. Nightingale had lost faith in Osburn when a family letter with newsy information on the care of Prince Alfred had been copied and circulated by one of Osburn's cousins. Schultz, *A Tapestry of Service*, 82.

101. Public Charities Commission, *First Report*, 30.

102. Ibid., 76.

103. Mother Mary Aikenhead, in *A Century of Service*, 24.

104. St. Vincent's proudly claims a few "firsts." For instance, it was the first hospital to employ a chloroformist, Richard Bailey. See *Australia's Quest for Colonial Health* (Brisbane: University of Queensland, Department of Child Health, RCH, 1983), 91.

105. See Miller, *Earlier Days*, 66–67 and Sisters of Charity, "A History of the Sisters of Charity," 104.

106. Miller, *Earlier Days*, 24.

107. In 1886 the university senate accepted these rules for medical appointments, and in 1891 St. Vincent's expanded its role as a teaching hospital for the Faculty of Medicine at the University of Sydney. See Miller, *Earlier Days*, 24.

108. Ibid., 105.

109. O'Sullivan, *A Cause of Trouble?*, 20.

110. Ibid., 303.

111. Sisters of Charity, "A History of the Sisters of Charity in Australia," 117.

112. The conversion claims so common in the North American hospital annals are conspicuously absent from those of the Sydney Sisters of Charity.

113. Training at St. Vincent's was at a cost to the nurses — ten guineas in 1888. This provided workers and income for the sisters. The sisters could honestly claim that by necessity they attracted a "better class of girl." Training of secular women commenced in 1882. The first sister to be trained was Ann Cunningham in 1857. First Register, St. Vincent's Hospital, Darlinghurst, Sydney.

114. Above all, it was difficult to find a neat nurse, nor was neatness an easy attribute to instill. "It was very difficult to teach the novices to be neat. Miss Osburn found a pretty Irish girl had tied up the holes in her frock with string, and she slipped off her shoes and stockings when in the wards." Training was possible, however, and in spite of these defects Osburn claimed that this recruit went on to become "a kind and capital nurse." See M. Salmon, "A Pioneer of Trained Nurses," *Australasian Trained Nurses Journal* (15 November 1911): 365.

115. Lucy Osburn's sisters became matrons of Mudgee Hospital (1870), Tarbon Creek (1873), Orange (1877), Parramatta (1879), (1880), Children's Glebe (1880), Launceston (1880), Hobart (1881), Bathurst (1881), Ballarat (1885), and Young (1885). See R. Lynette Russell, "Lucy Osburn: The First of Many," *First National Nursing History Conference*, Melbourne, May 1993 (Melbourne: Royal College of Nursing, Australia, 1993), 68.

Chapter 6. Frontier

1. Chronicles of the Sisters of Providence, 3 May 1876–July 1878, vol. 1, 1 (56), trans. Sister Dorothy Lentz. Providence Seattle Medical Center Collection, Sisters of Providence Archives, Sacred Heart Province, Seattle, Washington (hereafter SPA; numbers in parentheses are collection numbers).

2. Of course the notion of "frontier" is far from problematic. Since Frederick Jackson Turner's famous 1893 essay, "The Significance of the Frontier in American History," the concept has been important in American historiography. Recent years have witnessed a critique of the race, gender, and class assumptions that underpinned white America's view of the so-called "empty" wilderness. See, for instance, Susan Armitage and Elizabeth Jameson, eds., *The Women's West* (Norman: University of Oklahoma Press, 1987). Without attempting to oversimplify the concept of "frontier," the missionary nuns expressed the romantic challenge of pioneering in a wild place. Their diaries touch on the beauty of the wilderness, their wonder at the strangeness of native American culture, and their horror at the barbarity of men. In short, they were touched by their environment and aware of their setting, and they were building empires in the new land. The notion of frontier, then, is useful when examining this chapter of their work in America.

3. The American Protective Association, or APA, was a secret national organization that aimed to keep all government posts in the hands of Protestants. It was very popular in the 1890s and very powerful in Seattle. The Ku Klux Klan was also very active against Catholics, and crosses were burned on hospital lawns in Oregon and in San Antonio. See Ellis Lucia, *Seattle's Sisters of Providence* (Seattle: Providence Medical Center, 1978), 57; and Sister Margaret Patricia Slattery, *Promises to Keep: A History of the Sisters of Charity of the Incarnate Word, San Antonio, Texas*, 2nd ed., 2 vols. (San Antonio: Sisters of the Incarnate Word, 1998), vol. 2, 227.

4. Mother Saint Pierre Cinquin, cited in Slattery, *Promises to Keep*, vol. 1, 7.

5. This was a community fully in the spirit of St. Vincent's Daughters of Charity. For instance, the Customary of the Daughters of Charity Servants of the Poor includes traditional Vincentian exercises such as recollection of prayer with the

striking of the clock; see General Chapter, 1938 Montreal, 12, SPA. Daughters of Charity Servants of the Poor was the original official title for the community, although the sisters had other common names. In 1970 the official title was changed to Sisters of Providence. This title is still used to refer to the early community when they were officially Daughters of Charity, Sisters of Providence; their French name was Filles de Charité Servantes des Pauvres.

6. That said, a rich mix of women became Sisters of Providence. The register of entrants for the three western provinces shows Irish, English, American, German (and even an Australian!) women trained in Montreal. Nonetheless, Montreal women predominate even in the 1900s. In fact it is not until the 1930s that there are more U.S. than Quebec women on the register. Register Secretary General Office, SPA.

7. Letters of Mother Saint Pierre Cinquin, trans. Sister Kathleen Garvey (1977), 6. Motherhouse of the Incarnate Word, San Antonio, Texas (hereafter LMSP, AMIW).

8. Patricia Slattery's two-volume history of the community provides detailed background on the mother community in France, see. See Slattery, *Promises to Keep*, vol. 1, 11–17.

9. Ibid., 208.

10. Ibid, 134.

11. Non-Mexican religious were expelled from Mexico in 1917. Slattery, *Promises to Keep*, vol. 2, 227 shows the list of college principals in Mexico—the names change to Spanish by 1909. Vol. 1, 135 lists recruits by nationality—Mexican women entrants rise from four in 1911 to fifteen in 1922.

12. Ibid., 61.

13. Ibid., 23.

14. There is ample evidence that the first leader, Mother Madeleine Chollet (1869–72), who was again leader at the end of her life in 1894–1906, was illiterate. See Slattery, *Promises to Keep*, vol. 1, 22–23. The charge for private patients was $1.00 to $2.50 per day, city patients 50 cents per day, and there were a large number of free patients. 29, AMIW. At Fort Worth there were three classes of patient: private, city (charity and employee), and railroad. Slattery, vol. 2, 91.

15. Slattery, vol. 2, 3.

16. Santa Rosa Infirmary Remark Book, June 1892–October 1892, January 1896–December 1898. AMIW.

17. Mother Saint Pierre to Lyons. LSPC, AMIW.

18. Mother Saint Pierre to Lyons 19 July, 1884, 117. LSPC, AMIW.

19. The county hospital closed down after five years, following devastation in a storm, and the sisters had great difficulty getting money owed them by the county. See Slattery, *Promises to Keep*, vol. 2, 11.

20. For instance, the St. Louis hospital led to the establishment of a major foundation in Missouri, which eventually became a separate province. Slattery, vol. 1, 53.

21. The story of the Amarillo Hospital, St. Anthony's, is a good example of the leverage applied to attract the sisters. The town of Amarillo had no hospital in 1898, but the local doctors banded together and tried to persuade the Sisters of the Incarnate Word to establish one. The missionary argument—that the town would build a Catholic church if that was what it took to get the sisters to come, was what finally swayed Mother Madeleine. Slattery, vol. 2, 123–29.

22. Slattery, vol. 1, 59.

23. This training program went on to become one of the first baccalaureate programs in the country. Slattery, vol. 2, 16.

24. Slattery, vol. 1, 91.

25. 14 September 1882, 53. LSPC, AMIW.

26. 19 July 1884. LSPC, AMIW.

27. Mother Saint Pierre Cinquin to Mother Mary de Sales, Superior of Presentation Convent Sneem, Kerry, 2 May 1883, 77. LSPC, AMIW.

28. Bishops were not keen on losing much needed sisters to foreign missions. Finally in 1913 the Sisters of the Incarnate Word, San Antonio were able to open a house in Holland for the reception of German women (the bishop prohibited recruitment of Dutch women). This house fell victim to World War I and closed in 1924. Finally, in 1924, some forty years after Mother Saint Pierre's attempt, a house in Galway, Ireland was opened that prepared women for the mission in Texas. Slattery, vol. 1, 147.

29. The first of five letters from Chief Seltice in 1870 to the sisters is addressed to Sister Catherine Ennis: "Rev Sister, Since the time you passed by this place, all my people have been greatly wishing to have amongst us some of your Sisters for the education of our girls. The fathers [Jesuits] here are doing their best to teach our boys, and we are glad of it, but our girls are orphans, and if you or some other sisters do not come, they will always be so, because nobody will take care of them." The girls were not orphans in the family sense of the word; they were "orphans" in the educational sense because the boys had teachers but the girls did not. Helen Mason, S.P., *History of St. Ignatius Province of the Sisters of Providence* (Spokane, Wash.: Providence Administration, 1997), 12. SPA.

30. They remained the principal health care providers for the northwest well into the twentieth century. As late as 1954 a Sister of Providence was president of the Washington Hospitals Association. Today Providence Health System is the largest nonprofit health care provider on the west coast. See Mason, *History of St. Ignatius.*

31. Mason, *History of St. Ignatius,* 6.

32. Lucille Dean, S.P., "Special Feature Mother Joseph of Providence," Part I, 1. SPA.

33. Ibid., Part II, 1.

34. Correspondence, Mother Joseph to Mother Godfrey, Superior General, discussing building repairs at Providence Hospital, Seattle, 2 September 1895 (13), Mother Joseph of the Sacred Heart Personal Papers Collection (hereafter MJSH), letters, trans. Sister Mary Leopoldine, vol. 2. Mother Joseph discusses elevator design with Mother Mary Antoinette, Superior General, in Montreal, 14 February 1900 (13). MJSH, translated letters, vol. 2, 282. Mother Philomene to Mother Joseph, compliments her on the altar she built at Walla Walla, 12 February 1880 (13). MJSH, Correspondence, Box 3, Personal Papers of Mother Philomene, trans. Sister Therese Carignan.

35. Sister Praxedes placed a letter under the statue of St. Joseph the day before the telegram arrived. Western Union Telegraph Company, 6 March 1877. SPA. The telegram is filed in a collection with a curious title: Correspondence — Other Missions. Correspondence between Emil Kauten and Mother Praxedes, trans. Sister Therese Carignan.

36. Chronicles 1894–95, 36 (56). Providence Seattle Medical Center Collection, SPA. Other secret baptisms are recorded at 16, 31.

37. Register of patients, St. Joseph Hospital, Vancouver, Washington, 1858 (23). St. Joseph Hospital, Vancouver, Washington Collection, SPA.

38. It was said that "Freemasons need extraordinary grace." (23) Chronicles 1871–72, trans. Sister Dorothy Lentz, vol. 8, 18. St. Joseph Hospital, Vancouver, Washington Collection, SPA.

39. Letter from Mother Joseph of the Sacred Heart to parishes being visited, 18 December 1876, (13). MJSH, Correspondence, Box 2: Letters of Introduction for Mother Joseph, trans. Sister Therese Carignan, 13.

40. Christopher J. Kauffman, *Ministry and Meaning: A Religious History of Catholic Health Care in the United States* (New York: Crossroad, 1995),100.

41. Chronicles, 1883, 37–38, 36 (56), Providence Seattle Medical Center Collection, SPA.

42. "Si non pavisti, occidisti" — if you have not fed them, you have killed them. See Elizabeth Rapley, *The Dévotes: Women and Church in Seventeenth-Century France* (Montreal: McGill University Press, 1990), 80.

43. Barbra Mann Wall, "Constancy Amid Change: Catholic Nuns and the Development of Health Care Institutions," PhD dissertation, University of Notre Dame, 2000.

44. Articles of Incorporation, Sisters of Charity of the House of Providence, Vancouver, Washington, 19 March 1869.

45. Chronicles, 1 July 1878, vol. 1, 5, 36 (56). Providence Seattle Medical Center Collection, SPA.

46. Ibid., 25.

47. Rev. Alfred Archambeault, Ecclesiastical Superior to Mother Joseph, 1 December 1894. MJSH, Correspondence, trans. Sister Mary Leopoldine, vol. 2, 260–66 (13). SPA.

48. Lucia, *Cornerstone*, 83.

49. *Little Medical Guide of the Sisters of Providence* (Montreal: Providence Maison-Mère, 1889), 15.

50. Ibid.

51. Chronicles, 1 July 1878, vol. 1, 5 36 (56). Providence Seattle Medical Center Collection, SPA.

52. Chronicles, 24 July 1885 (56). Providence Seattle Medical Center Collection, SPA.

53. Chronicles, 1871–72, St. Joseph Hospital, Vancouver, Washington Collection, vol. 8, 18. SPA

54. Chronicles, 24 July 1885 (56). Providence Seattle Medical Center Collection, SPA. Providence Hospital.

55. Lucia, *Cornerstone*, 83.

56. A typical story relates how individuals who were opposed to the sisters and worked against the hospital could be transformed by their care. One woman was so hostile to the sisters that her doctor arranged for her to have a private secular nurse when she was admitted. However, she dismissed her nurse and then her doctor and became a firm friend of the sisters. Chronicles, 1896–97, 40 (56). Providence Seattle Medical Center Collection, SPA.

57. The 1926 customary deals very clearly with the mix of professional and spiritual duties and decorum issues for sisters, and gives an unambiguous account of their professional/spiritual responsibilities.

58. Chronicles, 24 July 1885 (56). Providence Seattle Medical Center Collection, SPA.

59. Sister Blandine to Mother Joseph, 14 February 1897 (13), MJSH Personal Papers Collection, Correspondence, Box 1, 1856–1901.

60. *Régistre des missions démandées à la Province du Sacred Coeur des Soeurs de Charité Servantes des Pauvres, Vancouver, Washington, depuis l'époque de la Fondation 1856.* SPA

61. Foundation Requests, A–Z, Rev. A. Parodi, S.J., Request for a school and hospital in Ellensburg, Washington, 5 March 1884. SPA.

62. Foundation Requests, A–Z, Rev. William H. Judge, S.J., Request for a school in Dawson (Circle City), North West Territories, 28 December 1896. SPA.

63. Referred to another Province and accepted. Foundation Requests, A–Z, Request from Father Hartleib, S.J., Moscow, Idaho, 9 May 1892. SPA

64. Lucia, *Cornerstone*, 95.

65. Clara S. Weeks wrote *Textbook of Nursing*, the first textbook for nurses to be published in the United States (New York: Appleton, 1885).

66. Notes from a collection of papers by Miss Margaret Tynan, RN entitled *St. Vincent's School of Nursing of the Institute of Providence: Its History and Alumnae* (Portland: School of Nursing, St. Vincent's, 1930), 53, 1–3. SPA.

67. Slattery, *Promises to Keep*, vol. 1, 36.

68. Suzy Farren, *A Call to Care: The Women Who Built Catholic Healthcare in America* (St. Louis: Catholic Association of the United States, 1996), 139.

69. Slattery, *Promises to Keep*, vol. 1, 35.

70. Sister Blandina's recollections were published as Blandina Segale, *At the End of the Santa Fe Trail* (Columbus, Ohio: Columbian Press, 1932; rpt. Albuquerque: University of New Mexico Press, 1999).

71. "If those who came after us could only realize what the first sisters went through to build up the different houses in the West, they would not so easily find fault with what they find there." "Sister Catherine Mallon's Journal," ed. Thomas Richter, Part Two, *New Mexico History Review* 52, 3 (1977): 246.

72. Slattery, *Promises to Keep*, vol. 1, 38.

73. An early party of sisters from Montreal (1852) attempted to return to Canada via Cape Horn from an ill-fated expedition to the northwest. After a hair-raising trip they ended up in Chile, where they remained. Sister Peter of Alcantara to Mother Amable, Superior General, 18 February 1880 (13). MJSH, Personal Papers Collection, Correspondence, Box 2: Notes of trip to Chile. SPA

74. "We did not find there the kind generous Irish heart that we had met in other camps." "Sister Catherine Mallon's Journal," 151.

75. Letter from Mother Joseph of the Sacred Heart to parishes being visited, Montreal, 18 December 1876 (13). MJSH, Personal Papers Collection, Correspondence Box 1, 1856–1901. SPA. It was not always profitable, however, and circumstances changed dramatically from one year to the next. In 1876, for instance, a begging trip in Portland produced little because the local mine had gone bankrupt. See Lucia, *Cornerstone*, 63.

76. The trip from Fort Vancouver to St. Ignatius, Montana was 650 miles, 400 on horseback, and Sister Mary Edward had been kicked by a horse and was unable to ride for the last section of the journey. See Mason, *History of St. Ignatius Province*, 2.

77. Apparently at night the sisters in training slept in tents with handbags or saddles for pillows and cooked in the open. Mother Joseph of the Sacred Heart to Bishop Ignatius Bourget, 10 May 1864. MJSH, Personal Papers Collection, Correspondence, Box 1, 1856–1901, vol. 1, 132–36. SPA.

78. Lucille Dean, S.P., "Special Feature Mother Joseph of Providence," Part 3. SPA.

79. Chronicles, 24 July 1885, vol. 1, 21 (56). Providence Seattle Medical Center Collection. SPA.

80. Ibid., 21.

81. Ibid, 23.

82. Richard Berner, "Port Blakely Mill Company 1876–89," *Pacific Northwest Quarterly* (October 1966): 153–71.

83. Sister Eugene, Superior of Providence Hospital, Seattle to Mr. J. Campbell, 12 August 1895. Port Blakely Mill Co. Collection.

84. The sisters were certainly keen to formalize arrangements between the Mill and the hospital. Sister Eugene to Port Blakely Mill, 7 October 1898, addressed simply to "Gentlemen" seeking to meet with them to negotiate rates. Port Blakely Mill Co. Collection, SPA. By the 1920s this practice was challenged as exploitative of casual workers, whose single day's pay was being docked for a week's insurance coverage. The Bureau of Labor Statistics, State of Washington, *9th Biennial Report*, 1913–14, 64 states that the "hospital fee system is too often abused" and that it constitutes "an onerous tax upon the workingman." Providence Health System Corporation Records, Tickets—General. SPA.

85. Deliberations of the Corporation, 1859–1941. Providence Health System Corporation Records, SPA.

86. *Régistre des missions démandées*. SPA. They reported regularly to Montreal. Mother Joseph was instructed to "establish a fixed rule of correspondence" and to write monthly. Mother Philomene to Mother Joseph, 4 June 1863 (13). MJSH, Personal Papers Collection, Correspondence, Box 1, 1856–1901, vol. 1, 79. SPA.

87. *Inventaires des immeubles de la Province du Sacre Coeur*, SPA.

88. Mary Ewens, "The Leadership of Nuns in Immigrant Catholicism," in *Women and Religion in America*, vol. 1, *The Nineteenth Century*, ed. Rosemary Radford Ruether and Rosemary Skiller Keller (San Francisco: Harper and Row, 1981), 105.

89. Slattery, *Promises to Keep*, vol. 1, 19–22.

90. Since the habit had been revealed to the founder Jeanne de Chantal in a vision, this was a serious breach of the rule. Slattery, vol. 1, 13.

91. "Rule given to our first mothers on leaving France," 1869, 5. AMIW.

92. Ibid., 3–5.

93. Constitutions of the Sisters of Charity of the Incarnate Word, 1872, 20. AMIW.

94. Ibid., 57.

95. Ibid., 56.

96. Slattery, vol. 1, 31.

97. Mother Saint Pierre to the Very Rev. Mother Marie of Jesus, 14 September 1882, 51–52. AMIW.

98. Slattery, vol. 1, 134.

99. Ibid., 77.

100. In fact, Mother Mary Godfrey, Superior General, urged them to plan their week around French and English, so that the Canadian sisters would learn English and the American sisters learn French—"the language sacrifice will be blessed and will create unity among the sisters"; see Lucia, *Cornerstone*, 72.

101. See the Customary of the Sisters of Providence, Circulars of the Superior General, vol. 1, 1898–1904 (Providence Mother House, Montreal, 1910), 11.

102. "Our strength comes from our motherhouse." Mother Praxedes to Father Kauten in response for request to take over hospital in Seattle House of Providence, 7 March 1877, Vancouver. Correspondence, SPA.

103. The Chronicles celebrate occasions of renewal, retreats, foundress day, visits from Montreal, etc. See for instance Chronicles, vol. 1, 34 (56). Providence Seattle Medical Center Collection SPA.

104. Chronicles, May 1886–July 1879, vol. 1 (56). Providence Seattle Medical Center Collection, SPA.

105. Sister Saint Pierre to Sister Alphonse, 5 February 1889. Correspondence, 314. AMIW.

Chapter 7. Crossing the Confessional Divide

1. See Ralph Gibson, "Female Religious Orders in Nineteenth-Century France: Catholicism in Britain and France Since 1789," in *Catholicism in Britain and France Since 1789*, ed. Frank Tallett and Nicholas Atkin (London: Hambledon, 1996). The Ultramontane revolution in Ireland is classically reviewed in Emmet Larkin, "Devotional Revolution in Ireland," *American Historical Review* 80 (1972): 625–52. Mary Peckham Magray gives the women a more central role in this transformation in *The Transforming Power of the Nuns: Women, Religion, and Cultural Change in Ireland, 1750–1900* (New York: Oxford University Press, 1998).

2. See Rev. W. A. Passavant, "The Deaconess and the Professional Nurse," *Proceedings and Papers of the Third Conference of Evangelical Lutheran Deaconess Mother-houses in the United States* (Omaha, Neb., 1899), 333–35.

3. As discussed earlier, the French Daughters of Charity were formed in the seventeenth century; however it was not until the nineteenth century that this community and its many clones moved beyond the French world. New France was of course a major site of the expansion of these orders and its influence on American nursing sisterhoods particularly relevant. See Christine Allen, "Women in Colonial French America," in *Women and Religion in America*, vol. 2, *The Colonial and Revolutionary Periods*, ed. Rosemary Radford Ruether and Rosemary Skinner Keeler (San Francisco: Harper and Row, 1983), 79–131, for a survey of the French American experience. However, in general the most influential nursing communities, such as the American Daughters of Charity, the Irish Sisters of Charity, and the Sisters of Mercy were nineteenth-century developments.

4. The 1815 Congress of Vienna realigned state and confessional boundaries Meanwhile, Catholic workers moved to industrializing Protestant areas, while Protestants moved into Catholic areas forming a Protestant bourgeoisie in the Catholic Lower Rhine and Ruhr. See Jonathan Sperber, *Popular Catholicism in Nineteenth-Century Germany* (Princeton, N.J.: Princeton University Press, 1984), 45–46.

5. Sperber cites clerical complaints to police, 15.

6. This influence is suggestive of a flow-on effect of religious revival from France. Ibid., 93.

7. Mass pilgrimages heavily orchestrated by Catholic clergy became a gesture of resistance to the Prussian state in the early 1870s. They were also de facto rallies for the Center Party. Demonstrations, boycotts of state holidays, and mass celebrations on Catholic festivals were also a feature of this period. Ibid., 223–29.

8. Stanley Nadel argues that the New York German community was distinguished by its "overwhelming predominance of secular subcommunities over its religious ones. In 1860, half of New York's Germans were without religious affiliation." See Nadel, *Little Germany: Ethnicity, Religion, and Class in New York City, 1845–1880* (Urbana: University of Illinois Press, 1990), 91.

9. Sister Mary Gabriel Henninger, *Sisters of St. Mary and Their Healing Mission* (St. Louis: Sisters of St. Mary of the Third Order of Saint Francis, 1979), 4. Katharina Berger is variously known as Sister (later Mother) Odilia, Odelia, and Ottilia.

10. Women represented only 41 percent of total German migrants, Irish women 52.9 percent. The proportion increased through the century, from 35 percent in 1830 to 53.8 percent in 1900. Hasia Diner, *Erin's Daughters in America: Irish Immigrant Women in the Nineteenth Century* (Baltimore: Johns Hopkins University Press, 1983), 30–33.

11. According to Sperber, the tavern was the center of town and village life in these years, with little respect among rural and urban common people for the church. The illegitimacy rates are commonly cited as an indicators of unreligiousness. See Catherine M. Prelinger, *Charity, Challenge, and Change: Religious Dimensions of the Mid-Nineteenth-Century Women's Movement in Germany* (New York: Greenwood Press, 1987), 18 and Sperber, *Popular Catholicism*, 93–94. More striking are numerous complaints from clergy of abuse and insults during religious service and the busy trade of taverns on Sundays.

12. Rev. William Keuenhof, Chaplain of the Sisters of St. Mary's Infirmary, Kansas City, Foreword to the 1921 silver jubilee history of the hospital, Sisters of St. Mary, *The Sisters of St. Mary and Their Hospital Work in Kansas City, Missouri, 1895–1920* (Kansas City: St. Mary's Hospital, 1921), 6.

13. Henninger, *Sisters of Saint Mary and Their Healing Mission*, 2.

14. Ibid., 10.

15. Henninger cites the annals of the Servants of the Sacred Heart, which state, "Father Braun moved his community . . . the good will of the Archbishop which had cooled towards him following the recent dispute with the elderly religious [Mother Odilia]" (3).

16. Sister Louise Hirner, *Called to Be Faithful: A History of the Sisters of St. Francis, Maryville, Missouri* (Maryville, Mo.: Sisters of St. Francis, Mount Alverno Convent, Maryville, 1984), 10, argues that they could have been immunized by the Prussian Army as this was widespread during the Franco-Prussian War.

17. There was a general call for nurses, doctors, and medical supplies from the Howard corps of physicians. Ibid., 14.

18. Letter from Mother Odilia to Sister Margaret Mary Noelkner during the yellow fever epidemic in Memphis, 1878, cited in Henninger, *Sisters of Saint Mary and Their Healing Mission*, 16. Mother Odilia began her letter to the nursing sister, "Greetings from all your companion Sisters who are continually praying and weeping for you." The obituary list is available in Wilhelm Faerber, *The Sisters of St. Mary of St. Louis: In Commemoration of the Silver Jubilee of the Order, 1872–16 November 1897* (St. Louis: Amerika Printing House, 1897), 25.

19. Henninger, *Sisters of Saint Mary and Their Healing Mission*, 17.

20. This Franciscan training was the eventual cause of discord. See Hirner, *Called to Be Faithful*, 22.

21. Other clergy also acted as chaplains and conducted retreats. Ibid., 11.

22. According to Faerber's history, 26, the Sisters of St. Mary nursed 4,213 families in their homes in St. Louis between 1872 and 1897.

23. St. Mary's Hospital, St. Louis, *Annual Report*, 1896 (included at the back of Faerber, 28) lists patients as 968 Catholic, 284 Protestant, 53 no religion, 5 Hebrew. Nationality is listed as 627 United States, 371 Ireland, 164 Germany, 26 England, and thereafter numbers decreasing to one. The 1897 *Annual Report* (Faerber, 27) lists numbers of charity and private patients since 1877, showing

twice as many private as charity patients consistently over that period. The ratio varies with institutions; St. Joseph's Hospital, St. Charles in 1887–97 had between 80 and 100 percent charity patients (29).

24. Henninger, *Sisters of Saint Mary and Their Healing Mission*, 21.

25. Ibid., 113. See Faerber, *Sisters of St. Mary of St. Louis*, 6, for a list of institutions.

26. This hospital, St. Mary's, Kansas City, was dedicated in 1909. See Henninger, *Sisters of Saint Mary and Their Healing Mission*, 115.

27. See ibid., 352 for a full list of superiors at Sisters of St. Mary institutions.

28. Ibid., 11.

29. While this "impression" may well be completely misleading, it is worth noting that it is in sharp distinction to that offered in the annual reports of American Daughters of Charity, or Sisters of Providence annual reports and brochures (see chapters 3 and 6).

30. This was the case at St. Mary's, Kansas City, according to Joseph G. Webster, "The Staff of St. Mary's Hospital," *Jackson County Medical Society Weekly Bulletin* 50 (30 June 1965): 1570–71. Finally, under the leadership of Mother Mary Concordia in 1921 (who had all foreign-born sisters naturalized), St. Mary's embraced the Catholic Hospital Association, entered into contractual arrangements with the Jesuit fathers at St. Louis University and established St. Mary's Group of Hospitals as university teaching hospitals. Henninger, *Sisters of St. Mary and Their Healing Mission*, 39.

31. Ibid., 37.

32. Hirner, *Called to Be Faithful*, 14.

33. Henninger, *Sisters of Saint Mary and Their Healing Mission*, 116.

34. A school of nursing at St. Mary's, Kansas City was not opened until 1916, under the leadership of Sister Mary Marcellina, RN, B.S., in *St. Mary's Hospital School of Nursing, Kansas City Missouri, 1964–65* (Kansas City: St. Mary's Hospital, 1965), 6.

35. Henninger, *Sisters of Saint Mary and Their Healing Mission*, 31.

36. The Sisters of St. Mary and the Sisters of St. Francis reunited as the Franciscan Sisters of Mary in 1987, honoring both Mother Odilia and their American-born Mother Augustine. See *Franciscan Sisters of Mary: Priceless Heritage, 1823–1988* (St. Louis: Franciscan Sisters of Mary, 1988).

37. Ibid., 19.

38. Ibid., 11.

39. Even the historian of the Sisters of St. Mary concedes these points; ibid., 27.

40. Hirner, *Called to Be Faithful*, 22.

41. Ibid., 13.

42. Ibid., 27.

43. Ibid., 22.

44. Ibid., 47.

45. Ibid., 14.

46. By 1927 the Sisters of St. Francis owned and conducted four hospitals: St. Francis, Maryville; St. Anthony's, Oklahoma City; St. Elizabeth's, Hannibal; and St. Mary's, Nebraska City. In 1906 the Sisters of St. Francis took charge of Wabash Railroad hospitals at Moberly, Missouri, Peru, Indiana, and Decatur, Illinois. Hirner, *Called to Be Faithful*, 22, 147–49.

47. Prayers were said in German, French, English, and Latin however, reflecting the sisters' religious training. Official documentation was in German. Ibid., 44.

48. Ibid., 16.

49. Although there is much talk of the Kaiserswerth model in nineteenth-

century nursing, and reformers such as Elizabeth Fry and Florence Nightingale were profoundly influenced by Fliedner, there is remarkably little detail, especially in recent scholarship in the field. One exception is Irene Schuessler Poplin's study, "Nursing Uniforms: Romantic Idea, Functional Attire, or Instrument of Social Change," *Nursing History Review* 2 (1994): 153–67.

50. The Dutch Mennonite example was the official inspiration published by the Kaiserswerth Institute in the important history compiled by Isabel Hampton Robb, *Nursing the Sick: Papers from the International Congress of Charities, Correction, and Philanthropy* (Chicago, 1893; rpt. New York: McGraw-Hill, 1949), 57–59.

51. Catherine Prelinger's work is one of the few scholarly sources available in English on women and religion in nineteenth-century Germany. See *Charity, Challenge, and Change: Religious Dimensions of the Mid-Nineteenth-Century Women's Movement in Germany* (New York: Greenwich Press, 1987), 10.

52. Ibid., 19.

53. Ibid.

54. Ibid., 11; Frederick S. Weiser, "Serving Love" (Degree of Divinity thesis, Church History, Lutheran Theological College, Gettysburg, Pennsylvania, 1960), 21.

55. Abdel Ross Wentz, *Fliedner the Faithful* (Philadelphia: Board of Publication of the United Lutheran Church in America, 1936), 35.

56. Ibid., 56.

57. This was the standard Kaiserswerth deaconess model; there were variations, particularly when formal nursing or teacher training became compulsory.

58. Poplin, "Nursing Uniforms," 155, gives extensive detail on the outfitting and uniforms at Kaiserswerth.

59. Most notably, Prussian minister of state Freiherr vom Stein had voiced praise for the Sisters of Charity in the 1810s and called for a Lutheran equivalent. See Weiser, "Serving Love," 17.

60. Catherine Prelinger, "Prelude to Consciousness," in *German Women in the Nineteenth Century: A Social History,* ed. John C. Fout (New York, Holmes and Meier, 1984), 126.

61. The Synods of the Rhineland and of Westphalia were the first to take official action to restore the role of deaconess. Wentz, *Fliedner the Faithful,* 79.

62. According to Prelinger, the Prussian king, Frederick William IV, had not supported the deaconess notion at first, preferring a society of male nurses for the Berlin hospital. *Charity, Challenge, and Change,* 2.

63. Isabel Hampton Robb et al., "The Work of Deaconesses in Germany from the Fliedner Institute," in *Nursing the Sick,* 99.

64. Fliedner was originally influenced by Elizabeth Fry's prison work, but the nursing side of the operation dominated from the early days. Wentz, *Fliedner the Faithful,* 34.

65. "Would You Like to be a Deaconess?" (Cincinnati: Bethesda Hospital, 1922).

66. Ann Doyle, "Nursing by Religious Orders in the United States, Part IV — Lutheran Deaconesses, 1849–1928," *American Journal of Nursing* 10 (1929): 1197–1207, 1200.

67. Marie Kruger had originally been at Kaiserswerth but had resigned. Roberta Mayhew West, *History of Nursing in Pennsylvania, Lankenau Hospital, Formerly German Hospital, Philadelphia* (Harrisburg: Pennsylvania State Nurses Association, 1939), 441.

68. Lankenau's support was critical. Lankenau, a wealthy banker and a widower

who had lost both his children, channeled all his energies and ample funds into the deaconess movement and the German Hospital. Weiser, "Serving Love," 50.

69. It should be remembered that the Daughters of Charity who influenced Kaiserswerth were a less "ecclesiastical" version of sisterhood than their Irish or American counterparts. They took only annual vows and were free to leave.

70. This makes it quite difficult to track their presence in state nursing organizations or licensing bodies. Another group, Mennonite deaconesses, did not establish hospitals until the twentieth century.

71. Usually the first twelve months involved religious and nursing training.

72. Meyer had been instrumental in locating a group of deaconesses prepared to come to America. See Doyle, "Nursing by Religious Orders, Part IV," 1201.

73. Charles H. Meyer, Letter to the Board of Trustees of the German Hospital of Philadelphia to the Members of the Medical Board, 14 December 1885, Wm. N. Mencke, Secretary. 268.0B1.1, F3. Archives of the Deaconess Community of the Evangelical Lutheran Church in America (hereafter ADCELCA).

74. Ibid.

75. *History of the German Hospital* (Philadelphia: German Hospital of Philadelphia, 1895; 1, 1, f1, CSNH). The *History* does not mention deaconesses until page 29, and then only for one paragraph. In the 1911 Annual Report there are no deaconesses on the hospital board and the chair of the nursing committee is both a board member and a clergyman. *52nd Annual Report of the Trustees of the German Hospital* (Philadelphia: Steen and Co., 1911).

76. Flyer, Donation Day at the German Hospital, Thanksgiving Day, 27 November 1884. 268.0 61.1 f3, ADCELCA.

77. Mary Drexel was the aunt of St. Katherine Drexel, foundress of the (Catholic) Sisters of the Blessed Sacrament for Indians and Colored People.

78. "Agreement," German Hospital of the City of Philadelphia and the Mary Drexel Home and Philadelphia Mother House of Deaconesses, 21 March 1899, 7–9. 268.0 B1, F3. ADCELCA.

79. Frederick S. Weiser, *To Serve the Lord and His People, 1884–1984: Celebrating the Heritage of a Century of Lutheran Deaconesses in America* (Gladwyne, Pa.: Deaconess Community of the Lutheran Church in America, 1984).

80. Weiser, "Serving Love," 70. Non-German entrants remained rarities until World War II (124).

81. British and American German Methodists evangelized back to Germany; the latter focused particularly on the Hamburg area. See Rupert E. Davies, *Methodism* (London: Epworth Press, 1963), 140.

82. Methodists split into separate conferences (democratic conventions/administrative units) along racial and language/ethnic lines. See James Kirby, Russell E. Richey, and Kenneth E. Rowe, *The Methodists* (Westport, Conn.: Greenwood Press, 1996), 90–92.

83. The Conference was the administrative and organizational meeting of Methodist and Lutheran churches. Deaconesses formed their own Kaiserswerth Conference in 1861. See Wentz, *Fliedner the Faithful*, 94.

84. The first German Methodist church in America was founded in 1838 in Cincinnati. Historical Sketches and Nine Lives of the Organization, n.d., c. 1948. 2, 2–3, f11, CHSNCGM.

85. Clara M. Bay of Ohio agonizes over whether to go into the German deaconesses because she does not have the language — though her parents do. 1897. 2, 2–15, f11, CHSNCGM.

86. In the 1922 pamphlet "Would You Like to Be a Deaconess?" the training,

lack of drudgery, career opportunities, and comfort and security of the deaconess life are strongly emphasized for those whom God calls. 2, 2–22, 515. CHSNCGM.

87. Clara M. Bay of Ohio.

88. Louise Golder, "The Deaconess Motherhouse," in *The Deaconess and Her Work* (Cincinnati: Bethesda Hospital, n.d.). 2, 2–1, f2, CHSNCGM. Rev. Christian Golder, *History of the Deaconess Movement in the Christian Church* (New York: Eaton and Mains, 1903).

89. A Report to the Second National Deaconess Conference, Ocean Grove, New Jersey, 7–9 August 1889, shows Bethesda Hospital, Cincinnati conducted by a Board president, a bishop; vice president, clergyman; second vice president, clergyman; third vice president, Miss Isabella Thoburn; 3 women secretaries (one an MD); a male treasurer; and an executive committee of 5 men (2 clergy) and 4 women. 2, 2–22, f2. CHSNCGM.

90. No deaconess is a signatory on the articles of incorporation of the German Methodist Deaconess Home in 1896. Even the revised constitution (1934, in English) clearly shows that the Deaconess Committee is dominated by the hospital: "The Deaconess Committee shall consist of seven (7) members, the chairman of which shall be the President of the Organization. This committee shall have supervision of the admission, the training and the maintenance of the deaconesses, and it shall report these matters to the Board of Managers or the Executive Committee. It shall also report with recommendations on the conduct and appointment of each deaconess to her Conference Deaconess Board. The Superintendent of the Motherhouse and the chaplain shall be members of this committee." Articles of Incorporation of the German Methodist Deaconess Home, p. 6. 2, 2–1, f2, CHSNCGM.

91. The 1902 publication *Diakonissen-Mutterhaus und Bethesda Hospital* lists Miss Louise Golder (*Oberin*) as an ex officio member of the board. *Diakonissen Mutterhaus und Bethesda Hospital* (Pittsburgh: City Mission Publishing Company, 1902), 47. CHSNCGM.

92. Weiser, *To Serve the Lord,* 15.

93. Weiser, "Serving Love," 158. Weiser's list of deaconesses records whether they left to marry. From this record, marriages to pastors were not infrequent.

94. Leslie Larson, "Fogelstrom and the Diaconate," *Augustinian Quarterly* 5, 26, 4 (October 1947): 347–54. Archives of the Deaconess Motherhouse, Gladwyne, Pennsylvania, United Lutheran Church in America.

95. E. A. Fogelstrom, *Autobiography,* trans. Sister Elfrida Sandberg, Immanuel, 1957–58, 3.

96. Ibid., 350.

97. The Immanuel Deaconess Institute was eventually accepted in the American Augustana Synod and the Kaiserswerth Conference of Europe. See Fogelström, *Autobiography,* 3–4.

98. Fogelstrom, *Autobiography,* 31.

99. "Fogelstrom and the Diaconate," 351.

100. Prelinger, *Charity, Challenge, and Change.* 19.

101. Weiser, "Serving Love," 21–23.

102. Fogelstrom, *Autobiography.* The joy of God's work is a powerful motif in Fogelstrom's writing, see 26–28.

103. Carol K. Coburn's study of Miami County, Kansas gives detailed background to the establishment of the Synod and its central position in this rural community's identity. See Coburn, *Life at Four Corners: Religion, Gender, and Educa-*

tion in a German-Lutheran Community, 1868–1945 (Lawrence: University Press of Kansas, 1992), 25–30.

104. Ibid., 56–57.

105. But the maintenance of tradition relies on education, and so education and the establishment of a network of German schools and colleges were central to their efforts over this period. The synod created a system of elementary schools, junior colleges, colleges, and seminaries that until World War I was the largest Protestant educational system in America. Ibid., 27.

106. Ibid., 50.

107. Weiser, "Serving Love," 119–20. Two hospitals were the beginning of deaconess work for the Missouri Synod: Fort Wayne, Indiana and Beaver Dam, Wisconsin. There was no motherhouse and they did not join the Deaconess Conference.

108. Moves to eradicate non-English educational systems occurred again in 1890. Coburn, *Life at Four Corners,* 176.

109. Those who remained suffered badly under Stalin. 92,000 were moved from Bessarabia to settle Poland, and following the war many were herded to Siberia by the Red Army. See Shirley Fischer Arends, *The Central Dakota Germans: Their History, Language, and Culture* (Washington, D.C.: Georgetown University Press, 1989), 63–65.

110. At the end of the nineteenth century hospitals were founded by deaconesses in Grafton, North Dakota, Fargo, North Dakota, and throughout Minnesota. Doyle, "Nursing by Religious Orders," 1204.

111. Mass, of course, was in Latin until Vatican II in the 1960s. Nonetheless, prayers, Bible lessons, hymns, and the many complex festivals and devotions were all in German.

112. Hirner, *Called to Be Faithful,* 9.

113. Jay P. Dolan, *The American Catholic Experience: A History from Colonial Times to the Present* (Garden City, N.Y.: Doubleday, 1987), 297. See also Dolan, *The Immigrant Church: New York's Irish and German Catholics, 1815–1865* (Baltimore: Johns Hopkins University Press, 1975).

114. George C. Stewart, *Marvels of Charity: History of American Sisters and Nuns* (Huntington, Ind.: Our Sunday Visitor, 1994), 412 records that Franciscans were the fastest growing communities of women in the United States between 1918 and 1945. They grew from 6,461 sisters in 1900 to 30,241 in 1945.

115. Henninger, *Sisters of St. Mary and Their Healing Mission,* 10, 116.

116. The young sisters were relieved when Mother Seraphia Scholctemeyer fell asleep and they eventually made themselves comfortable on their nine-hour journey. Ibid., 117.

117. Both rules are quite clear on this, forbidding fasting, night prayers, etc., which are common Franciscan practices. See Chapter 6.

118. This changed in the twentieth century, when many Franciscan communities became teaching communities. Stewart, *Marvels of Charity,* 412.

119. These sanguine comments were in Keuenhof's Foreword to *The Sisters of St. Mary and Their Hospital Work.* He was far more glowing in his praise of the late Father Faerber, spiritual director of the community in St. Louis.

120. Christian Golder's *History of the Deaconess Movement* is the only source of photographs and profiles of the early deaconesses. It is the source for Doyle's "Nursing by Religious Orders, Part V."

121. Ibid.

122. Prelinger, *Charity, Challenge, and Change,* 18.

123. Ibid.

124. Catherine Prelinger, "The Nineteenth-Century Deaconessate in Germany: The Efficacy of the Family Model," in *German Women in the Eighteenth and Nineteenth Centuries: A Social and Literary History*, ed. Ruth-Ellen B. Joeres and Mary Jo Maynes (Bloomington: Indiana University Press, 1986), 215–29.

125. Ibid., 15–16.

126. At least, this is how the situation appears. Research in German, Swedish, Danish, and Norwegian hospital archives would really need to be done to say whether that rule applied throughout all deaconess hospitals in the United States. It certainly applied in the notable hospitals that have been examined, and the Catholic sisterhoods were the exceptions to the rule. Catholic religious communities have controlled their own assets in Catholicism throughout the history of the monastic movement, these immigrant Catholic women in the United States merely followed customary practice.

127. Suzy Farren, *A Call to Care: The Women Who Built Catholic Healthcare in America* (St. Louis: Catholic Association of the United States, 1996).

128. Weiser, "Serving Love," 69, cites Sister Julie Mergner's letter to *The Lutheran* (21 April 1904): 504–5. Sister Julie is adamant: "We are convinced this is not the remedy to our difficulties. We need workers"; but so do the English and German-English using houses in Baltimore and Milwaukee, she points out. "Why should we throw away a treasure [German language] before there is the least necessity for doing so? Let those who desire an English-speaking house go where there is one."

129. Golder, *History of the Deaconess Movement*, 133. In 1924 only 124 of 810 active deaconesses were listed as serving in hospitals, whereas all deaconesses in Germany were graduate nurses. Doyle, "Nursing by Religious Orders in the United States, Part V—Deaconesses, 1855–1928," *American Journal of Nursing* 19, 11 (1929): 1336.

Chapter 8. The Twentieth Century

1. Kathleen M. Joyce, *Medicine, Markets, and Morals: Catholic Hospitals and the Ethics of Abortion in Early 20th-Century America*, Working Papers series 29, 2 (South Bend, Ind.: Cushwa Center for the Study of American Catholicism, University of Notre Dame, Fall 1997), 7.

2. This is Anne Summers's argument, see "The Mysterious Demise of Sarah Gamp: The Domiciliary Nurse and Her Detractors," *Victorian Studies* 32 (1989): 365–86 and "Ministering Angels," *History Today* 39 (February 1989): 31–37.

3. See Christine Allen, "Women in Colonial French America," in *Women and Religion in America*, vol. 2, *The Colonial and Revolutionary Periods*, ed. Rosemary Radford Ruether and Rosemary Skinner Keller (San Francisco: Harper and Row, 1983), 80–83, 111–17. See also Pauline Pauls, "A History of the Edmonton General Hospital, 1895–1970," PhD dissertation, University of Alberta, 1994.

4. Susan M. Reverby, *Ordered to Care: The Dilemma of American Nursing, 1850–1945* (Cambridge: Cambridge University Press, 1987). Celia Davies makes this point too in her conclusion to *Gender and the Professional Predicament in Nursing* (Buckingham: Open University Press, 1995), 180.

5. Margaret MacCurtain, "Godly Burden: Catholic Sisterhoods in 20th-Century Ireland," in *Gender and Sexuality in Modern Ireland*, ed. Anthony Bradley and Maryann Gialanella Valiulis (Amherst: University of Massachusetts Press, 1997), 248.

6. Anne Summers, "The Costs and Benefits of Caring: Nursing Charities, c.1830–1860," in *Medicine and Charity Before the Welfare State*, ed. Jonathan Barry and Colin Jones (London: Routledge, 1991), 133–48.

7. Sue Ellen Hoy, "The Journey Out: The Recruitment and Emigration of Irish Religious Women to the United States, 1812–1914," *Journal of Women's History* 6, 4 (1995): 64–98.

8. Mary E. Daly, "Women in the Irish Workforce from Pre-Industrial to Modern Times," *SOATHAR* 7 (1981): 77.

9. Margaret MacCurtain, "Late in the Field: Catholic Sisters in Twentieth-Century Ireland and the New Religious History," *Journal of Women's History* 6, 4/7, 1 (Winter/Spring 1995): 54.

10. For a discussion of the Irish takeover of the Sisters of the Holy Cross and the Sisters of St. Joseph of Carondelet — two French communities — see Barbra Mann Wall, "Religion, Ethnicity, and Nursing: The Americanization of Irish Catholic Sister Nurses," *Proceedings of the Conference on the History of Women Religious*, Loyola University, Chicago, 24 June 1998, 2–3; and Wall, "Unlikely Entrepreneurs: Nuns, Nursing, and Hospital Development in the West and Midwest, 1805–1915," PhD dissertations, University of Notre Dame, 2000.

11. Byrne, "In the Parish But Not of It: Sisters," 139, cites Mary Schneider.

12. Patricia Byrne, "In the Parish But Not of It: Sisters," in *Transforming Parish Ministry: The Changing Roles of Catholic Clergy, Laity, and Women Religious*, ed. Jay P. Dolan, R. Scott Appleby, Patricia Byrne, and Debra Campbell (New York: Cross-road, 1990), 155, cites Joan A. Chittister's comment that prior to Vatican II "every day life got smaller. Religious life had become the celebration of the trivial."

13. The Second Vatican Council (1962–65) resulted in a dramatic transformation of Catholic liturgy and life.

14. The codification of canon law covered every aspect of church law, not simply matters pertaining to religious women. It was the result of a massive consultative project with the entire episcopate — all the bishops in the world. Needless to say, women were not consulted.

15. See Byrne, "In the Parish But Not of It: Sisters," for a discussion of these changes and their implications.

16. This is not to say that some women did not manage to overcome restrictions and maintain a high professional profile. The trend, however, was to move sisters out of the limelight.

17. Byrne, "In the Parish But Not of It: Sisters," 113.

18. Helen R. Ebaugh, "Patriarchal Bargains and Latent Avenues of Social Mobility: Nuns in the Roman Catholic Church," *Gender and Society* 7, 3 (September 1993): 400–414, 403.

19. For a brief discussion of the impact of these changes on the Sisters of St. Joseph of Carondelet see Carol K. Coburn and Martha Smith, *Spirited Lives: How Nuns Shaped Catholic Culture and American Life, 1836–1920* (Chapel Hill: University of North Carolina Press, 1999), 224–25.

20. Byrne, "In the Parish But Not of It: Sisters," 131.

21. The incongruous existence of religious women in the twentieth century before Vatican II is discussed by Elizabeth Kolmer, *Religious Women in the United States: A Survey of the Influential Literature from 1950 to 1983* (Wilmington, Del.: Michael Glazier, 1984); Helen Rose Fuchs Ebaugh, *Out of the Cloister: A Study of Organizational Dilemmas* (Austin: University of Texas Press, 1977); Byrne, "In the Parish But Not of It: Sisters," 115–33.

22. Of course its patient base did not necessarily follow suit. The patient base of

a hospital followed the social and demographic profile of its constituency, and location rather than religion was the primary reason for hospital use. See Bernadette McCauley, "Sublime Anomalies: Women Religious and Roman Catholic Hospitals in New York City, 1850–1920," *Journal of the History of Medicine and Allied Sciences* 52 (1997): 304.

23. "Sisters should be trained in these matters and instruct students properly however, it is best if they do not perform such indelicate tasks 'as a rule,'" Customary, 1928, Sisters of Providence Archives, Seattle, Washington, 106. This rule is in common with usual practice — trained nurses did supervise the hands-on works of trainees and the sister-nurses were no different in this respect.

24. Ibid., 105.

25. Joyce, "Medicine, Markets, and Morals," 7.

26. Sisters of St. Francis founder Mother Augustine Giesen lost her arm in the laundry mangle. See Sister Louise Hirner, *Called to Be Faithful: A History of the Sisters of St. Francis, Maryville, Missouri* (Maryville, Mo.: Sisters of St. Francis, Mount Alverno Convent, Maryville, 1984).

27. Joyce, "Medicine, Markets, and Morals," 7.

28. Jean Richardson, "Catholic Religious Women as Institutional Innovators: the Sisters of Charity and the Rise of the Modern Urban Hospital in Buffalo, N.Y., 1848–1900," PhD dissertation, State University of New York at Buffalo, 1996, 233–39.

29. See Kathleen M. Joyce, "Science and the Saints: American Catholics and Health Care, 1880–1930," PhD dissertation, Princeton University, 1995, 227–32.

30. Bernadette McCauley argues that in New York the diocesan hierarchy "supported reform criticisms of sisters and in so doing assumed a new, proactive role in Catholic health care." See "Sublime Anomalies," 305.

31. Sisters delivered babies in San Antonio and Seattle. Daughters of Charity conducted maternity hospitals in Buffalo, although doctors performed deliveries — as was the norm in the northeast. Sisters attended unexpected arrivals.

32. Sister Mary Gabriel Henninger, *Sisters of Saint Mary and Their Healing Mission* (St. Louis: Sisters of St. Mary of the Third Order of Saint Francis, 1979), 171.

33. Teresa Keaney, who established the Franciscan Missionaries to Africa, campaigned tirelessly for permission to train and practice as midwives. When in 1936 Pius IX capitulated with Canon 489, "Maternity Training for Midwifery Sisters," she opened a midwifery school in Uganda. See MacCurtain, "Godly Burden," 251.

34. Christopher J. Kauffman, *Ministry and Meaning: A Religious History of Catholic Health Care in the United States* (New York: Crossroad, 1995), 171.

35. Joyce, *Medicine, Markets, and Morals*, 24.

36. Ibid., 6.

37. In 1873 there were only three schools; in 1880 only 560 trained nurses scattered through the entire country; by 1890 only thirty-five schools. Barbara Melosh, *"The Physician's Hand": Work Culture and Conflict in American Nursing* (Philadelphia: Temple University Press, 1982), 25–26. 30. Ann Doyle, "Nursing by Religious Orders in the United States, Part III — 1871–1928," *American Journal of Nursing* 19, 9 (1929): 1085 cites the three quoted Catholic hospitals.

38. Ibid., 1092.

39. Ibid., 1090.

40. The first nurse to be registered in Alabama was Sister Chrysostom of St. Vincent's Hospital. Ibid., 1093.

41. Ibid., 1094. Even in the 1950s the Daughters of Providence in Seattle pro-

vided the president of the state hospital association. See *History of the Washington State Hospital Association* (Seattle: Washington State Hospital Association, 1958).

42. Elizabeth Smyth develops the idea of dual professional engagement and cites a 1965 census of religious women in Canada that demonstrates the high level of professional education and training of sisters. See Smyth, "Professionalization Among the Professed: The Case of Roman Catholic Women Religious," in *Challenging Professions: Historical and Contemporary Perspectives on Women's Professional Work*, ed. Smyth, Sandra Acker, Sandra Bourne, and Alison Prentice (Toronto: University of Toronto Press, 1999), 248. MacCurtain describes the nuns as the "pioneering graduate elite" of Ireland after they were permitted to attend university in the 1940s. MacCurtain, "Godly Burden," 249.

43. Anne Marie Rafferty, *The Politics of Nursing Knowledge* (London: Routledge, 1996), 40; Susan Reverby supports this idea in her depiction of character as skill in *Ordered to Care*, as does Celia Davies in *Gender and the Professional Predicament*.

44. Melosh, *"The Physician's Hand"*, 23.

Bibliography

Archives

This research has relied upon a range of both primary and secondary texts. I believe that, given the unfamiliar nature of the primary and archival sources to historians of nursing, it is worthwhile providing a brief explanation of the material used.

Archives of religious women generally include the following types of information:

Annals. These are in-house accounts of events. They may be authored by a sequence of non-named members of the community, or written for many years by a single hand. They may be handwritten, in English or other languages. Originals may have been typed and translated. The annals often include extensive necrologies, or accounts of important community members on the occasion of their death.

Letters. Letters relevant to the foundation of a community or institution are often kept in the archives. In the nineteenth century letters to and from the motherhouse, letters between community members, between the confessor (priest) and the mother superior, between the community and the diocese, affectionate newsy letters, business letters, and so on are all found in archives. As with annals, these letters may be handwritten and in various languages, or they may have been collated, edited, typed, and translated.

Religious materials. Prayer books, pious literature, sermons, and lessons are sometimes available. Outlines of religious training are particularly revealing of the religious life and the religious tradition a community follows.

Rules. Each community had its own special rule, often modified over the years. This rule and its various editions are always available in the archives.

Membership details. These details can be quite extensive. Some archives hold full lists of all members, their home address, their father's occupation, and so on. Dowry lists may be available. Full lists of members including women who left the community and why may be available. Country of origin of members, their age, and previous life experience may be on record.

Financial details. Property lists, deeds, mortgage documents, bequests, debts and debtors, even everyday financial transactions may be available.

Unpublished histories. Histories were often undertaken by sisters or their pastor to commemorate an anniversary such as the community's or hospital's fiftieth anniversary. Twentieth-century master's and PhD dissertations on the community's history are often also available in community archives as well as in routine sources.

Archives (religious and other) used for this study:

British Library, London (BL)

Cincinnati Historical Society, Cincinnati, Ohio, Nippert Collection of German Methodism (CHSNCGM)

Daughters of Charity, Albany, New York (DOCA)

Dublin Archdiocese, Bishop's Palace, Dublin

Deaconess Community of the Evangelical Lutheran Church of America (AD-CELCA), Gladwyne, Pennsylvania

Mitchell Library, State Library of New South Wales

Notre Dame University, South Bend, Indiana

Sisters of Charity, Harold's Cross, Dublin

Sisters of the Incarnate Word, Motherhouse, San Antonio Texas (AMIW)

Sisters of Mercy, Bermondsey, London

Sisters of Providence, Sacred Heart Province, Seattle, Washington (SPA)

St. Joseph's Hospital, Vancouver

St. Vincent's Hospital, Sydney

Sydney Diocese, St. Mary's Cathedral, Sydney

Sydney Hospital, Sydney

Wellcome Institute for the History of Medicine Library, London

Published and Other Sources

Agnew, Sister Clare. *Geraldine, a Tale of Conscience.* Philadelphia: E. Cummiskey, 1819.

Allen, Christine. "Women in Colonial French America." In *Women and Religion in America,* vol. 2, *The Colonial and Revolutionary Periods,* ed. Rosemary Radford Ruether and Rosemary Skinner Keller. San Francisco: Harper and Row, 1983. 79–131.

Allchin, A. M. *The Silent Rebellion: Anglican Religious Communities, 1845–1900.* London: SCM, 1958.

Anson, Peter Frederick. *The Call of the Cloister: Religious Communities and Kindred Bodies in the Anglican Communion.* London: SPCK, 1955.

Arends, Shirley Fischer. *The Central Dakota Germans: Their History, Language, and Culture.* Washington, D.C.: Georgetown University Press, 1989.

Armiger, Sister Bernadette. "The History of the Hospital Work of the Daughters of Charity of St. Vincent de Paul in the Eastern Province of the United States, 1823–1860." Master of Science in Nursing Education thesis, Catholic University of America, 1947.

Armitage, Susan and Elizabeth Jameson, eds. *The Women's West.* Norman: University of Oklahoma Press, 1987.

Arnstein, Walter L. *Protestant Versus Catholic in Mid-Victorian England: Mr. Newdegate and the Nuns.* Columbia: University of Missouri Press, 1982.

Baly, Monica E. *Florence Nightingale and the Nursing Legacy.* London: Croom Helm, 1986.

———. "The Nightingale Nurses: The Myth and the Reality." In *Nursing His-*

tory: The State of the Art, ed. Christopher Maggs. London: Croom Helm, 1987. 33–59.

Bartlett, Alan. "From Strength to Strength: Roman Catholicism in Bermondsey up to 1939." In *The Church and the People: Catholics and Their Church in Britain, c.1880–1939.* Warwick: Centre for the Study of Social History, University of Warwick, 1988. 30.

Berner, Richard. "Port Blakely Mill Company 1876–89." *Pacific Northwest Quarterly* (October 1966): 153–71.

Blackwell, Elizabeth and Emily Blackwell. *Medicine as a Profession for Women.* New York: W.H. Tinson, 1860.

Blessing, J. Patrick. "Irish Emigration to the United States, 1800–1920: An Overview." In *The Irish in America: Emigration, Assimilation, and Impact,* ed. P. J. Drudy. New York: Cambridge University Press, 1985.

Bolster, Evelyn. *The Sisters of Mercy in the Crimean War.* Cork: Mercier Press, 1964.

Bossy, John. *The English Catholic Community, 1570–1850.* London: Darton, Longman, and Todd, 1976.

Boud, D. G. *Lucy Osburn, 1836–1891.* Windsor: Hawksbury Press, 1968.

Brown, Peter. *The Body and Society: Men, Women, and Sexual Renunciation in Early Christianity.* London: Faber and Faber, 1990.

Brynn, Edward. *The Church of Ireland in the Age of Catholic Emancipation.* New York: Garland, 1982.

Byrne, Patricia. "In the Parish But Not of It: Sisters." In *Transforming Parish Ministry: The Changing Roles of Catholic Clergy, Laity, and Women Religious,* ed. Jay P. Dolan, R. Scott Appleby, Patricia Byrne, and Debra Campbell. New York: Crossroad, 1990.

Campion, Edmund. *Rockchoppers: Growing Up Catholic in Australia.* Melbourne: Penguin, 1982.

Carroll, Mary Austin, RSM. *Leaves from the Annals of the Sisters of Mercy,* 4 vols., vol. 2, *England, Crimea, Scotland, Australia, and New Zealand.* New York: Catholic Publication Society, 1883.

Casteras, Susan P. "Virgin Vows." In *Religion in the Lives of English Women, 1760–1930,* ed. Gail Malmgreen. London: Croom Helm, 1986. 129–60.

Casterline, Gail Farr. "St. Joseph's and St. Mary's: The Origins of Catholic Hospitals in Philadelphia." *Pennsylvania Magazine of History and Biography* 108, 3 (1984): 291–314.

A Century of Service: The Record of One Hundred Years. Published for the Centenary of St. Vincent's Hospital, 23 January 1934. Dublin: Browne and Nolan, 1934.

Clark, Manning. *A Short History of Australia.* Melbourne: Penguin, 1995.

Clear, Caitrona. *Nuns in Nineteenth Century Ireland.* Dublin: Gill and Macmillan, 1897.

Coburn, Carol K. *Life at Four Corners: Religion, Gender, and Education in a German-Lutheran Community, 1868–1945.* Lawrence: University Press of Kansas, 1992.

Coburn, Carol K. and Martha Smith. " 'Pray for Your Wanderers': Women Religious on the Colorado Mining Frontier, 1877–1917." *Frontiers* 15, 3 (1995): 27–52.

Coburn, Carol K. and Martha Smith. *Spirited Lives: How Nuns Shaped Catholic Culture and American Life, 1836–1920.* Chapel Hill: University of North Carolina Press, 1999.

Coleman, Rev. Leighton. "English Sisterhoods and Deaconesses." *Church Magazine* (1886).

Connolly, Gerard. "Irish Catholic Myth or Reality? Another Sort of Irish and the

Renewal of Catholic Professional Among Catholics in England, 1791–1918." In *The Irish in the Victorian City,* ed. Roger Swift and Sheridan Gilley. London: Croom Helm, 1985. 225–54.

"Convent of Mercy, Bermondsey." *Southwark Record,* January 1932, 15–19.

Cook, Edward. *The Life of Florence Nightingale.* 2 vols. London: Macmillan, 1913.

Copy of correspondence between the Colonial government and Miss Florence Nightingale and others with reference to the Introduction of Trained Nurses for the Sydney Infirmary and Dispensary. Sidney: Joseph Cook, 1867.

Cott, Nancy F. *The Bonds of Womanhood: "Woman's Sphere" in New England, 1780–1835.* New Haven, Conn.: Yale University Press, 1977.

Cummings, Sister Celeste. "History of the Hospital Work and the Development of the Schools of Nursing of the Sisters of Charity in the Eastern Province (1860–1900)." Master's thesis, Catholic University of America, 1948.

Cummins, C. J. "The Colonial Medical Service." *Modern Medicine of Australia* (7 January 1974).

Curtis, L. P., Jr. *Anglo-Saxons and Celts: A Study of Anti-Irish Prejudice in Victorian England.* Bridgeport, Conn: University of Bridgeport Conference on British Studies, 1968.

———. *Apes and Angels: The Irishman in Victorian Caricature.* Washington, D.C.: Smithsonian Institution Press, 1971.

Daly, Mary W. "Women in the Irish Workforce from Pre-Industrial to Modern Times." *SOATHAR* 7 (1981).

Davies, Celia. *Gender and the Professional Predicament in Nursing.* Buckingham: Open University Press, 1995.

Davies, Rupert E. *Methodism.* London: Epworth Press, 1963.

Davis, Elizabeth. *The Autobiography of Elizabeth Davis, a Balaclava Nurse, Daughter of Dafydd Cadwaladyr.* 2 vols. Ed. Jane Williams. London: Hurst and Blackett, 1857.

Davis, Graham. *The Irish in Britain, 1815–1914.* Dublin: Gill and Macmillan, 1991.

Dean, Mitchell. *The Constitution of Poverty: Towards a Genealogy of Liberal Governance.* London: Routledgel, 1994.

Delumeau, Jean. *Catholicism Between Luther and Voltaire: A New View of the Counter-Reformation.* Trans. John Bossy. London: Burns and Oates, 1977.

Diakonissen Mutterhaus und Bethesda Hospital. Pittsburgh: City Mission Publishing Company, 1902.

Dickey, Brian. "St. Vincent's Hospital, Sydney: A Note." *Journal of the Royal Australian Historical Society* (8 September 1978): 131–33.

Diner, Hasia. *Erin's Daughters in America: Irish Immigrant Women in the Nineteenth Century.* Baltimore: Johns Hopkins University Press, 1983.

Dixson, Miriam. *The Real Matilda: Women and Identity in Australia, 1788–1975.* Sydney: Penguin Books, 1976.

Dolan, Jay P. *The American Catholic Experience: A History from Colonial Times to the Present.* Garden City, N.Y.: Doubleday, 1987.

———. *The Immigrant Church: New York's Irish and German Catholics, 1815–1865.* Baltimore: Johns Hopkins University Press, 1975.

Doona, Mary Ellen. "Sister Mary Joseph Croke: Another Voice from the Crimean War, 1854–1856." *Nursing History Review* 3 (1995): 3–41.

Doyle, Ann. "Nursing by Religious Orders in the United States, Part III — 1871–1928." *American Journal of Nursing* 19, 9 (1929): 1085–95.

———. "Nursing by Religious Orders in the United States, Part IV — Lutheran Deaconesses, 1849–1928." *American Journal of Nursing* 19, 10 (1929): 1197–1207.

———. "Nursing by Religious Orders in the United States, Part V—Deaconesses, 1855–1928." *American Journal of Nursing* 19, 11 (1929): 1331–43.

Ebaugh, Helen Rose Fuchs. *Out of the Cloister: A Study of Organizational Dilemmas.* Austin: University of Texas Press, 1977.

———. "Patriarchal Bargains and Latent Avenues of Social Mobility: Nuns in the Roman Catholic Church." *Gender and Society* 7, 3 (September 1993): 400–414.

Edward-Rees, Desiree. *The Story of Nursing.* London: Constable Young Books, 1965.

Engels, Friedrich. *The Condition of the Working Class in England.* 1844; Oxford: Blackwell, 1971.

Ewens, Mary. "The Leadership of Nuns in Immigrant Catholicism." In *Women and Religion in America,* vol. 1, *The Nineteenth Century,* ed. Rosemary Radford Ruether and Rosemary Skinner Keller. San Francisco: Harper and Row, 1981.

Ewens, Mary. *The Role of the Nun in Nineteenth-Century America.* New York: Arno Press, 1978.

Faerber, Wilhelm. *The Sisters of St. Mary of St. Louis: In Commemoration of the Silver Jubilee of the Order, 1872–16 November 1897.* St. Louis: Amerika Printing House, 1897.

Farren, Suzy. *A Call to Care: The Women Who Built Catholic Healthcare in America.* St. Louis: Catholic Hospitals Association, 1996.

Fielding, Steven. *Class and Ethnicity: Irish Catholics in England, 1880–1939.* Buckingham: Open University Press, 1993.

Fitzgerald, Shirley, *Rising Damp: Sydney 1870–90.* Melbourne: Oxford University Press, 1987.

Fitzpatrick, David. "A Curious Middle Place: The Irish in Britain, 1871–1920." In *The Irish in Britain, 1815–1939,* ed. Roger Swift and Sheridan Gilley. Savage, Md.: Barnes and Noble, 1989.

Fogelström, E. A. *Autobiography.* Trans. Sister Elfrida Sandberg, Immanuel, 1957–58, 31.

Foucault, Michel. "Governmentality." In *The Foucault Effect: Studies in Governmentality,* ed. Graham Burchill, Colin Gordon, and Vear Miller. Chicago: University of Chicago Press, 1991.

Franchot, Jenny. *Roads to Rome: The Antebellum Protestant Encounter with Catholicism.* Berkeley: University of California Press, 1994.

Franciscan Sisters of Mary: Priceless Heritage, 1823–1988. St. Louis: Franciscan Sisters of Mary, 1988.

Frederick S. Weiser and His People, 1884–1984: Celebrating the Heritage of a Century of Lutheran Deaconesses in America. Gladwyne, Pa.: Deaconess Community of the Lutheran Church in America, 1984.

Gerber, David. *The Making of an American Pluralism, Buffalo, New York, 1825–60.* Urbana: University of Illinois Press, 1989.

Gerber, Linda. "Separate Spheres, Female Worlds, Women's Place: The Rhetoric of Women's History." *Journal of American History* 75, 1 (1988): 9–39.

Gibson, Ralph. "Female Religious Orders in Nineteenth-Century France: Catholicism in Britain and France Since 1789." In *Catholicism in Britain and France Since 1789,* ed. Frank Tallet and Nicholas Atkin. London: Hambledon, 1996.

———. *A Social History of French Catholicism, 1789–1914.* London: Routledge, 1989.

Gill, Sean. *Women and the Church of England: From the Eighteenth Century to the Present.* London: SPCK, 1994.

Gilley, Sheridan. "Garibaldi Riots of 1862." *Historical Journal* 16, 4 (1973): 697–732.

——. "Heretic London, Holy Poverty, and the Irish Poor, 1830–1870. *Downside Review* 89 (1971): 64–89.

——. "Irish Catholicism in Britian." In *Religion, State, and Ethnic Groups,* ed. Donal A. Kerr. Aldershot: Dartmouth Publishing, 1992.

——. "Protestant London, No-Popery and the Irish Poor, 1830–1860." *Recusant History* 10, 4 (1969): 210–30.

——. "The Roman Catholic Church and the Nineteenth Century Irish Diaspora." *Journal of Ecclesiastical History* 35, 2 (1984).

——. "The Roman Catholic Mission to the Irish in London." *Recusant History* 10, 3 (1969): 123–45

Ginzberg, Lori D. *Women and the Work of Benevolence: Morality, Politics, and Class in the Nineteenth-Century United States.* New Haven, Conn.: Yale University Press, 1990.

Godden, Judith and Sue Forsyth. "Defining Relationships and Limiting Power: Two Leaders of Australian Nursing, 1868–1904." *Nursing Inquiry* 7 (2000).

Golder, Christian, ed. *The Deaconess Motherhouse, in Its Relation to the Deaconess Work.* Pittsburgh: Pittsburgh Printing Co., 1907.

Golder, Christian. *History of the Deaconess Movement in the Christian Church.* New York: Eaton and Mains, 1903.

Golder, Louise. "The Deaconess Motherhouse." In *The Deaconess and Her Work.* Bethesda Hospital, Cincinnati, Ohio.

Gusfield, Joseph R. *Symbolic Crusade: Status Politics and the American Temperance Movement.* Urbana: University of Illinois Press, 1986.

Hampton, Isobel A. et al. *Nursing of the Sick, 1893.* New York: McGraw-Hill, 1949.

Helmstadter, Carol. "Old Nurses and New: Nursing in the London Teaching Hospitals Before and After the Mid-Nineteenth-Century Reforms." *Nursing History Review* 1 (1993): 43–70.

——. "Robert Bentley Todd, Saint John's House, and the Origins of the Modern Trained Nurse." *Bulletin of the History of Medicine* 67, 3 (1993): 282–319.

Helmstadter, Richard and Paul T. Phillips, eds. *Religion in Victorian Society: A Sourcebook of Documents.* Lanham, Md.: University Press of America, 1985.

Henninger, Sister Mary Gabriel. *Sisters of St. Mary and Their Healing Mission.* St. Louis: Sisters of St. Mary of the Third Order of St. Francis, 1979.

Hirner, Sister Louise. *Called to Be Faithful: A History of the Sisters of St. Francis, Maryville, Missouri.* Maryville, Mo.: Sisters of St. Francis, Mount Alverno Convent, Maryville, 1984.

History of the Washington State Hospital Association. Seattle: Washington State Hospital Association, 1958.

Hobbs, Colleen Adele. *Florence Nightingale.* New York: Twayne, 1997.

Hogan, Michael. "Whatever Happened to Australian Sectarianism." *Journal of Religious History* 13, 1 (1984–85): 83–91.

House Surgeon and Physician's Semi-Annual Report to the Board of Physicians and Surgeons, and staff of the Buffalo Hospital of the Sisters of Charity, Oct 1 1856–April 1, 1856. *Buffalo Medical Journal* 12 (June 1856): 62.

Hoy, Suellen. "The Journey Out: The Recruitment and Emigration of Irish Religious Women to the United States, 1812–1914." *Journal of Women's History* 6, 7/7, 1 (Winter/Spring 1995): 64–98.

Hudson, Winthrop S. *Religion in America: An Historical Account of the Development of American Religious Life.* New York: Scribner's, 1981.

Hufton, Olwen and Frank Tallet, "Communities of Women, the Religious Life, and Public Service in Seventeenth-/Eighteenth-Century France." In *Connecting Spheres: Women in the Western World, 1500 to the Present,* ed. Marilyn H. Boxer and Jean H. Quatraert. New York: Oxford University Press, 1987. 75–85.

Ignatiev, Noel. *How the Irish Became White.* New York: Routledge, 1995.

James, Lillian. "Horse-Breaking Preferred! Lucy Osburn of Sydney Hospital." In *Lives Obscurely Great: Historical Essays on Women of New South Wales,* ed. Patricia Thompson and Susan Yorke. Sydney: Society of Women Writers (Australia) New South Wales Branch, 1980.

Jameson, Anna. *Sisters of Charity, Catholic and Protestant, Abroad and at Home.* London: Longmans, 1855.

Jensen, John. "Before the Surgeon General: Marine Hospitals in Mid-19th Century America." *Public Health Reports* (November–December 1997): 112, 525–27.

Johnson, Dale A., ed. *Women in English Religion, 1700–1925.* New York: Edwin Mellen, 1983.

Jones, Colin. *The Charitable Imperative: Hospitals and Nursing in Ancien Régime and Revolutionary France.* London: Routledge, 1989.

Joyce, Kathleen M. *Medicine, Markets, and Morals: Catholic Hospitals and the Ethics of Abortion in Early 20th-Century America.* Working Papers series 29, 2. South Bend, Ind.: Cushwa Center for the Study of American Catholicism, Fall 1997.

Joyce, Kathleen M. "Science and the Saints: American Catholics and Health Care, 1880–1930." PhD dissertation, Princeton University, 1995.

Kauffman, Christopher J. *Ministry and Meaning: A Religious History of Catholic Health Care in the United States.* New York: Crossroad, 1995.

Kelly, Gerald A. *The Life of Mother Hieronymo.* Rochester, N.Y.: Christopher Press, 1900.

Kingston, Beverley. *My Wife, My Daughter, and Poor Mary Ann: Women and Work in Australia.* Sydney: Nelson, 1975.

Kirby, James, Russell E. Richey, and Kenneth E. Rowe. *The Methodists.* Westport, Conn: Greenwood Press, 1996.

Kolmer, Elizabeth. *Religious Women in the United States: A Survey of the Influential Literature from 1950 to 1983.* Wilmington, Del.: Michael Glazier, 1984.

Langlois, Claude. *Le Catholicisme au féminin: Les congrégations françaises à supérieure générale au XIXe siècle.* Paris: Cerf, 1984.

Larkin, Emmet. "Devotional Revolution in Ireland." *American Historical Review* 80 (1972): 625–52.

———. *The Roman Catholic Church and the Creation of the Irish State.* Philadelphia: American Philosophical Society, 1975.

Larson, Leslie. "Fogelström and the Diaconate." *Augustinian Quarterly* 5, 26, 4 (October 1947): 347–54.

Little Medical Guide of the Sisters of Providence. Montreal: Providence Maison-Mère, 1889.

Lucia, Ellis. *Cornerstone: The Story of St. Vincent—Oregon's First Permanent Hospital, Its Formative Years.* Portland, Ore.: St. Vincent's Medical Foundation, 1975.

———. *Seattle's Sisters of Providence.* Seattle: Providence Medical Center, 1978.

Luddy, Maria. *Women and Philanthropy in Nineteenth-Century Ireland.* Cambridge: Cambridge University Press, 1995.

Lynaugh, Joan. *The Community Hospitals of Kansas City, Missouri, 1870–1915.* New York: Garland Press, 1989.

McCauley, Bernadette. "'Sublime Anomalies': Women Religious and Roman

Catholic Hospitals in New York City, 1850–1920." *Journal of the History of Medicine and Allied Sciences* 52 (July 1997): 289–309.

MacCurtain, Margaret. "Godly Burden: Catholic Sisterhoods in 20th-Century Ireland." In *Gender and Sexuality in Modern Ireland,* ed. Anthony Bradley and Maryann Gialanella Valiulis. Amherst: University of Massachusetts Press, 1997.

———. "Late in the Field: Catholic Sisters in Twentieth-Century Ireland and the New Religious History." *Journal of Women's History* 6, 4/7, 1 (Winter/Spring 1995): 54.

MacGinley, Rosa. *A Dynamic of Hope: Women Religious Institutes in Australia.* Sydney: Crossing Press, 1996.

Magray, Mary Peckham. *The Transforming Power of the Nuns: Women, Religion, and Cultural Change in Ireland, 1750–1900.* New York: Oxford University Press, 1998.

Maher, Mary Denis. *To Bind Up the Wounds: Catholic Sister Nurses in the U.S. Civil War.* New York: Greenwood Press, 1989.

Mallon, Sister Catherine. "Sister Catherine Mallon's Journal. Part Two." Ed. Thomas Richter. *New Mexico History Review* 52, 3 (1977).

Mannard, Joseph G. "Converts in Convents: Protestant Women and the Social Appeal of Catholic Religious Life in Antebellum America." *Records of the American Catholic Historical Society of Philadelphia* 104, 1–4 (1993): 79–90.

Mansell, S. B. *English Sisterhoods: An Address Delivered at the Re-opening and Benediction of St. Peter's Home, Brompton Square, 5 May 1863.* London: Joseph Masters Aldergate Street, 1863.

Marteau, Louis. *The Hospital of St. John and St. Elizabeth, 1856–1992.* London: Hospital of St. John and St. Elizabeth, 1992.

Martin, Allan William. *Henry Parkes: A Biography.* Melbourne: Melbourne University Press, 1980.

Martin, R. "They Served the Sick, in North and South." *Military Medicine* (July 1961): 575

Mason, Helen, S.P. *History of St. Ignatius Province of the Sisters of Providence.* Spokane, Wash.: Sisters of Providence, 1997.

Master, J. "A Few Words to Some of the Women of the Church of God." London, 1850. Reprinted in *Women in English Religion, 1700–1925,* ed. Dale A. Johnson. New York: Edwin Mellen, 1983. 17–23.

Mayhew, Henry. *London Labour and the London Poor.* 1861–12; Harmondsworth: Penguin, 1985.

McDonnell, Freda. *Miss Nightingale's Young Ladies.* Sydney: Angus and Robertson, 1970.

McGinley, M. R. *A Dynamic of Hope: Institutes of Women Religious in Australia.* Sydney: Crossing Press, 1996.

McLeod, Hugh. *Religion and Society in England, 1850–1914.* New York: St. Martin's Press, 1996.

McNamara, Jo Ann Kay. *Sisters in Arms: Catholic Nuns Through Two Millennia.* Cambridge, Mass: Harvard University Press, 1996.

Melosh, Barbara. *"The Physician's Hand": Work Culture and Conflict in American Nursing.* Philadelphia: Temple University Press, 1982.

Miller, Douglas. *Earlier Days: A Story of St. Vincent's.* Sydney: Angus and Robertson, 1969.

Mitchell, B. R. *International Historical Statistics: Africa, Asia and Oceania, 1750–1988.* 2nd rev. ed. New York: Stockton, 1995.

————. *International Historical Statistics: The Americas and Australasia.* Detroit: Gale Research, 1983.

Monk, Maria. *The Awful Disclosures of Maria Monk, or the Secrets of a Nun's Life in a Convent Exposed.* 1836. New York: D.M. Bennett, 1878.

Moore, Judith. *A Zeal for Responsibility: The Struggle for Professional Nursing in Victorian England, 1868–1883.* Athens: University of Georgia Press, 1988.

Morris, Charles. *Saints and Sinners.* New York: Times Books, 1997.

Muhlenberg, William Augustus, ed. *Thoughts on Evangelical Sisterhoods.* London: S.W. Partridge and Co, 1872.

Mumm, Susan. *Stolen Daughters, Virgin Mothers: Anglican Sisterhoods in Victorian Britain.* London: Leicester University Press, 1999.

Murphy, Denis G. *Terra Incognita or the Convents of the United Kingdom.* London: Longmans, 1873.

————. *They Did Not Pass By: The Story of the Early Pioneers of Nursing.* London: Longmans, 1956.

Nadel, Stanley. *Little Germany: Ethnicity, Religion, and Class in New York City, 1845–80.* Urbana: University of Illinois Press, 1990.

Neale, John Mason. *Letters of John Mason Neale.* Ed. Mary Sackville Lawson. London: Longmans, 1920.

Nelson, Sioban. "Entering the Professional Domain in 17th Century France." *Nursing History Review* 7 (1999): 171–88.

————. "Reading Nursing History." *Nursing Inquiry* 4, 4 (1997): 229–36.

Newman, John Henry. *Apologia Pro Vita Sua.* 1864. New York: Penguin, 1994.

Nightingale, Florence. *As Miss Nightingale Said: Florence Nightingale Through Her Sayings: A Victorian Perspective.* Ed. Monica Baly. London: Scutari Press, 1991.

————. "On Different Systems of Hospital Nursing." Appendix to *Notes on Hospitals,* 1859, reprinted in *Florence Nightingale on Hospital Reform,* ed. Charles E. Rosenberg. New York: Garland, 1989.

————. *Ever Yours, Florence Nightingale: Selected Letters.* Ed. Martha Vicinus and Bea Nergaard. London: Virago Press, 1989.

North London Deaconess Institution. *Second Annual Report.* London: Varty Printers, 1803.

O'Brien, Susan. "French Nuns in Nineteenth Century England." *Past and Present* 154 (1997): 142–80.

O'Carrigan, Catherine. "Australian Catholic Hospitals in the Nineteenth Century." *Journal of the Australian Catholic Historical Society* 7, 4 (1964): 20–36.

————. "St. Vincent's Hospital, Sydney, Pioneer in Nineteenth Century Health Care." MA thesis, University of Sydney, 1986.

O'Connell, Marvin. "The Roman Catholic Tradition Since 1545." In *Caring and Curing: Health and Medicine in the Western Religious Traditions,* ed. Ronald L. Numbers and Darrel W. Amundsen. New York: Macmillan, 1986. 108–45.

O'Farrell, Patrick. *The Irish in Australia,* rev. ed. Kensington: New South Wales University Press, 1993.

O'Sullivan, Maureen M. K. *A Cause of Trouble? Irish Nuns and English Clerics.* Sydney: Crossing Press, 1995.

Parkes, Henry. *Fifty Years of Australian History.* 2 vols. London: Longmans, 1892.

Partington, Geoffrey. *The Australian Nation: Its British and Irish Roots.* Melbourne: Australian Scholarly Publishing, 1994.

Passavant, W. A. "The Deaconess and the Professional Nurse." *Proceedings and Papers of the Third Annual Conference of Evangelical Deaconess Motherhouses.* Omaha, Neb., 1899.

Pauls, Pauline. "A History of the Edmonton General Hospital, 1895–1970." PhD dissertation, University of Alberta, 1994.

Phillips, Paul T. "Converting the Working Classes." In *Religion in Victorian Society: A Sourcebook of Documents,* ed. Richard T. Helms — *and Paul T. Phillips. Lanham, Md.: University Press of America, 1985. 211–63.

Polding, John Bede. *The Letters of John Bede Polding.* Ed. M. Xavier Compton et al. Sydney: Good Samaritan Sisters, 1994.

Poovey, Mary. *Uneven Developments: The Ideological Work of Gender in Mid-Victorian England.* Chicago: University of Chicago Press, 1988.

Poplin, Irene Schuessler. "Nursing Uniforms: Romantic Idea, Functional Attire, or Instrument of Social Change." *Nursing History Review* 2 (1994): 153–67.

Prelinger, Catherine M. *Charity, Challenge, and Change: Religious Dimensions of the Mid-Nineteenth-Century Women's Movement in Germany.* New York: Greenwood Press, 1987.

——. "The Nineteenth-Century Deaconessate in Germany: The Efficacy of a Family Model." In *German Women in the Eighteenth and Nineteenth Centuries: A Social and Literary History,* ed. Ruth-Ellen B. Joeres and Mary Jo Maynes. Bloomington: Indiana University Press, 1986. 215–30

——. "Prelude to Consciousness." In *German Women in the Nineteenth Century: A Social History,* ed. John C. Fout. New York, Holmes and Meier, 1984.

Prochaska, F. K. "Body and Soul: Bible Nurses and the Poor in Victorian London." *Historical Research* 60, 143 (1987): 336–34.

Public Charities Commission. *Commission Appointed to Inquire into and Report Upon the Working and Management of the Public Charities, First Report,* 18 September 1873. Sydney: Thomas Richards, 1973.

Rafferty, Anne Marie. *The Politics of Nursing Knowledge.* London: Routledge, 1996.

Rapley, Elizabeth. *The Dévotes: Women and Church in Seventeenth-Century France.* Montreal: McGill University Press, 1990.

Reverby, Susan M. *Ordered to Care: The Dilemma of American Nursing, 1850–1945.* Cambridge: Cambridge University Press, 1987.

Reynolds, Henry. *Dispassion: Black Australians and White Invaders.* Sydney: Allen and Unwin, 1989.

Richardson, Jean. "Catholic Religious Women as Institutional Innovators: The Sisters of Charity and the Rise of the Modern Urban Hospital in Buffalo, N.Y., 1848–1900." PhD dissertation, State University of New York at Buffalo, 1996.

——. "A Tale of Two Nineteenth Century Hospitals: Buffalo Hospital of the Sisters of Charity and Buffalo General Hospital." In *Medical History in Buffalo, 1846–1996: Collected Essays,* ed. Lilli Stentz. Buffalo: School of Medicine and Biomedical Services, State University of New York at Buffalo, 1996. 47–60.

Robb, Isabel Hampton, ed., *Nursing of the Sick: Papers from the International Congress of Charities, Correction, and Philanthropy.* Chicago, 1893; rpt. New York: McGraw-Hill, 1949.

Rose, Nicolas. *Governing the Soul: The Shaping of Private Life.* London: Routledge, 1990.

Rosenberg, Charles E. *The Care of Strangers: The Rise of America's Hospital System.* New York: Basic Books, 1987.

——. *The Cholera Years: The United States in 1832, 1849, and 1866.* Chicago: University of Chicago Press, 1962.

Russell, R. Lynette. "Lucy Osburn: The First of Many." *First National Nursing History Conference: Australian Nursing — The Story.* Melbourne, May 1993. Melbourne: Royal College of Nursing, Australia, 1993.

Salmon, M. "A Pioneer of Trained Nurses." *Australasian Trained Nurses Journal* (15 November 1911): 365.

Schell, E. "Nurses Under Attack: The Lewes Riot and the Society of St. Margaret." *Nursing Research* 41, 1 (1992): 33–38.

Schultheiss, Katrin. " 'La Véritable médicine des femmes': Anna Hamilton and the Politics of Nursing Reform in Bordeaux, 1900–1914." *French Historical Studies* 19, 1 (Spring 1995).

Schultz, Bartz. *A Tapestry of Service: The Evolution of Nursing in Australia.* Melbourne: Churchill Livingstone, 1991.

Schultz, Jane E. "The Inhospitable Hospital: Gender and Professionalism in Civil War Medicine." *Signs* (Winter 1992): 367.

Schultz, Rima Lunin. "Woman's Work and Woman's Calling in the Episcopal Church: Chicago, 1880–1989." In *Episcopal Women: Gender, Spirituality, and Commitment in an American Mainline Denomination,* ed. Catherine M. Prelinger. New York: Oxford University Press, 1992. 19–71.

Segale, Blandina. *At the End of the Santa Fe Trail.* Columbus, Ohio: Columbian Press, 1932; reprint Albuquerque: University of New Mexico Press, 1999.

Serle, Geoffrey. *The Golden Age: A History of the Colony of Victoria, 1851–1861.* Melbourne: Melbourne University Press, 1971.

Seymer, Lucy Ridgely. *A General History of Nursing.* New York: Macmillan, 1932, 73.

Showalter, Elaine. "Florence Nightingale's Feminist Complaint: Women, Religion, and *Suggestions for Thought.*" *Signs: Journal of Women in Culture and Society* 6, 3 (1981): 395–412

Sisters of Mercy. *Harvest of Mercy.* Convent of Mercy, Bermondsey. London: Winchester Press, 1978.

Sisters of St. Mary. *The Sisters of St. Mary and Their Hospital Work in Kansas City, Missouri, 1895–1920.* Kansas City: Sisters of St. Mary, 1921.

Slattery, Sister Margaret Patrice. *Promises to Keep: A History of the Sisters of Charity of the Incarnate Word, San Antonio, Texas.* 2 vols. 2nd ed. San Antonio: Sisters of the Incarnate Word, San Antonio, 1998.

Smith, F. B. *Florence Nightingale: Reputation and Power.* London: Croom Helm, 1982.

Smyth, Elizabeth. "Professionalization Among the Professed: The Case of Roman Catholic Women Religious." In *Challenging Professions: Historical and Contemporary Perspectives on Women's Professional Work,* ed. Elizabeth Smyth, Sandra Acker, Sandra Bourne, and Alison Prentice. Toronto: University of Toronto Press, 1999. 234–54.

Sperber, Jonathon. *Popular Catholicism in Nineteenth-Century Germany.* Princeton, N.J.: Princeton University Press, 1984.

Stephenson, T. Bowman. *Concerning Sisterhoods.* London: C.H. Kelly, 1890.

Stepsis, Ursula and Dolores Liptak, eds. *Pioneer Healers: The History of Women Religious in American Health Care.* New York: Crossroad, 1989.

Stevens, Rosemary. *In Sickness and in Wealth: American Hospitals in the Twentieth Century.* New York: Basic Books, 1989.

St. Mary's Hospital School of Nursing, Kansas City Missouri, 1964–65. Kansas City: St. Mary's Hospital, 1955.

St. Vincent's Hospital, Sydney. *Annual Reports of St Vincent's Hospital Sydney Under the Care of the Sisters of Charity, 1857–1900.* Sydney: Cook and Co., 1900.

Stewart, George C., Jr. *Marvels of Charity: History of American Sisters and Nuns.* Huntington, Ind.: Our Sunday Visitor, 1994.

Sullivan, Mary C. *The Friendship of Florence Nightingale and Mary Clare Moore.* Philadelphia: University of Pennsylvania Press, 1999.

Summers, Anne. *Angels and Citizens: British Women as Military Nurses, 1854–1915.* London: Routledge, 1988.

Summers, Anne. "The Cost and Benefits of Caring: Nursing Charities, c 1830–1860." In *Medicine and Charity Before the Welfare State,* ed. Jonathan Barry and Colin Jones. London: Routledge, 1991. 133–48.

——. "Frameworks or Straitjackets? Secular and Religious Models in the Historiography of Nursing. *Past Is Present: The CAHN/ACHN Keynote Presentations, 1988–1996,* ed. Sheila J. Rankin Zerr. Vancouver: Canadian Association for the History of Nursing, 1997. 215–39.

——. "Ministering Angels." *History Today* 39 (February 1989): 31–37.

——. "The Mysterious Demise of Sarah Gamp: The Domiciliary Nurse and Her Detractors." *Victorian Studies* 32 (1989): 365–86.

Taylor, Fanny M. et al. *Eastern Hospitals and English Nurses, the Narrative of Twelve Months' Experience in the Hospitals of Koulali and Scutari.* 2 vols. London: Hurst and Blackett, 1856.

Taylor, Philip. *The Distant Magnet: European Emigration to the U.S.A.* London: Eyre & Spottiswoode, 1971.

Teale, Ruth, ed. *Colonial Eve: Sources on Women in Australia, 1788–1914.* Melbourne: Oxford University Press, 1978.

Thompson, Margaret Susan. *To Serve the People of God: Nineteenth Century Sisters and the Creation of a Religious Life.* Working Papers ser. 18, 2. South Bend, Ind.: Cushwa Center for the Study of American Catholicism, University of Notre Dame, Spring 1987.

——. "Women, Feminism, and the New Religious History: Catholic Sisters as a Case Study." In *Belief and Behavior: Essays in the New Religious History,* ed. Philip R. VanderMeer and Robert P. Swierenga. New Brunswick, N.J.: Rutgers University Press, 1991.

Tranter, Janice. "The Irish Dimension of an Australian Religious Sisterhood: The Sisters of St. Joseph." In *The Irish World Wide,* vol. 5, *Religion and Identity,* ed. Patrick O'Sullivan. London: Leicester University Press, 1996. 234–55.

O'Tuathraigh, M. A. G. "The Irish in Nineteenth-Century Britain, Problems of Integration." In *The Irish in Britain, 1815–1939,* ed. Roger Swift and Sheridan Gilley. Savage, Md.: Barnes and Noble, 1989. 13–36.

"200 Years of Nursing, a Photographic History." Bicentennial lift out, *The Lamp,* April 1988.

Tynan, Margaret, RN. *St. Vincent's School of Nursing of the Institute of Providence: Its History and Alumnae.* Portland: School of Nursing, St. Vincent's, 1930.

Vicinus, Martha. *Independent Women: Work and Community for Single Women, 1850–1920.* Chicago: University of Chicago Press, 1985.

Wall, Barbra Mann. "Religion, Ethnicity, and Nursing: The Americanization of Irish Catholic Sister Nurses." In *Proceedings of the Conference on the History of Women Religious,* Loyola University, Chicago, June 1998.

——. "Unlikely Entrepreneurs: Nuns, Nursing, and Hospital Development in the West and Midwest, 1865–1915." PhD dissertation, University of Notre Dame, 2000.

Ward, David. *Cities and Immigrants: A Geography of Change in Nineteenth-Century America.* New York: Oxford University Press, 1978.

Watson, J. Frederick. *The History of the Sydney Hospital from 1811 to 1911.* Sydney: W.A. Gullick, 1911.

Webster, Joseph G. "The Staff of St. Mary's Hospital." *Jackson County Medical Society Weekly Bulletin* 50 (30 June 1965): 1570–71.

Weeks, Clara S. *A Text-book of Nursing.* New York: Appleton, 1885.

Weiner, Dora B. *The Citizen-Patient in Revolutionary and Imperial Paris.* Baltimore: Johns Hopkins University Press, 1993, 110.

——. "The French Revolution, Napoleon, and the Nursing Profession." *Bulletin of the History of Medicine* 46, 3 (1972): 274–305.

Weiser, Frederick S. *To Serve the Lord and His People, 1884–1984: Celebration of the Heritage of a Century of Lutheran Deaconesses in America.* Gladwyne, Pa.: Deaconess Community of the Lutheran Church in America, 1984.

——. "Serving Love." Degree of Divinity thesis, Church History, Lutheran Theological College, Gettysburg, Pennsylvania, 1960.

Wentz, Abdel Ross. *Fliedner the Faithful.* Philadelphia: Board of Publications of the United Lutheran Church in America, 1936.

West, Roberta Mayhew. *History of Nursing in Pennsylvania, Lankenau Hospital, Formerly German Hospital, Philadelphia.* Harrisburg: Pennsylvania State Nurses Association, 1939.

Westerkamp, Marilyn J. *Women and Religion in Early America, 1600–1850: The Puritan and Evangelical Traditions.* London: Routledge, 1999.

Whitaker, Anne-Maree. "The Convict Priests: Irish Catholicism in Early Colonial New South Wales." In *The Irish World Wide: History, Heritage, Identity,* vol. 5, *Religion and Identity,* ed. Patrick O'Sullivan. London: Leicester University Press, 1996, 25–40.

Widerquist, JoAnn G. "Dearest Rev'd Mother." In *Florence Nightingale And Her Era: A Collection of New Scholarship,* ed. Vern Bullough, Bonnie Bullough, and Marietta P. Stanton. New York: Garland, 1990.

Williamson, Thomas Jay. *Priscilla Sellon, the Restorer After Three Centuries of the Religious Life in the Anglican Church.* London: SPCK, 1950.

Wiseman, Patrick Stephen Cardinal. Address to the Catholic Congress of Malines, Belgium, 21 August 1864. In *The Religious and Social Position of Catholics in England.* Dublin: James Duffy, 1864.

Wordsworth, Christopher. *On Sisterhoods and Vows: A Letter to the Ven. Sir George Provost.* London: Rivingtons, 1879.

"Would You Like to be a Deaconess?" Cincinnati: Bethesda Hospital, 1922.

Index

Acknowledgments

In the pursuit of this endeavor I have incurred many debts — material, intellectual, and personal. I need first to acknowledge the funding sources that have made this ambitious project possible. In 1997 I was fortunate to receive a three-year postdoctoral fellowship from the Faculty of Medicine, Dentistry, and Health Sciences at the University of Melbourne. This fellowship provided me with both the time and the financial support to research in far-flung archives. In 1997 the university also provided funds to support Sydney-based research. In 1998, the Australian Research Council funded more research in Sydney and also in Dublin. In 1999 the Australian Research Council further funded an extensive visit to the United States and Canada. The Wellcome Trust, London enabled me to visit the Bermondsey archives of the Sisters of Mercy in the East End of London and to spend time in the manuscript collection of the British Library and the Wellcome Library in 1998. The Cushwa Center for the Study of American Catholicism was also generous in its support, providing access to the excellent archive repository at Notre Dame University, South Bend, Indiana, and financial assistance for two trips to the United States in 1998 and 1999.

In addition to funding assistance I have also depended on the intellectual generosity of friends and colleagues throughout the world. Research is always a collective endeavor. Over the course of this project I have relied on scholars with far greater expertise than mine in the religious, nursing, or medical history of their respective countries, and they have been, without exception, overwhelmingly generous with their knowledge and advice. The many scholars who have replied to my emails, introduced me to experts and sources, and provided criticism and support are simply too numerous to mention. I have further taxed the good will of colleagues by involving them in the review of draft material, and the book is immeasurably the better for it. Joan Lynaugh, Center for the Study of

Nursing History, University of Pennsylvania, has been an enthusiastic champion of this project from beginning to end. Joan Lynaugh and another great supporter, Judith Parker, University of Melbourne, both read the entire manuscript and their comments were insightful and encouraging. Barbra Mann Wall, Purdue University, carefully read all the United States material, and has been a great ally throughout. The following colleagues commented on relevant sections: Jean Richardson, State University of New York at Buffalo; Carol Coburn, University of Kansas; Christine Anderson, Xavier College, Cincinnati; Geertje Boschma, University of Calgary; Anita Specht, Kansas Wesleyan University; Judith Godden, University of Sydney; Sister Rosa McGinley, (formerly) Institute of Religious Studies, Macquarie University, Sydney; Carol Helmstadter, Toronto; Janet McCalman, University of Melbourne; Pat D'Antonio, University of Pennsylvania; Sister Catherine O'Corrigan, Sisters of Charity, Potts Point, Sydney. Needless to say, all remaining errors in this text are mine alone.

In addition to those mentioned above, others have patiently feigned an interest in nuns over these three years to help me talk aloud my thesis, and to overcome my methodological challenges. I am grateful to Suzanne Gordon, Boston; Anne Marie Rafferty, University of London; Mary Ellen Purkis, University of Victoria, British Columbia; Denise Gastaldo, University of Toronto; and Hilda Smith, University of Cincinnati for their kindness and willingness to become interested in religious history in the cause of friendship.

Archivists have been an enormous support to the project and I have been amazed by their preparedness to go to any lengths to provide assistance. I have received generous support at the Daughters of Charity Archives, Albany, New York; the Archives of the Sisters of Providence, Seattle, Washington; the Archives of the Deaconesses of the Evangelical Lutheran Church of America, Gladwyne, Pennsylvania; and the Archives of the Sisters of the Incarnate Word, San Antonio, Texas. I am grateful also to the archivists at the Sydney Diocesan Archive; the Sisters of Charity Generalate, Harold's Cross, Dublin; the Dublin Diocesan Archive, Bishop's Palace, Dublin; Notre Dame University, South Bend, Indiana; the Cincinnati Historical Society, Cincinnati, Ohio; and staff at the Wellcome Institute for the History of Medicine and the British Library, London.

The following archivists have also provided feedback on draft material: Sister Elaine Wheeler, Daughters of Charity Archives; Loretta Green, Archives of the Sisters of Providence; Sister Louise Burroughs, Archives of the Deaconesses of the Evangelical Lutheran Church of America; and Sister Francesca Eikan, Sisters of the Incarnate Word.

This research has relied on the stalwart efforts of Marie Rogers, my research assistant for the duration of this project. Marie's invaluable contribution has covered every aspect of research and production.

Finally, my ever supportive family have endured my many absences and unsettling preoccupations with matters religious over the past three years — they are pleased it's over.